Atlas of
Common Pain
Syndromes

Atlas of Common Pain Syndromes

Second Edition

Steven D. Waldman, MD, JD

Clinical Professor, Department of Anesthesiology
University of Missouri–Kansas City School of Medicine
Kansas City, Missouri
Director, Headache and Pain Center
Leawood, Kansas

**Color illustrations by
Lauren Shavell and Pat Carico for Medical Imagery**

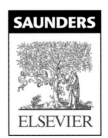

SAUNDERS

ELSEVIER

SAUNDERS
ELSEVIER

1600 John F. Kennedy Boulevard
Suite 1800
Philadelphia, Pennsylvania 19103-2899

Atlas of Common Pain Syndromes   ISBN: 978-1-4160-4675-2

Copyright © 2008, 2002 by Saunders, an imprint of Elsevier Inc.

Notice

Knowledge and best practice in this field are constantly changing. As new research and experience broaden our knowledge, changes in practice, treatment, and drug therapy may become necessary or appropriate. Readers are advised to check the most current information provided (i) on procedures featured or (ii) by the manufacturer of each product to be administered, to verify the recommended dose or formula, the method and duration of administration, and contraindications. It is the responsibility of the practitioner, relying on his or her own experience and knowledge of the patient, to make diagnoses, to determine dosages and the best treatment for each individual patient, and to take all appropriate safety precautions. To the fullest extent of the law, neither the publisher nor the author assumes any liability for any injury and/or damage to persons or property arising out or related to any use of the material contained in this book.

The Publisher

Library of Congress Cataloging-in-Publication Data

Waldman, Steven D.
    Atlas of common pain syndromes/Steven D. Waldman; color illustrations by Lauren Shavell and Pat Carico for Medical Imagery.—2nd ed.
        p; cm.
    Includes bibliographical references and index.
    ISBN 978-1-4160-4675-2
    1. Pain—Atlases. I. Title.
    [DNLM: 1. Pain—Atlases. 2. Syndrome—Atlases.   WL 17 W164ab 2008]
    RB127.W347   2008
    616′.0472—dc22   2007025632

Executive Publisher: Natasha Andjelkovic
Publishing Services Manager: Tina Rebane
Design Direction: Louis Forgione
Printed in China

Working together to grow
libraries in developing countries

www.elsevier.com | www.bookaid.org | www.sabre.org

ELSEVIER   BOOK AID International   Sabre Foundation

Last digit is the print number: 9 8 7 6 5 4 3 2 1

In memory of William T. Sirridge, MD—mentor, teacher, caring physician, and, most importantly, friend

Preface

As I noted in the Preface to the first edition of *Atlas of Common Pain Syndromes,* the work represented a departure from the standard pain management texts and atlases of its vintage. Published in 2001, it was the first pain management work to focus primarily on the diagnosis of pain rather than primarily on its treatment. With any departure from the tried and true, there is always the concern that the new approach may miss the mark. Fortunately, that has not been the case and I was pleased to see that the first edition of *Atlas of Common Pain Syndromes* was extremely well received by the medical community and became one of the best-selling pain management atlases to date.

Embarking on the writing of the second edition of such a successful book is very challenging in that the author must be careful not to alter the aspects of the atlas that made it popular to begin with while at the same time making the new edition even better than the old one. To that end, I conceived the following format.

To preserve the popular elements of the first edition, we made sure that the second edition of the atlas:

- Follows the "how-to-do-it" format that has become the hallmark of all of the texts I have written.
- Includes full-color illustrations for each chapter that visually depict the signs and symptoms of each pain syndrome being presented.
- Highlights pathognomonic physical, laboratory, and radiographic findings that help the clinician streamline the diagnostic process.

- Provides a *Clinical Pearls* section for each chapter to outline the most current tricks of the trade and make caring for the pain patient easier.
- Provides the most up-to-date ICD-9 codes for each pain syndrome presented to help the clinician obtain proper reimbursement.

To make the second edition even better than the first one, we have added the following features:

- Twenty-eight completely new chapters highlighting other common pain syndromes not included in the first edition.
- Greatly expanded physical examination sections with many new full-color photographs and illustrations to make it easier for the clinician to make the correct pain diagnosis.
- Greatly expanded use of radiographic imaging, including many new plain radiographs and nuclear medicine, CT, and MR images, to help the clinician better understand the pathophysiology and anatomy responsible for the patient's pain.
- An image-bank CD-ROM that allows the reader to browse through all the illustrations featured in the atlas and download them to PowerPoint for lectures and presentations.

It is my hope that the second edition of *Atlas of Common Pain Syndromes* will continue to help clinicians more effectively care for patients in pain.

STEVEN D. WALDMAN, MD, JD

Acknowledgment
A special thanks to Natasha Andjelkovic, my publisher at Elsevier,
for her keen insights, great advice, amazing work ethic, and great editing.

Contents

Section 15

Pain Syndromes of the Ankle

Section 16

Pain Syndromes of the Foot

Section 1

Headache Pain Syndromes

Chapter 1

Acute Herpes Zoster of the Trigeminal Nerve

ICD-9 CODE 053.12

THE CLINICAL SYNDROME

Herpes zoster is an infectious disease caused by the varicella-zoster virus (VZV). Primary infection with VZV in a nonimmune host manifests clinically as the childhood disease chickenpox (varicella). It is postulated that during the course of this primary infection, the virus migrates to the dorsal root or cranial ganglia, where it remains dormant, producing no clinically evident disease. In some individuals, the virus reactivates and travels along the sensory pathways of the first division of the trigeminal nerve, producing the characteristic pain and skin lesions of herpes zoster, or shingles.

Why reactivation occurs in some individuals but not in others is not fully understood, but it is theorized that a decrease in cell-mediated immunity may play an important role in the evolution of this disease by allowing the virus to multiply in the ganglia and spread to the corresponding sensory nerves, producing clinical disease. Patients who are suffering from malignancy (particularly lymphoma) or chronic disease and those receiving immunosuppressive therapy (chemotherapy, steroids, radiation) are generally debilitated and thus much more likely than the healthy population to develop acute herpes zoster. These patients all have in common a decreased cell-mediated immune response, which may also explain why the incidence of shingles increases dramatically in patients older than 60 years and is relatively uncommon in those younger than 20.

The first division of the trigeminal nerve is the second most common site for the development of acute herpes zoster, after the thoracic dermatomes. Rarely, the virus attacks the geniculate ganglion, resulting in hearing loss, vesicles in the ear, and pain (Fig. 1-1). This constellation of symptoms is called Ramsay Hunt syndrome and must be distinguished from acute herpes zoster involving the first division of the trigeminal nerve.

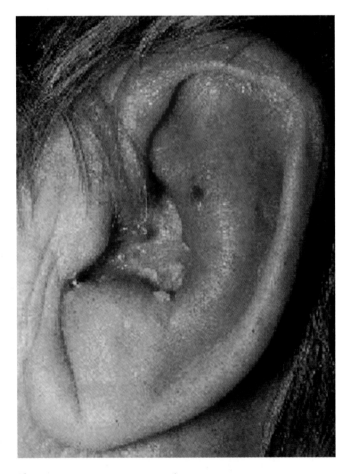

Figure 1–1. Ramsay Hunt syndrome.

SIGNS AND SYMPTOMS

As viral reactivation occurs, ganglionitis and peripheral neuritis cause pain that may be accompanied by flulike symptoms. The pain generally progresses from a dull, aching sensation to dysesthetic or neuritic pain in the distribution of the first division of the trigeminal nerve. In most patients, the pain of acute herpes zoster precedes the eruption of rash by 3 to 7 days, often leading to an erroneous diagnosis (see Differential Diagnosis). However, in most patients, the clinical diagnosis of shingles is readily made when the characteristic rash appears. Like chicken-pox, the rash of herpes zoster appears in crops of macular lesions that rapidly progress to papules and then to vesicles (Fig. 1-2). Eventually, the vesicles coalesce, and crusting occurs. The affected area can be extremely painful, and the pain tends to be exacerbated by any movement or contact (e.g., with clothing or sheets). As the lesions heal, the crust falls away, leaving pink scars that gradually become hypopigmented and atrophic.

In most patients, the hyperesthesia and pain resolve as the skin lesions heal. In some, however, pain persists beyond lesion healing. This common and feared complication of acute herpes zoster is called postherpetic neuralgia, and the elderly are affected at a higher rate than is the general population suffering from acute herpes zoster (Fig. 1-3). The symptoms of postherpetic neuralgia can vary from a mild, self-limited condition to a debilitating, constantly burning pain that is exacerbated by light touch, movement, anxiety, or temperature change. This unremitting pain may be so severe that it completely devastates the patient's life; ultimately, it can lead to suicide. To avoid this disastrous sequela to a usually benign, self-limited disease, the clinician must

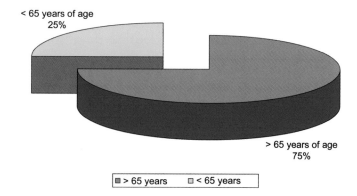

Figure 1-3. Age of patients suffering from acute herpes zoster.

use all possible therapeutic efforts in patients with acute herpes zoster of the trigeminal nerve.

TESTING

Although in most instances the diagnosis is easily made on clinical grounds, confirmatory testing is occasionally required. Such testing may be desirable in patients with other skin lesions that confuse the clinical picture, such as those with acquired immunodeficiency syndrome who are suffering from Kaposi's sarcoma. In such patients, the diagnosis of acute herpes zoster may be confirmed by obtaining a Tzanck smear from the base of a fresh vesicle, which reveals multinucleated giant cells and eosinophilic inclusions (Fig. 1-4). To differentiate acute herpes zoster from localized herpes simplex infection, the clinician can obtain fluid from a fresh vesicle and submit it for immunofluorescent testing.

DIFFERENTIAL DIAGNOSIS

A careful initial evaluation, including a thorough history and physical examination, is indicated in all patients suffering from acute herpes zoster of the trigeminal nerve. The goal is to rule out occult malignancy or systemic disease that may be responsible for the patient's immunocompromised state. A prompt diagnosis allows early recognition of changes in clinical status that may presage the development of complications, including myelitis or dissemination of the disease. Other causes of pain in the distribution of the first division of the trigeminal nerve include trigeminal neuralgia, sinus disease, glaucoma, retro-orbital tumor, inflammatory disease (e.g., Tolosa-Hunt syndrome), and intracranial pathology, including tumor.

TREATMENT

The therapeutic challenge in patients presenting with acute herpes zoster of the trigeminal nerve is twofold: (1) the immediate relief of acute pain and symptoms, and

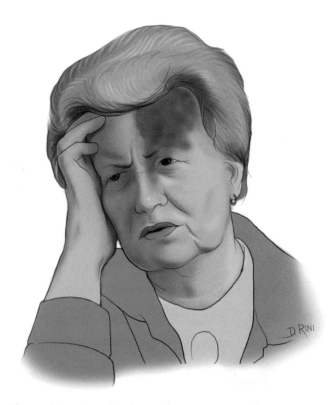

Figure 1-2. The pain of acute herpes zoster of the trigeminal nerve often precedes the characteristic vesicular rash.

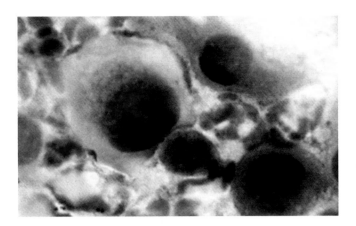

Figure 1–4. Tzanck smear showing giant multinucleated cells. (Courtesy of Dr. John Minarcik.)

(2) the prevention of complications, including postherpetic neuralgia. It is the consensus of most pain specialists that the earlier treatment is initiated, the less likely it is that postherpetic neuralgia will develop. Further, because older individuals are at the highest risk for developing postherpetic neuralgia, early and aggressive treatment of this group of patients is mandatory.

Nerve Block

Sympathetic neural blockade with local anesthetic and steroid via stellate ganglion block is the treatment of choice to relieve the symptoms of acute herpes zoster of the trigeminal nerve, as well as to prevent postherpetic neuralgia. As vesicular crusting occurs, the steroid may also reduce neural scarring. Sympathetic nerve block is thought to achieve these goals by blocking the profound sympathetic stimulation caused by viral inflammation of the nerve and gasserian ganglion. If untreated, this sympathetic hyperactivity can cause ischemia secondary to decreased blood flow of the intraneural capillary bed. If this ischemia is allowed to persist, endoneural edema forms, increasing endoneural pressure and causing a further reduction in endoneural blood flow, with irreversible nerve damage.

These sympathetic blocks should be continued aggressively until the patient is pain free and should be reimplemented if the pain returns. Failure to use sympathetic neural blockade immediately and aggressively, especially in the elderly, may sentence the patient to a lifetime of suffering from postherpetic neuralgia. Occasionally, some patients do not experience pain relief from stellate ganglion block but do respond to blockade of the trigeminal nerve.

Opioid Analgesics

Opioid analgesics can be useful to relieve the aching pain that is common during the acute stages of herpes zoster, while sympathetic nerve blocks are being implemented.

Opioids are less effective in relieving neuritic pain, which is also common. Careful administration of potent, long-acting narcotic analgesics (e.g., oral morphine elixir, methadone) on a time-contingent rather than an as-needed basis may be a beneficial adjunct to the pain relief provided by sympathetic neural blockade. Because many patients suffering from acute herpes zoster are elderly or have severe multisystem disease, close monitoring for the potential side effects of potent narcotic analgesics (e.g., confusion or dizziness, which may cause a patient to fall) is warranted. Daily dietary fiber supplementation and milk of magnesia should be started along with opioid analgesics to prevent constipation.

Adjuvant Analgesics

The anticonvulsant gabapentin represents a first-line treatment for the neuritic pain of acute herpes zoster of the trigeminal nerve. Studies suggest that gabapentin may also help prevent postherpetic neuralgia. Treatment with gabapentin should begin early in the course of the disease; this drug may be used concurrently with neural blockade, opioid analgesics, and other adjuvant analgesics, including antidepressants, if care is taken to avoid central nervous system side effects. Gabapentin is started at a bedtime dose of 300 mg and is titrated upward in 300-mg increments to a maximum of 3600 mg given in divided doses, as side effects allow.

Carbamazepine should be considered in patients suffering from severe neuritic pain who fail to respond to nerve blocks and gabapentin. If this drug is used, strict monitoring of hematologic parameters is indicated, especially in patients receiving chemotherapy or radiation therapy. Phenytoin may also be beneficial to treat neuritic pain, but it should not be used in patients with lymphoma; the drug may induce a pseudolymphoma-like state that is difficult to distinguish from the actual lymphoma.

Antidepressants may also be useful adjuncts in the initial treatment of patients suffering from acute herpes zoster. On an acute basis, these drugs help alleviate the significant sleep disturbance that is commonly seen. In addition, antidepressants may be valuable in ameliorating the neuritic component of the pain, which is treated less effectively with narcotic analgesics. After several weeks of treatment, antidepressants may exert a mood-elevating effect, which may be desirable in some patients. Care must be taken to observe closely for central nervous system side effects in this patient population. In addition, these drugs may cause urinary retention and constipation, which may mistakenly be attributed to herpes zoster myelitis.

Antiviral Agents

A limited number of antiviral agents, including famciclovir and acyclovir, can shorten the course of acute herpes zoster and may even help prevent its development. They are probably useful in attenuating the disease in immunosuppressed patients. These antiviral agents can be used in conjunction with the aforementioned treatment modalities. Careful monitoring for side effects is mandatory.

Adjunctive Treatments

The application of ice packs to the lesions of acute herpes zoster may provide relief in some patients. Application of heat increases pain in most patients, presumably because of the increased conduction of small fibers; however, it is beneficial in an occasional patient and may be worth trying if the application of cold is ineffective. Transcutaneous electrical nerve stimulation and vibration may also be effective in a limited number of patients. The favorable risk-benefit ratio of these modalities makes them reasonable alternatives for patients who cannot or will not undergo sympathetic neural blockade or cannot tolerate pharmacologic interventions.

Topical application of aluminum sulfate as a tepid soak provides excellent drying of the crusting and weeping lesions of acute herpes zoster, and most patients find these soaks soothing. Zinc oxide ointment may also be used as a protective agent, especially during the healing phase, when temperature sensitivity is a problem. Disposable diapers can be used as absorbent padding to protect healing lesions from contact with clothing and sheets.

COMPLICATIONS AND PITFALLS

In most patients, acute herpes zoster of the trigeminal nerve is a self-limited disease. In the elderly and the immunosuppressed, however, complications may occur. Cutaneous and visceral dissemination may range from a mild rash resembling chickenpox to an overwhelming, life-threatening infection in those already suffering from severe multisystem disease. Myelitis may cause bowel, bladder, and lower extremity paresis. Ocular complications from trigeminal nerve involvement may range from severe photophobia to keratitis with loss of sight.

Clinical Pearls

Because the pain of herpes zoster usually precedes the eruption of skin lesions by 3 to 7 days, some other painful condition (e.g., trigeminal neuralgia, glaucoma) may erroneously be diagnosed. In this setting, an astute clinician should advise the patient to call immediately if a rash appears, because acute herpes zoster is a possibility. Some pain specialists believe that in a small number of immunocompetent patients, when reactivation of VZV occurs, a rapid immune response attenuates the natural course of the disease, and the characteristic rash of acute herpes zoster may not appear. In this case, pain in the distribution of the first division of the trigeminal nerve without an associated rash is called zoster sine herpete and is, by necessity, a diagnosis of exclusion. Therefore, other causes of head pain must be ruled out before this diagnosis is invoked.

Chapter 2

Migraine Headache

ICD-9 CODE **346.1**

THE CLINICAL SYNDROME

Migraine headache is a periodic unilateral headache that may begin in childhood but almost always develops before age 30 years. Attacks occur with variable frequency, ranging from every few days to once every several months. More frequent migraine headaches are often associated with a phenomenon called analgesic rebound. Between 60% and 70% of patients who suffer from migraine are female, and many report a family history of migraine headache. The personality type of migraineurs has been described as meticulous, neat, compulsive, and often rigid in nature. They tend to be obsessive in their daily routines and often find it hard to cope with the stresses of everyday life. Migraine headache may be triggered by changes in sleep patterns or diet or by the ingestion of tyramine-containing foods, monosodium glutamate, nitrates, chocolate, or citrus fruits. Changes in endogenous and exogenous hormones, such as with the use of birth control pills, can also trigger migraine headache. Approximately 20% of patients suffering from migraine headache also experience a neurologic event before the onset of pain called an aura. The aura most often takes the form of a visual disturbance, but it may also present as an alteration in smell or hearing; these are called olfactory and auditory auras, respectively.

SIGNS AND SYMPTOMS

Migraine headache is, by definition, a unilateral headache. Although the headache may change sides with each episode, the headache is never bilateral. The pain of migraine headache is usually periorbital or retroorbital. It is pounding in nature, and its intensity is severe. The time from onset to peak of migraine pain is short, ranging from 20 minutes to 1 hour. In contradistinction to tension-type headache, migraine headache is often associated with systemic symptoms, including nausea and vomiting, photophobia, and sonophobia, as well as alterations in appetite, mood, and libido. Menstruation is a common trigger of migraine headache.

As mentioned, in about 20% of patients, migraine headache is preceded by an aura (called migraine with aura). The aura is thought to be the result of ischemia of specific regions of the cerebral cortex. A visual aura often occurs 30 to 60 minutes before the onset of headache pain; this may take the form of blind spots, called scotoma, or a zigzag disruption of the visual field, called fortification spectrum. Occasionally, migraine patients lose an entire visual field during the aura. Auditory auras usually take the form of hypersensitivity to sound, but other alterations of hearing, such as sounds being perceived as farther away than they actually are, have also been reported. Olfactory auras may take the form of strong odors of substances that are not actually present or extreme hypersensitivity to otherwise normal odors, such as coffee or copy machine toner. Migraine that presents without other neurologic symptoms is called migraine without aura.

Rarely, patients who suffer from migraine experience prolonged neurologic dysfunction associated with the headache pain. Such neurologic dysfunction may last for more than 24 hours and is termed migraine with prolonged aura. These patients are at risk for the development of permanent neurologic deficit, and risk factors such as hypertension, smoking, and oral contraceptives must be addressed. Even less common than migraine with prolonged aura is migraine with complex aura. Patients suffering from migraine with complex aura experience significant neurologic dysfunction that may include aphasia or hemiplegia. As with migraine with prolonged aura, patients suffering from migraine with complex aura may develop permanent neurologic deficits.

Patients suffering from all forms of migraine headache appear systemically ill (Fig. 2-1). Pallor, tremulousness, diaphoresis, and light sensitivity are common physical findings. The temporal artery and the surrounding area may be tender. If an aura is present, results of the neurologic examination will be abnormal; otherwise, the neurologic examination is usually within

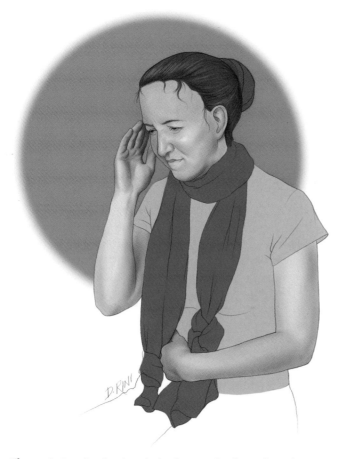

Figure 2–1. Migraine headache is an episodic, unilateral headache that occurs more commonly in females.

normal limits before, during, and after migraine without aura.

TESTING

There is no specific test for migraine headache. Testing is aimed primarily at identifying occult pathology or other diseases that may mimic migraine headache (see Differential Diagnosis). All patients with a recent onset of headache thought to be migraine should undergo magnetic resonance imaging (MRI) of the brain. If neurologic dysfunction accompanies the patient's headache symptoms, MRI should be performed with and without gadolinium contrast medium (Fig. 2-2); magnetic resonance angiography should be considered as well. MRI should also be performed in patients with previously stable migraine headaches who experience an inexplicable change in symptoms. Screening laboratory tests, including an erythrocyte sedimentation rate, complete blood count, and automated blood chemistry, should be performed if the diagnosis of migraine is in question. Ophthalmologic evaluation is indicated in patients who experience significant ocular symptoms.

DIFFERENTIAL DIAGNOSIS

The diagnosis of migraine headache is usually made on clinical grounds by obtaining a targeted headache history. Tension-type headache is often confused with migraine headache, which can lead to illogical treatment plans because these two headache syndromes are managed quite differently. Table 2-1 distinguishes migraine headache from tension-type headache and should help clarify the diagnosis.

Diseases of the eyes, ears, nose, and sinuses may also mimic migraine headache. The targeted history and physical examination, combined with appropriate testing, should allow the clinician to identify and properly treat any underlying diseases of these organ systems. Glaucoma; temporal arteritis; sinusitis; intracranial pathology, including chronic subdural hematoma, tumor (see Fig. 2-2), brain abscess, hydrocephalus, and pseudotumor cerebri; and inflammatory conditions, including sarcoidosis, may all mimic migraine and must be considered when treating headache patients.

TREATMENT

When deciding how best to treat a patient suffering from migraine, the clinician should consider the frequency and severity of the headaches, their effect on the patient's lifestyle, the presence of focal or prolonged neurologic disturbances, the results of previous testing and treatment, any history of previous drug abuse or misuse, and the presence of other systemic diseases (e.g., peripheral vascular or coronary artery disease) that might preclude the use of certain treatment modalities.

If the patient's migraine headaches occur infrequently, a trial of abortive therapy may be warranted. However, if the headaches occur with greater frequency or cause the patient to miss work or be hospitalized, prophylactic therapy is warranted.

Table 2–1. Comparison of Migraine Headache and Tension-Type Headache

	Migraine Headache	Tension-Type Headache
Onset-to-peak interval	Minutes to 1 hr	Hours to days
Frequency	Rarely >1/wk	Often daily or continuous
Location	Temporal	Nuchal or circumferential
Character	Pounding	Aching, pressure, bandlike
Laterality	Always unilateral	Usually bilateral
Aura	May be present	Never present
Nausea and vomiting	Common	Rare
Duration	Usually <24 hr	Often days

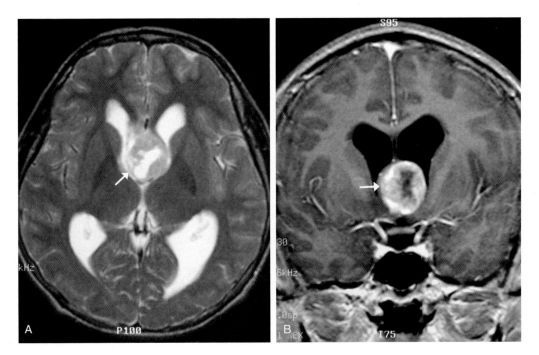

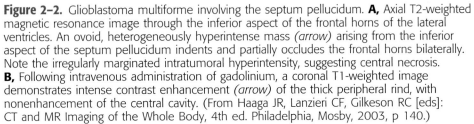

Figure 2–2. Glioblastoma multiforme involving the septum pellucidum. **A,** Axial T2-weighted magnetic resonance image through the inferior aspect of the frontal horns of the lateral ventricles. An ovoid, heterogeneously hyperintense mass *(arrow)* arising from the inferior aspect of the septum pellucidum indents and partially occludes the frontal horns bilaterally. Note the irregularly marginated intratumoral hyperintensity, suggesting central necrosis. **B,** Following intravenous administration of gadolinium, a coronal T1-weighted image demonstrates intense contrast enhancement *(arrow)* of the thick peripheral rind, with nonenhancement of the central cavity. (From Haaga JR, Lanzieri CF, Gilkeson RC [eds]: CT and MR Imaging of the Whole Body, 4th ed. Philadelphia, Mosby, 2003, p 140.)

Abortive Therapy

For abortive therapy to be effective, it must be initiated at the first sign of headache. This is often difficult because of the short interval between the onset and peak of migraine headache, coupled with the fact that migraine sufferers often experience nausea and vomiting that may limit the use of oral medications. By altering the route of administration to parenteral or transmucosal, this problem can be avoided.

Abortive medications that can be considered in migraine headache patients include compounds that contain isometheptene mucate (e.g., Midrin); the non-steroidal anti-inflammatory drug naproxen; ergot alkaloids; the triptans, including sumatriptan; and intravenous lidocaine combined with antiemetic compounds. The inhalation of 100% oxygen may abort migraine headache, and sphenopalatine ganglion block with local anesthetic may be effective. Caffeine-containing preparations, barbiturates, ergotamines, triptans, and narcotics have a propensity to cause a phenomenon called analgesic rebound headache, which may ultimately be more difficult to treat than the original migraine. The ergotamines and triptans should not be used in patients with coexistent peripheral vascular disease, coronary artery disease, or hypertension.

Prophylactic Therapy

For most patients with migraine headache, prophylactic therapy is a better option than abortive therapy. The mainstay of prophylactic therapy is β-blocking agents. Propranolol and most other drugs in this class can control or decrease the frequency and intensity of migraine headache and help prevent auras. An 80-mg daily dose of the long-acting formulation is a reasonable starting point for most patients with migraine. Propranolol should not be used in patients with asthma or other reactive airway diseases.

Valproic acid, calcium channel blockers (e.g., verapamil), clonidine, tricyclic antidepressants, and nonsteroidal anti-inflammatory drugs have also been used for the prophylaxis of migraine headache. Each of these drugs has advantages and disadvantages, and the clinician should tailor a treatment plan that best meets the needs of the individual patient.

COMPLICATIONS AND PITFALLS

In most patients, migraine headache is a painful but non-life-threatening disease. However, patients who suffer from migraine with prolonged aura or migraine with complex aura are at risk for the development of permanent neurologic deficits. Such patients are best treated by headache specialists who are familiar with these unique risks and are better equipped to deal with them. Occasionally, prolonged nausea and vomiting associated with severe migraine headache may result in dehydration that necessitates hospitalization and treatment with intravenous fluids.

Clinical Pearls

The most common reason for a patient's lack of response to traditional treatment for migraine headache is that the patient is actually suffering from tension-type headache, analgesic rebound headache, or a combination of headache syndromes. The clinician must be sure that the patient is not taking significant doses of over-the-counter headache preparations containing caffeine or other vasoactive drugs such as barbiturates, ergots, or triptans that may cause analgesic rebound headache. Until these drugs are withdrawn, the patient's headache will not improve.

Chapter 3

Tension-Type Headache

ICD-9 CODE 307.81

THE CLINICAL SYNDROME

Tension-type headache, formerly known as muscle contraction headache, is the most common type of headache that afflicts humankind. It can be episodic or chronic, and it may or may not be related to muscle contraction. Significant sleep disturbance usually occurs. Patients with tension-type headache are often characterized as having multiple unresolved conflicts surrounding work, marriage, social relationships, and psychosexual difficulties. Testing with the Minnesota Multiphasic Personality Inventory in large groups of tension-type headache patients revealed not only borderline depression but somatization as well. Most researchers believe that this somatization takes the form of abnormal muscle contraction in some patients; in others, it results in simple headache.

SIGNS AND SYMPTOMS

Tension-type headache is usually bilateral but can be unilateral, and it often involves the frontal, temporal, and occipital regions (Fig. 3-1). It may present as a bandlike, nonpulsatile ache or tightness in the aforementioned anatomic areas. Associated neck symptoms are common. Tension-type headache evolves over a period of hours or days and then tends to remain constant, without progression. There is no associated aura, but significant sleep disturbance is usually present. This may manifest as difficulty falling asleep, frequent awakening at night, or early awakening. These headaches most frequently occur between 4 and 8 AM and 4 and 8 PM. Although both sexes are affected, females predominate. There is no hereditary pattern to tension-type headache, but it may occur in family clusters as children mimic and learn the pain behavior of their parents.

The triggering event for acute, episodic tension-type headache is invariably either physical or psychological stress. This may take the form of a fight with a coworker or spouse or an exceptionally heavy workload. Physical

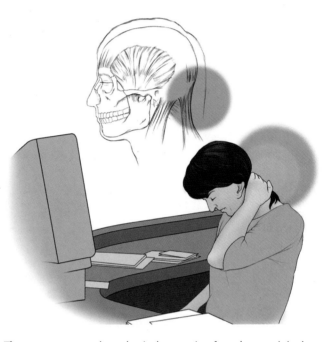

Figure 3-1. Mental or physical stress is often the precipitating factor in tension-type headache.

stress such as a long drive, working with the neck in a strained position, acute cervical spine injury due to whiplash, or prolonged exposure to the glare from a cathode ray tube may precipitate a headache. A worsening of preexisting degenerative cervical spine conditions, such as cervical spondylosis, can also trigger a tension-type headache. The pathology responsible for the development of tension-type headache can produce temporomandibular joint dysfunction as well.

TESTING

There is no specific test for tension-type headache. Testing is aimed primarily at identifying occult pathology or other diseases that may mimic tension-type headache (see Differential Diagnosis). All patients with the recent onset of headache that is thought to be tension type should undergo magnetic resonance imaging (MRI) of the brain and, if significant occipital or nuchal symptoms are present, of the cervical spine. MRI should also be

Table 3-1. Comparison of Tension-Type Headache and Migraine Headache

	Tension-Type Headache	Migraine Headache
Onset-to-peak interval	Hours to days	Minutes to 1 hr
Frequency	Often daily or continuous	Rarely >1/wk
Localization	Nuchal or circumferential	Temporal
Character	Aching, pressure, bandlike	Pounding
Laterality	Usually bilateral	Always unilateral
Aura	Never present	May be present
Nausea and vomiting	Rare	Common
Duration	Often days	Usually <24 hr

performed in patients with previously stable tension-type headaches who have experienced a recent change in symptoms. Screening laboratory tests consisting of a complete blood count, erythrocyte sedimentation rate, and automated blood chemistry should be performed if the diagnosis of tension-type headache is in question.

DIFFERENTIAL DIAGNOSIS

Tension-type headache is usually diagnosed on clinical grounds by obtaining a targeted headache history. Despite their obvious differences, tension-type headache is often incorrectly diagnosed as migraine headache. Such misdiagnosis can lead to illogical treatment plans and poor control of headache symptoms. Table 3-1 helps distinguish tension-type headache from migraine headache and should aid the clinician in making the correct diagnosis.

Diseases of the cervical spine and surrounding soft tissues may also mimic tension-type headache. Arnold-Chiari malformations may present clinically as tension-type headache, but these can be easily identified on images of the cervical spine. Occasionally, frontal sinusitis is confused with tension-type headache, although individuals with acute frontal sinusitis appear systemically ill. Temporal arteritis, chronic subdural hematoma, and other intracranial pathology such as tumor may be incorrectly diagnosed as tension-type headache.

TREATMENT

Abortive Therapy

In determining the best treatment, the physician must consider the frequency and severity of the headaches, their effect on the patient's lifestyle, the results of any previous therapy, and any prior drug misuse or abuse. If the patient suffers an attack of tension-type headache only once every 1 or 2 months, the condition can often be managed by teaching the patient to reduce or avoid stress. Analgesics or nonsteroidal anti-inflammatory drugs (NSAIDs) can provide symptomatic relief during acute attacks. Combination analgesic drugs used concomitantly with barbiturates or narcotic analgesics have no place in the management of headache patients. The risk of abuse and dependence more than outweighs any theoretical benefit. The physician should also avoid an abortive treatment approach in patients with a prior history of drug misuse or abuse. Many drugs, including simple analgesics and NSAIDs, can produce serious consequences if they are abused.

Prophylactic Therapy

If the headaches occur more frequently than once every 1 or 2 months or are so severe that the patient repeatedly misses work or social engagements, prophylactic therapy is indicated.

Antidepressants

Antidepressants are generally the drugs of choice for the prophylactic treatment of tension-type headache. These drugs not only help decrease the frequency and intensity of headaches but also normalize sleep patterns and treat any underlying depression. Patients should be educated about the potential side effects of this class of drugs, including sedation, dry mouth, blurred vision, constipation, and urinary retention. They should also be told that relief of headache pain generally takes 3 to 4 weeks. However, normalization of sleep occurs immediately, and this may be enough to provide a noticeable improvement in headache symptoms.

Amitriptyline, started at a single bedtime dose of 25 mg, is a reasonable initial choice. The dose may be increased in 25-mg increments as side effects allow. Other drugs that can be considered if the patient does not tolerate the sedative and anticholinergic effects of amitriptyline include trazodone (75 to 300 mg at bedtime) or fluoxetine (20 to 40 mg at lunchtime). Because of the sedating nature of these drugs (with the exception of fluoxetine), they must be used with caution in elderly patients and in others who are at risk for falling. Care should also be exercised when using these drugs in patients who are prone to cardiac arrhythmias, because these drugs may be arrhythmogenic. Simple analgesics or longer-acting NSAIDs may be used with antidepressant compounds to treat exacerbations of headache pain.

Biofeedback

Monitored relaxation training combined with patient education about coping strategies and stress-reduction techniques may be of value in some tension-type headache sufferers who are adequately motivated. Patient selection is of paramount importance if good results are to be achieved. If the patient is significantly depressed, it may be beneficial to treat the depression before trying biofeedback. The use of biofeedback may allow the patient to control the headaches while avoiding the side effects of medications.

Cervical Epidural Nerve Block

Multiple studies have demonstrated the efficacy of cervical epidural nerve block with steroid in providing long-term relief of tension-type headaches in patients for whom all other treatment modalities have failed. This treatment can also be used while waiting for antidepressant compounds to become effective. Cervical epidural nerve block can be performed on a daily to weekly basis, depending on clinical symptoms.

COMPLICATIONS AND PITFALLS

A small number of patients with tension-type headache have major depression or uncontrolled anxiety states in addition to a chemical dependence on narcotic analgesics, barbiturates, minor tranquilizers, or alcohol. Attempts to treat these patients in the outpatient setting is disappointing and frustrating. Inpatient treatment in a specialized headache unit or psychiatric setting results in more rapid amelioration of the underlying and coexisting problems and allows the concurrent treatment of headache. Monoamine oxidase inhibitors can often reduce the frequency and severity of tension-type headache in this subset of patients. Phenelzine, at a dosage of 15 mg three times a day, is usually effective. After 2 to 3 weeks, the dosage is tapered to an appropriate maintenance dose of 5 to 10 mg three times a day. Monoamine oxidase inhibitors can produce life-threatening hypertensive crises if special diets are not followed or if these drugs are combined with some commonly used prescription or over-the-counter medications. Therefore, their use should be limited to highly reliable and compliant patients. Physicians prescribing this potentially dangerous group of drugs should be well versed in how to use them safely.

Clinical Pearls

Although tension-type (muscle contraction) headache occurs frequently, it is commonly misdiagnosed as migraine headache. By obtaining a targeted headache history and performing a targeted physical examination, the physician can make a diagnosis with a high degree of certainty. The avoidance of addicting medications, coupled with the appropriate use of pharmacologic and nonpharmacologic therapies, should result in excellent palliation and long-term control of pain in the vast majority of patients suffering from this headache syndrome.

Chapter 4

Cluster Headache

ICD-9 CODE 346.2

THE CLINICAL SYNDROME

Cluster headache derives its name from the headache pattern—that is, headaches occur in clusters, followed by headache-free remission periods. Unlike other common headache disorders that affect primarily females, cluster headache is much more common in males, with a male-female ratio of 5:1. Much less common than tension-type headache or migraine headache, cluster headache is thought to affect approximately 0.5% of the male population. Cluster headache is most often confused with migraine by clinicians who are unfamiliar with the syndrome; however, a targeted headache history allows the clinician to easily distinguish these two distinct headache types (Table 4-1).

The onset of cluster headache occurs in the late third or early fourth decade of life, in contradistinction to migraine, which almost always manifests by the early second decade. Unlike migraine, cluster headache does not appear to run in families, and cluster headache sufferers do not experience auras. Attacks generally occur approximately 90 minutes after the patient falls asleep. This association with sleep is reportedly maintained when a shift worker changes from nighttime to daytime hours of sleep. Cluster headache also appears to follow a distinct chronobiologic pattern that coincides with seasonal changes in the length of the day. This results in an increased frequency of cluster headache in the spring and fall.

During a cluster period, attacks occur two or three times a day and last for 45 minutes to 1 hour. Cluster periods usually last for 8 to 12 weeks, interrupted by remission periods of less than 2 years. In rare patients, the remission periods become shorter and shorter, and the frequency may increase up to 10-fold. This situation is termed chronic cluster headache and differs from the more common episodic cluster headache described earlier.

Table 4–1. Comparison of Cluster Headache and Migraine Headache

	Cluster Headache	Migraine Headache
Gender	Male 5:1	Female 2:1
Age of onset	Late 30s to early 40s	Menarche to early 20s
Family history	No	Yes
Aura	Never	May be present (20% of the time)
Chronobiologic pattern	Yes	No
Onset-to-peak interval	Seconds to minutes	Minutes to 1 hr
Frequency	2 or 3/day	Rarely >1/wk
Duration	45 min	Usually <24 hr

SIGNS AND SYMPTOMS

Cluster headache is characterized as a unilateral headache that is retro-orbital and temporal in location. The pain has a deep burning or boring quality. Physical findings during an attack of cluster headache may include Horner's syndrome, consisting of ptosis, abnormal pupil constriction, facial flushing, and conjunctival injection (Fig. 4-1). Additionally, profuse lacrimation and rhinorrhea are often present. The ocular changes may become permanent with repeated attacks. Peau d'orange skin over the malar region, deeply furrowed glabellar folds, and telangiectasia may be observed.

Attacks of cluster headache may be provoked by small amounts of alcohol, nitrates, histamines, and other vasoactive substances, and occasionally by high altitude. When the attack is in progress, the patient may be unable to lie still and may pace or rock back and forth in a chair. This behavior contrasts with that characterizing other headache syndromes, during which patients seek relief by lying down in a dark, quiet room.

The pain of cluster headache is said to be among the worst pain a human being can suffer. Because of the severity of the pain, the clinician must watch closely for medication overuse or misuse. Suicide has been

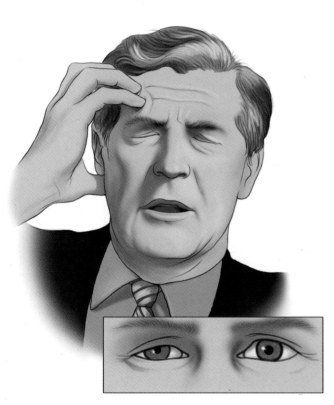

Figure 4-1. Horner's syndrome may be present during an acute attack of cluster headache.

associated with prolonged, unrelieved attacks of cluster headache.

TESTING

There is no specific test for cluster headache. Testing is aimed primarily at identifying occult pathology or other diseases that may mimic cluster headache (see Differential Diagnosis). All patients with a recent onset of headache thought to be cluster headache should undergo magnetic resonance imaging (MRI) of the brain. If neurologic dysfunction accompanies the patient's headache symptoms, MRI should be performed with and without gadolinium contrast medium (Fig. 4-2); magnetic resonance angiography should be considered as well. MRI should also be performed in patients with previously stable cluster headache who experience an inexplicable change in symptoms. Screening laboratory tests, including an erythrocyte sedimentation rate, complete blood count, and automated blood chemistry, should be performed if the diagnosis of cluster headache is in question. Ophthalmologic evaluation, including measurement of intraocular pressures, is indicated in patients who experience significant ocular symptoms.

DIFFERENTIAL DIAGNOSIS

Cluster headache is usually diagnosed on clinical grounds by obtaining a targeted headache history. Migraine headache is often confused with cluster headache, which can lead to illogical treatment plans because the management of these two headache syndromes is quite different. Table 4-1 distinguishes cluster headache from migraine headache and should help clarify the diagnosis.

Diseases of the eyes, ears, nose, and sinuses may also mimic cluster headache. The targeted history and physical examination, combined with appropriate testing, should help an astute clinician identify and properly treat any underlying diseases of these organ systems. Glaucoma; temporal arteritis; sinusitis (see Fig. 4-2); intracranial pathology, including chronic subdural hematoma, tumor, brain abscess, hydrocephalus, and pseudotumor cerebri; and inflammatory conditions, including sarcoidosis, may all mimic cluster headache and must be considered in headache patients.

TREATMENT

Whereas most patients with migraine headache experience improvement with β-blocker therapy, patients suffering from cluster headache usually require more individualized therapy. Initial treatment is commonly prednisone combined with daily sphenopalatine ganglion blocks with local anesthetic. A reasonable starting dose of prednisone is 80 mg given in divided doses and tapered by 10 mg/dose per day. If headaches are not rapidly brought under control, inhalation of 100% oxygen via a close-fitting mask is added.

If headaches persist and the diagnosis of cluster headache is not in question, a trial of lithium carbonate may be considered. The therapeutic window of lithium carbonate is small, however, and this drug should be used with caution. A starting dose of 300 mg at bedtime may be increased after 48 hours to 300 mg twice a day. If no side effects are noted after 48 hours, the dose may be increased again to 300 mg three times a day. The patient should stay at this dosage for a total of 10 days, after which the drug should be tapered over a 1-week period. Other medications that can be considered if these treatments are ineffective include methysergide and sumatriptan and sumatriptan-like drugs.

In rare patients, the aforementioned treatments are ineffective. In this setting, given the severity of the pain of cluster headache and the risk of suicide, more aggressive treatment is indicated. Destruction of the gasserian ganglion either by injection of glycerol or by radiofrequency lesioning may be a reasonable next step.

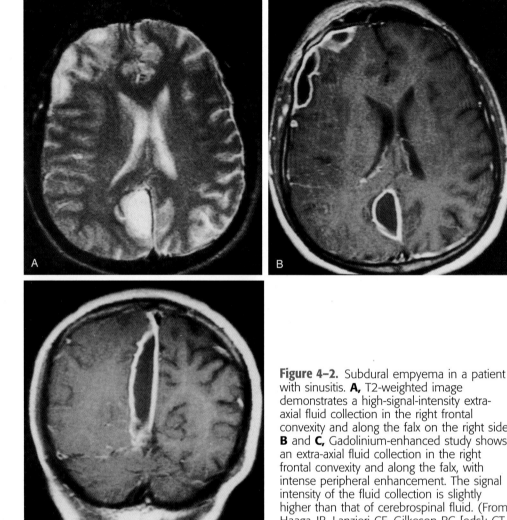

Figure 4–2. Subdural empyema in a patient with sinusitis. **A,** T2-weighted image demonstrates a high-signal-intensity extra-axial fluid collection in the right frontal convexity and along the falx on the right side. **B** and **C,** Gadolinium-enhanced study shows an extra-axial fluid collection in the right frontal convexity and along the falx, with intense peripheral enhancement. The signal intensity of the fluid collection is slightly higher than that of cerebrospinal fluid. (From Haaga JR, Lanzieri CF, Gilkeson RC [eds]: CT and MR Imaging of the Whole Body, 4th ed. Philadelphia, Mosby, 2003, p 209.)

COMPLICATIONS AND PITFALLS

The major risk in patients suffering from uncontrolled cluster headache is that they may become despondent owing to the unremitting, severe pain and commit suicide. Therefore, if the clinician has difficulty controlling the patient's pain, hospitalization should be considered.

Clinical Pearls

Cluster headache represents one of the most painful conditions encountered in clinical practice and must be viewed as a true pain emergency. In general, cluster headache is harder to treat than migraine headache and requires more individualized therapy. Given the severity of the pain associated with cluster headache, multiple modalities should be used early in the course of an episode of cluster headache. The clinician should beware of patients presenting with a classic history of cluster headache who request narcotic analgesics.

Chapter 5

Swimmer's Headache

ICD-9 CODE 350.8

THE CLINICAL SYNDROME

Swimmer's headache is seen with increasing frequency owing to the growing number of people who are swimming as part of a balanced program of physical fitness. Although an individual suffering from swimmer's headache most often complains of a unilateral frontal headache that occurs shortly after he or she begins to swim, this painful condition is more correctly characterized as a compressive mononeuropathy. Swim goggles that are either too large or too tight compress the supraorbital nerve as it exits the supraorbital foramen, causing swimmer's headache (Fig. 5-1). The onset of symptoms is insidious in most patients and usually occurs after the patient has been swimming for a while, caused by prolonged compression of the supraorbital nerve. There are several reported cases of acute-onset swimmer's headache, with a common history of the patient suddenly tightening one side of the goggles after experiencing a leak during his or her swim. In most cases, symptoms abate after use of the offending goggles is discontinued. However, with chronic compression of the supraorbital nerve, permanent nerve damage may result.

SIGNS AND SYMPTOMS

Swimmer's headache is usually unilateral and involves the skin and scalp subserved by the supraorbital nerve (Fig. 5-2). Swimmer's headache usually presents as cutaneous sensitivity above the affected supraorbital nerve, radiating into the ipsilateral forehead and scalp. This sensitivity may progress to unpleasant dysesthesias and allodynia, and the patient often complains that his or her hair hurts. With prolonged compression of the supraorbital nerve, a "woody" or anesthetized feeling of the supraorbital region and forehead may occur. Physical examination may reveal allodynia in the distribution of the compressed supraorbital nerve or, rarely, anesthesia. An occasional patient may present with edema of the eyelid due to compression of the soft tissues by the tight

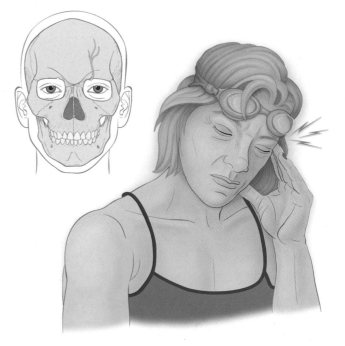

Figure 5–1. Swim goggles that are too tight can compress the supraorbital nerve and cause swimmer's headache.

goggles. Rarely, purpura may be present due to damage to the fragile blood vessels in the loose areolar tissue of the eyelid.

TESTING

There is no specific test for swimmer's headache. Testing is aimed primarily at identifying occult pathology or other diseases that may mimic swimmer's headache (see Differential Diagnosis). All patients with the recent onset of headache thought to be swimmer's headache should undergo magnetic resonance imaging (MRI) of the brain, and strong consideration should be given to obtaining computed tomography (CT) scanning of the sinuses, with special attention to the frontal sinuses, given the frequency of sinusitis in swimmers. Screening laboratory tests consisting of a complete blood count, erythrocyte sedimentation rate, and automated blood chemistry

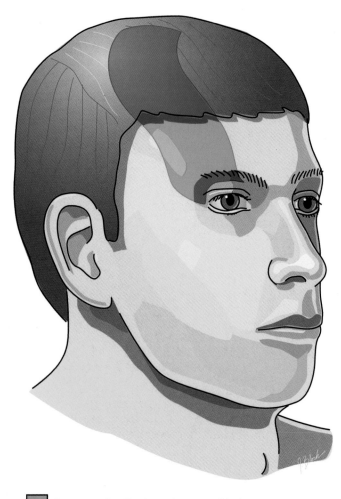

Sensory distribution of supraorbital nerve

Figure 5–2. Sensory distribution of the supraorbital nerve. (From Waldman SD: Atlas of Interventional Pain Management, 2nd ed. Philadelphia, Saunders, 2004, p 40.)

should be performed if the diagnosis of swimmer's headache is in question.

DIFFERENTIAL DIAGNOSIS

Swimmer's headache is usually diagnosed on clinical grounds by obtaining a targeted headache history.

Despite their obvious differences, swimmer's headache is often misdiagnosed as migraine headache. Such misdiagnosis leads to illogical treatment plans and poor control of headache symptoms. Table 5-1 distinguishes swimmer's headache from migraine headache and should aid the clinician in making the correct diagnosis.

As mentioned earlier, diseases of the frontal sinuses may mimic swimmer's headache and can be differentiated with MRI and CT scanning. Rarely, temporal arteritis may be confused with swimmer's headache, although individuals with temporal arteritis appear systemically ill. Intracranial pathology such as tumor may also be incorrectly diagnosed as swimmer's headache (Fig. 5-3).

TREATMENT

The mainstay of treatment of swimmer's headache is removal of the offending goggles. Often, simply substituting a new pair of goggles made of softer rubber does the trick, but occasionally, custom-fitted goggles that do not compress the supraorbital nerve but are large enough to avoid compressing the globe may be required. Analgesics or nonsteroidal anti-inflammatory drugs can provide symptomatic relief. However, even these drugs can lead to serious consequences if they are abused.

If the symptoms persist after removal of the offending goggles, gabapentin may be considered. Baseline blood tests should be obtained before starting therapy with 300 mg of gabapentin at bedtime for 2 nights. The patient should be cautioned about potential side effects, including dizziness, sedation, confusion, and rash. The drug is then increased, as side effects allow, in 300-mg increments given in equally divided doses over 2 days, until pain relief is obtained or a total dose of 2400 mg/day is reached. At this point, if the patient has experienced partial pain relief, blood values are measured, and the drug is carefully titrated upward using 100-mg tablets. Rarely is more than 3600 mg/day required. If significant sleep disturbance is present, amitriptyline at an initial bedtime dose of 25 mg and titrated upward, as side effects allow, may be beneficial.

In rare patients with persistent symptoms, supraorbital nerve block with local anesthetic and steroid may

Table 5–1. Comparison of Swimmer's Headache and Migraine Headache

	Swimmer's Headache	Migraine Headache
Onset-to-peak interval	Minutes	Minutes to 1 hr
Frequency	With swimming	Rarely >1/wk
Localization	Supraorbital radiating into the ipsilateral forehead and scalp	Temporal
Character	Cutaneous and scalp sensitivity progressing to painful dysesthesias and numbness	Pounding
Laterality	Usually unilateral	Always unilateral
Aura	Never present	May be present
Nausea and vomiting	Rare	Common
Duration	Usually subsides with removal of goggles, but may become chronic	Usually <24 hr

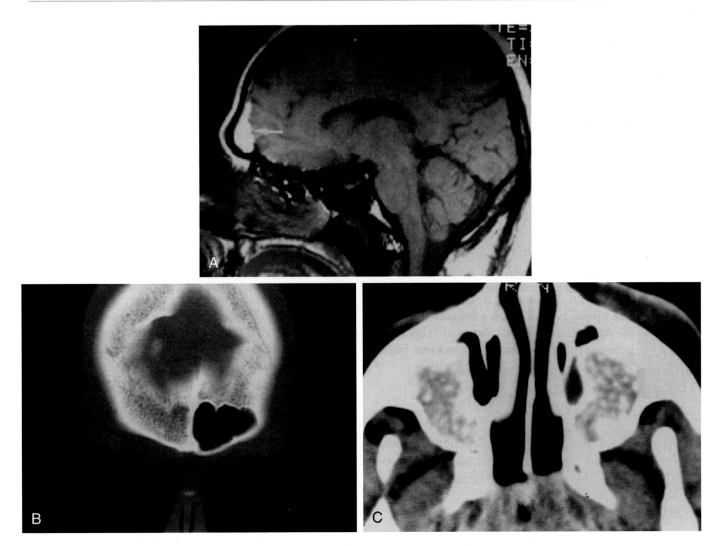

Figure 5–3. Intracranial pathology that may mimic swimmer's headache. **A,** Sagittal T1-weighted (TR 500, TE 32) magnetic resonance image in the midline. Increased signal is seen overlying the frontal sinus *(arrow)*. This may represent fat, hemorrhage, or a paramagnetic substance in a metastatic tumor such as melanoma. **B,** Accompanying coronal computed tomography scan shows a nonpneumatized and nondeveloped right frontal sinus. The marrow signal from this right frontal sinus was thought to produce the abnormal signal in the study in **A. C,** Non-contrast-enhanced axial computed tomography scan through the maxillary sinuses in a patient with sickle cell disease. The speckled pattern overlying the maxillary sinuses proved to be hyperactive marrow. (From Haaga JR, Lanzieri CF, Gilkeson RC [eds]: CT and MR Imaging of the Whole Body, 4th ed. Philadelphia, Mosby, 2003, p 565.)

be a reasonable next step. To perform supraorbital nerve block, the patient is placed supine with the head in the neutral position. The skin is prepared with povidone-iodine solution, being careful to avoid spilling solution into the eye. The supraorbital notch is identified by palpation. A 1½-inch, 25-gauge needle is advanced perpendicularly to the skin at the level of the supraorbital notch. Then, 3 to 4 mL of preservative-free local anesthetic and 40 mg of depot methylprednisolone are injected in a fan configuration to anesthetize the peripheral branches of the nerve (Fig. 5-4). To block the supratrochlear nerve, the needle is directed medially from the supraorbital notch toward the apex of the nose. Paresthesias are occasionally elicited.

COMPLICATIONS AND PITFALLS

In most cases, swimmer's headache is a painful but self-limited condition that is easily managed once it is diagnosed. Failure to promptly remove the offending goggles may result in permanent nerve damage with associated dysesthesias and numbness. Failure to recognize coexistent intracranial pathology or systemic diseases such as frontal sinusitis or tumor can have disastrous results.

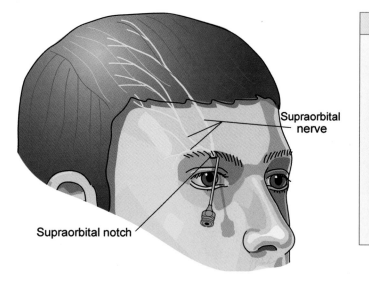

Figure 5–4. Correct needle placement for supraorbital nerve block. (From Waldman SD: Atlas of Interventional Pain Management, 2nd ed. Philadelphia, Saunders, 2004, p 40.)

Clinical Pearls

Although swimmer's headache is occurring with greater frequency owing to the increased interest in physical fitness, it is often misdiagnosed as sinus headache or occasionally migraine. By obtaining a targeted headache history and performing a targeted physical examination, the physician can make a diagnosis with a high degree of certainty. Avoidance of potentially addictive medications, coupled with the appropriate use of pharmacologic and nonpharmacologic therapies, should result in excellent palliation and long-term control of pain in the vast majority of patients suffering from this headache syndrome.

Chapter 6

Analgesic Rebound Headache

ICD-9 CODE 784.0

THE CLINICAL SYNDROME

Analgesic rebound headache is a recently identified headache syndrome that occurs in headache sufferers who overuse abortive medications to treat their symptoms. The overuse of these medications results in increasingly frequent headaches that become unresponsive to both abortive and prophylactic medications. Over a period of weeks, the patient's episodic migraine or tension-type headache becomes more frequent and transforms into a chronic daily headache. This daily headache becomes increasingly unresponsive to analgesics and other medications, and the patient notes an exacerbation of headache symptoms if abortive or prophylactic analgesic medications are missed or delayed (Fig. 6-1). Analgesic rebound headache is probably underdiagnosed by health care professionals, and its frequency is on the rise owing to the heavy advertising of over-the-counter headache medications containing caffeine.

SIGNS AND SYMPTOMS

Clinically, analgesic rebound headache presents as a transformed migraine or tension-type headache and may assume the characteristics of both these common headache types, blurring their distinctive features and making diagnosis difficult. Common to all analgesic rebound headaches is the excessive use of any of the following medications: simple analgesics, such as acetaminophen; sinus medications, including simple analgesics; combinations of aspirin, caffeine, and butalbital (Fiorinal); nonsteroidal anti-inflammatory drugs; opioid analgesics; ergotamines; and triptans, such as sumatriptan (Table 6-1). As with migraine and tension-type headache, the physical examination is usually within normal limits.

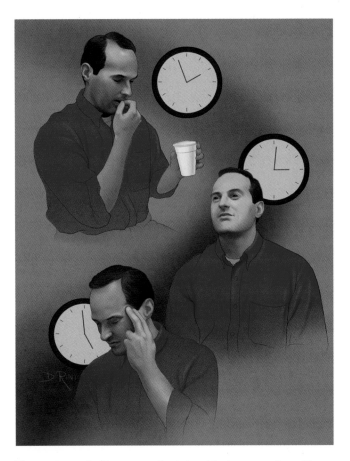

Figure 6–1. Classic temporal relationship between the taking of abortive medications and the onset of analgesic rebound headache.

TESTING

There is no specific test for analgesic rebound headache. Testing is aimed primarily at identifying occult pathology or other diseases that may mimic tension-type or migraine headaches (see Differential Diagnosis). All patients with the recent onset of chronic daily headaches thought to be analgesic rebound headaches should undergo magnetic resonance imaging (MRI) of the brain and, if

Table 6–1. Drugs Implicated in Analgesic Rebound Headache

Simple analgesics
Nonsteroidal anti-inflammatory drugs
Opioid analgesics
Sinus medications
Ergotamines
Combination headache medications that include butalbital
Triptans (e.g., sumatriptan)

significant occipital or nuchal symptoms are present, of the cervical spine. MRI should also be performed in patients with previously stable tension-type or migraine headaches who have experienced a recent change in headache symptoms. Screening laboratory tests consisting of a complete blood count, erythrocyte sedimentation rate, and automated blood chemistry should be performed if the diagnosis of analgesic rebound headache is in question.

DIFFERENTIAL DIAGNOSIS

Analgesic rebound headache is usually diagnosed on clinical grounds by obtaining a targeted headache history. Because analgesic rebound headache assumes many of the characteristics of the underlying primary headache, diagnosis can be confusing in the absence of a careful medication history, including specific questions regarding over-the-counter headache medications and analgesics. Any change in a previously stable headache pattern needs to be taken seriously and should not automatically be attributed to analgesic overuse without a careful reevaluation of the patient.

TREATMENT

Treatment of analgesic rebound headache consists of discontinuation of the overused or abused drugs and complete abstention for at least 3 months. Many patients cannot tolerate outpatient discontinuation of these medications and ultimately require hospitalization in a specialized headache unit. If outpatient treatment is being considered, the following points should be carefully explained to the patient:

- The headaches and associated symptoms will get worse before they get better.
- Any use, no matter how small, of the offending medications will result in continued analgesic rebound headaches.
- The patient cannot self-medicate with over-the-counter drugs.
- The significant overuse of opioids or combination medications containing butalbital or ergotamine can result in physical dependence, and discontinuation of such drugs must be done under the supervision of a physician familiar with the treatment of physical dependencies.
- If the patient follows the physician's orders regarding discontinuation of the offending medications, he or she can expect the headaches to improve.

COMPLICATIONS AND PITFALLS

Patients who overuse or abuse medications, including opioids, ergotamines, and butalbital, develop a physical dependence on these drugs, and their abrupt cessation results in a drug abstinence syndrome that can be life threatening if not properly treated. Therefore, most of these patients require inpatient tapering in a controlled setting.

Clinical Pearls

Analgesic rebound headache occurs much more commonly than was previously thought. The occurrence of analgesic rebound headache is a direct result of the overprescribing of abortive headache medications in patients for whom they are inappropriate. When in doubt, the clinician should avoid abortive medications altogether and treat most headache sufferers prophylactically.

Chapter 7

Occipital Neuralgia

ICD-9 CODE 723.8

THE CLINICAL SYNDROME

Occipital neuralgia is usually the result of blunt trauma to the greater and lesser occipital nerves (Fig. 7-1). The greater occipital nerve arises from fibers of the dorsal primary ramus of the second cervical nerve and, to a lesser extent, from fibers of the third cervical nerve. The greater occipital nerve pierces the fascia just below the superior nuchal ridge, along with the occipital artery. It supplies the medial portion of the posterior scalp as far anterior as the vertex. The lesser occipital nerve arises from the ventral primary rami of the second and third cervical nerves. The lesser occipital nerve passes superiorly along the posterior border of the sternocleidomastoid muscle, dividing into cutaneous branches that innervate the lateral portion of the posterior scalp and the cranial surface of the pinna of the ear.

Less commonly, repetitive microtrauma from working with the neck hyperextended (e.g., painting ceilings) or looking for prolonged periods at a computer monitor whose focal point is too high, causing extension of the cervical spine, may also cause occipital neuralgia. Occipital neuralgia is characterized by persistent pain at the base of the skull with occasional sudden shocklike paresthesias in the distribution of the greater and lesser occipital nerves. Tension-type headache, which is much more common, occasionally mimics the pain of occipital neuralgia.

SIGNS AND SYMPTOMS

A patient suffering from occipital neuralgia experiences neuritic pain in the distribution of the greater and lesser occipital nerves when the nerves are palpated at the level of the nuchal ridge. Some patients can elicit pain with rotation or lateral bending of the cervical spine.

TESTING

There is no specific test for occipital neuralgia. Testing is aimed primarily at identifying occult pathology or

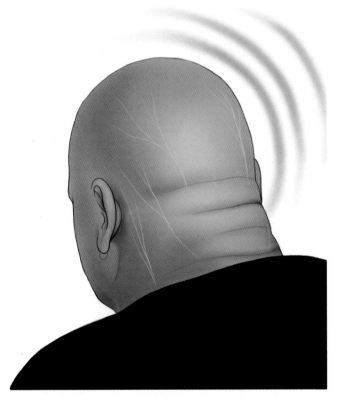

Figure 7–1. Occipital neuralgia is caused by trauma to the greater and lesser occipital nerves.

other diseases that may mimic occipital neuralgia (see Differential Diagnosis). All patients with the recent onset of headache thought to be occipital neuralgia should undergo magnetic resonance imaging (MRI) of the brain and cervical spine. MRI should also be performed in patients with previously stable occipital neuralgia who have experienced a recent change in headache symptoms. CT scanning of the brain and cervical spine may also be useful in identifying intracranial pathology that may mimic the symptoms of occipital neuralgia (Fig. 7-2). Screening laboratory tests consisting of a complete blood count, erythrocyte sedimentation rate, and automated blood chemistry should be performed if the diagnosis of occipital neuralgia is in question.

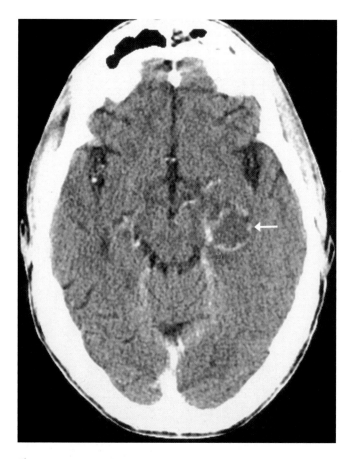

Figure 7-2. Supratentorial ependymoma. Axial computed tomography scan after intravenous contrast demonstrates a cystic-appearing, hypodense mass with irregular, rimlike contrast enhancement *(arrow)* in the medial aspect of the left temporal lobe. (From Haaga JR, Lanzieri CF, Gilkeson RC [eds]: CT and MR Imaging of the Whole Body, 4th ed. Philadelphia, Mosby, 2003, p 149.)

Neural blockade of the greater and lesser occipital nerves can help confirm the diagnosis and distinguish occipital neuralgia from tension-type headache. The greater and lesser occipital nerves can easily be blocked at the nuchal ridge.

DIFFERENTIAL DIAGNOSIS

Occipital neuralgia is an infrequent cause of headache and rarely occurs in the absence of trauma to the greater and lesser occipital nerves. More often, patients with headaches involving the occipital region are suffering from tension-type headache. Tension-type headache does not respond to occipital nerve blocks but is amenable to treatment with antidepressants such as amitriptyline, in conjunction with cervical epidural nerve block. Therefore, the clinician should reconsider the diagnosis of occipital neuralgia in patients whose symptoms are consistent with occipital neuralgia but

who fail to respond to greater and lesser occipital nerve blocks.

TREATMENT

The treatment of occipital neuralgia consists primarily of neural blockade with local anesthetic and steroid, combined with the judicious use of nonsteroidal anti-inflammatory drugs, muscle relaxants, tricyclic antidepressants, and physical therapy.

To perform neural blockade of the greater and lesser occipital nerves, the patient is placed in a sitting position with the cervical spine flexed and the forehead on a padded bedside table. A total of 8 mL of local anesthetic is drawn up in a 12-mL sterile syringe. When treating occipital neuralgia or other painful conditions involving the greater and lesser occipital nerves, a total of 80 mg methylprednisolone is added to the local anesthetic with the first block, and 40 mg of depot steroid is added with subsequent blocks. The occipital artery is palpated at the level of the superior nuchal ridge. After preparing the skin with antiseptic solution, a $1\frac{1}{2}$-inch, 22-gauge needle is inserted just medial to the artery and advanced perpendicularly until the needle approaches the periosteum of the underlying occipital bone. Paresthesias may be elicited, and the patient should be warned of this possibility. The needle is then redirected superiorly, and after gentle aspiration, 5 mL of solution is injected in a fanlike distribution, with care being taken to avoid the foramen magnum, which is located medially (Fig. 7-3). The lesser occipital nerve and a number of superficial branches of the greater occipital nerve are then blocked by directing the needle laterally and slightly inferiorly. After gentle aspiration, an additional 3 to 4 mL of solution is injected (see Fig. 7-3).

COMPLICATIONS AND PITFALLS

The scalp is highly vascular; this, coupled with the fact that both the greater and lesser occipital nerves are in close proximity to arteries, means that the clinician must carefully calculate the total dosage of local anesthetic that can be safely given, especially if bilateral nerve blocks are being performed. This vascularity and proximity to the arterial supply give rise to an increased incidence of postblock ecchymosis and hematoma formation. These complications can be decreased if manual pressure is applied to the area of the block immediately after injection. Application of cold packs for 20 minutes after the block can also decrease the amount of pain and bleeding. Care must be taken to avoid inadvertent needle placement into the foramen magnum, because the subarachnoid administration of local anesthetic in this region results in immediate total spinal anesthesia.

As with other headache syndromes, the clinician must be sure that the diagnosis is correct and that there is no coexistent intracranial pathology or disease of the cervical spine that may be erroneously attributed to occipital neuralgia.

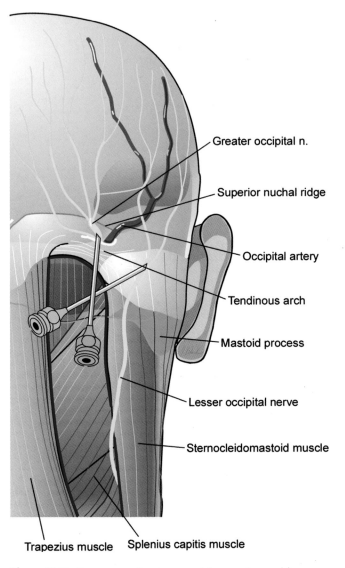

Figure 7–3. Proper needle placement for greater and lesser occipital nerve block. (From Waldman SD: Atlas of Interventional Pain Management, 2nd ed. Philadelphia, Saunders, 2004, p 25.)

Labels on figure:
- Greater occipital n.
- Superior nuchal ridge
- Occipital artery
- Tendinous arch
- Mastoid process
- Lesser occipital nerve
- Sternocleidomastoid muscle
- Trapezius muscle
- Splenius capitis muscle

Clinical Pearls

The most common reason that greater and lesser occipital nerve blocks fail to relieve headache pain is that the patient has been misdiagnosed. Any patient with headaches so severe that they require neural blockade should undergo MRI of the head to rule out unsuspected intracranial pathology. Further, cervical spine radiographs should be considered to rule out congenital abnormalities such as Arnold-Chiari malformations that may be the hidden cause of the patient's occipital headaches.

Section 2

Facial Pain Syndromes

Chapter 8

Trigeminal Neuralgia

ICD-9 CODE 350.1

THE CLINICAL SYNDROME

Trigeminal neuralgia occurs in many patients because of tortuous blood vessels that compress the trigeminal root as it exits the brainstem. Acoustic neuromas, cholesteatomas, aneurysms, angiomas, and bony abnormalities may also lead to compression of the nerve. The severity of the pain produced by trigeminal neuralgia is rivaled only by that of cluster headache. Uncontrolled pain has been associated with suicide and should therefore be treated as an emergency. Attacks can be triggered by daily activities involving contact with the face, such as brushing the teeth, shaving, and washing (Fig. 8-1). Pain can be controlled with medication in most patients. About 2% to 3% of patients with trigeminal neuralgia also have multiple sclerosis. Trigeminal neuralgia is also called tic douloureux.

SIGNS AND SYMPTOMS

Trigeminal neuralgia causes episodic pain afflicting the areas of the face supplied by the trigeminal nerve. The pain is unilateral in 97% of cases; when it does occur bilaterally, the same division of the nerve is involved on both sides. The second or third division of the nerve is affected in the majority of patients, with the first division being affected less than 5% of the time. The pain develops on the right side of the face in 57% of unilateral cases. The pain is characterized by paroxysms of electric shock–like pain lasting from several seconds to less than 2 minutes. The progression from onset to peak is essentially instantaneous.

Patients with trigeminal neuralgia go to great lengths to avoid any contact with trigger areas. In contrast, persons with other types of facial pain, such as temporomandibular joint dysfunction, tend to constantly rub the affected area or apply heat or cold to it. Patients with uncontrolled trigeminal neuralgia frequently require hospitalization for rapid control of pain. Between attacks, patients are relatively pain free. A dull ache remaining

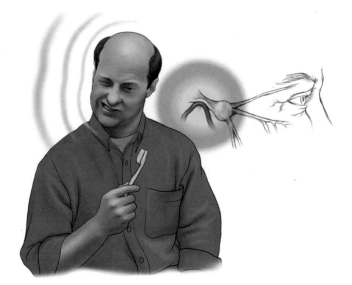

Figure 8–1. Paroxysms of pain triggered by brushing the teeth.

after the intense pain subsides may indicate persistent compression of the nerve by a structural lesion. This disease is almost never seen in persons younger than 30 years unless it is associated with multiple sclerosis.

Patients with trigeminal neuralgia often have severe depression (sometimes to the point of being suicidal), with high levels of superimposed anxiety during acute attacks. Both these problems may be exacerbated by the sleep deprivation that often accompanies painful episodes. Patients with coexisting multiple sclerosis may exhibit the euphoric dementia characteristic of that disease. Physicians should reassure persons with trigeminal neuralgia that the pain can almost always be controlled.

TESTING

All patients with a new diagnosis of trigeminal neuralgia should undergo magnetic resonance imaging (MRI) of the brain and brainstem, with and without gadolinium contrast medium, to rule out posterior fossa or brainstem lesions and demyelinating disease (Fig. 8-2). Magnetic resonance angiography is also useful to confirm vascular

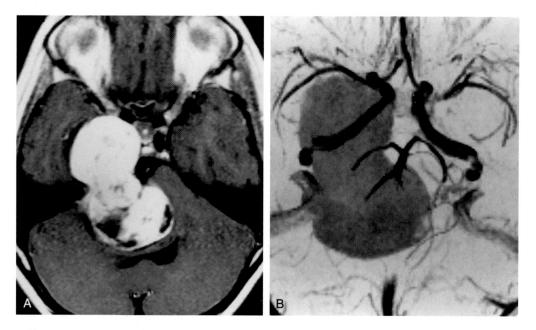

Figure 8–2. Cystic and solid schwannoma of the right trigeminal nerve and ganglion. **A,** Axial enhanced image showing a dumbbell-shaped tumor extending across the incisura from the posterior fossa into the medial portion of the right middle fossa. Note the heterogeneous enhancement of the tumor, suggesting areas of decreased cellularity and cystic change and a more solid component. **B,** Axial magnetic resonance angiogram performed after the magnetic resonance imaging examination showing near-homogeneous enhancement of the tumor because of the delay in imaging. Note the exquisite demonstration of the tumor in the skull base, including the displaced right petrous carotid artery. (From Stark DD, Bradley WG Jr: Magnetic Resonance Imaging, vol 3, 3rd ed. St Louis, Mosby, 1999, p 1218.)

compression of the trigeminal nerve by aberrant blood vessels (Fig. 8-3). Additional imaging of the sinuses should be considered if there is any question of occult or coexisting sinus disease. If the first division of the trigeminal nerve is affected, ophthalmologic evaluation to measure intraocular pressure and to rule out intraocular pathology is indicated. Screening laboratory tests consisting of a complete blood count, erythrocyte sedimentation rate, and automated blood chemistry should be performed if the diagnosis of trigeminal neuralgia is in question. A complete blood count is required for baseline comparisons before starting treatment with carbamazepine (see Treatment).

DIFFERENTIAL DIAGNOSIS

Trigeminal neuralgia is generally a straightforward clinical diagnosis that can be made on the basis of a targeted history and physical examination. Diseases of the eyes, ears, nose, throat, and teeth may all mimic trigeminal neuralgia or may coexist and confuse the diagnosis. Atypical facial pain is sometimes confused with trigeminal neuralgia, but it can be distinguished by the character of the pain: atypical facial pain is dull and aching, whereas the pain of trigeminal neuralgia is sharp and neuritic. Additionally, the pain of trigeminal neuralgia occurs in

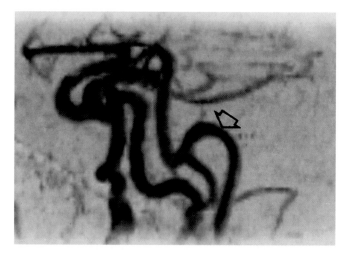

Figure 8–3. Vascular compression of the left trigeminal (fifth cranial) nerve in a 69-year-old man with trigeminal neuralgia. Three-dimensional time-of-flight magnetic resonance angiogram demonstrates that the compressive lesion is the markedly dominant right vertebral artery, which extends cephalad into the left cerebellopontine angle cistern *(open arrowhead).* (From Stark DD, Bradley WG Jr: Magnetic Resonance Imaging, vol 3, 3rd ed. St Louis, Mosby, 1999, p 1214.)

the distribution of the divisions of the trigeminal nerve, whereas the pain of atypical facial pain does not follow any specific nerve distribution. Multiple sclerosis should be considered in all patients who present with trigeminal neuralgia before the fifth decade of life.

TREATMENT

Drug Therapy

Carbamazepine

Carbamazepine is considered first-line treatment for trigeminal neuralgia. In fact, a rapid response to this drug essentially confirms the clinical diagnosis. Despite the safety and efficacy of carbamazepine, there has been some confusion and anxiety surrounding its use. This medication, which may be the patient's best chance for pain control, is sometimes discontinued because of laboratory abnormalities erroneously attributed to it. Therefore, baseline measurements consisting of a complete blood count, urinalysis, and automated blood chemistry profile should be obtained before starting the drug.

Carbamazepine should be initiated slowly if the pain is not out of control, with a starting dose of 100 to 200 mg at bedtime for 2 nights. The patient should be cautioned about side effects, including dizziness, sedation, confusion, and rash. The drug is increased in 100- to 200-mg increments given in equally divided doses over 2 days, as side effects allow, until pain relief is obtained or a total dose of 1200 mg/day is reached. Careful monitoring of laboratory parameters is mandatory to avoid the rare possibility of a life-threatening blood dyscrasia. *At the first sign of blood count abnormality or rash, this drug should be discontinued.* Failure to monitor patients on carbamazepine can be disastrous, because aplastic anemia can occur. When pain relief is obtained, the patient should be kept at that dosage of carbamazepine for at least 6 months before tapering of the medication is considered. The patient should be informed that under no circumstances should the drug dosage be changed or the drug refilled or discontinued without the physician's knowledge.

Gabapentin

In the uncommon event that carbamazepine does not adequately control a patient's pain, gabapentin may be considered. As with carbamazepine, baseline blood tests should be obtained before starting therapy, and the patient should be cautioned about potential side effects, including dizziness, sedation, confusion, and rash. The initial dose is 300 mg gabapentin at bedtime for 2 nights. The drug is then increased in 300-mg increments given in equally divided doses over 2 days, as side effects allow, until pain relief is obtained or a total dose of 2400 mg/

day is reached. At this point, if the patient has experienced only partial pain relief, blood values are measured, and the drug is carefully titrated upward using 100-mg tablets. Rarely is a dosage greater than 3600 mg/day required.

Baclofen

Baclofen may be of value in some patients who fail to obtain relief from carbamazepine or gabapentin. As with those drugs, baseline laboratory tests should be obtained before beginning baclofen therapy, and the patient should be warned about the same potential adverse effects. Start with a 10-mg dose at bedtime for 2 nights; then, increase the drug in 10-mg increments given in equally divided doses over 7 days, as side effects allow, until pain relief is obtained or a total dose of 80 mg/day is reached. This drug has significant hepatic and central nervous system side effects, including weakness and sedation. As with carbamazepine, careful monitoring of laboratory values is indicated when using baclofen.

When treating individuals with any of these drugs, the physician should make sure that the patient knows that premature tapering or discontinuation of the medication may lead to the recurrence of pain, which will be more difficult to control.

Invasive Therapy

Trigeminal Nerve Block

The use of trigeminal nerve block with local anesthetic and steroid is an excellent adjunct to drug treatment of trigeminal neuralgia. This technique rapidly relieves pain while medications are being titrated to effective levels. The initial block is carried out with preservative-free bupivacaine combined with methylprednisolone. Subsequent daily nerve blocks are carried out in a similar manner, using a lower dose of methylprednisolone. This approach may also be used to control breakthrough pain.

Retrogasserian Injection of Glycerol

The injection of small quantities of glycerol into the area of the gasserian ganglion can provide long-term relief for patients suffering from trigeminal neuralgia who have not responded to optimal drug therapy. This procedure should be performed only by a physician well versed in the problems and pitfalls associated with neurodestructive procedures.

Radiofrequency Destruction of the Gasserian Ganglion

The gasserian ganglion can be destroyed by creating a radiofrequency lesion under biplanar fluoroscopic guidance. This procedure is reserved for patients who have failed all the previously mentioned treatments for intractable trigeminal neuralgia and are not candidates for microvascular decompression of the trigeminal root.

Microvascular Decompression of the Trigeminal Root

This technique, which is also called Jannetta's procedure, is the major neurosurgical treatment of choice for intractable trigeminal neuralgia. It is based on the theory that trigeminal neuralgia is in fact a compressive mononeuropathy. The operation consists of identifying the trigeminal root close to the brainstem and isolating the compressing blood vessel. A sponge is then interposed between the vessel and the nerve, relieving the compression and thus the pain.

COMPLICATIONS AND PITFALLS

The pain of trigeminal neuralgia is severe and can lead to suicide; therefore, it must be considered a medical emergency, and strong consideration should be given to hospitalizing such patients. If a dull ache remains after the intense pain of trigeminal neuralgia subsides, this is highly suggestive of persistent compression of the nerve by a structural lesion such as a brainstem tumor or schwannoma. Trigeminal neuralgia is almost never seen in persons younger than 30 years unless it is associated with multiple sclerosis, and all such patients should undergo MRI to identify demyelinating disease.

Clinical Pearls

Trigeminal nerve block with local anesthetic and steroid is an excellent stopgap measure for patients suffering from the uncontrolled pain of trigeminal neuralgia while waiting for drug treatments to take effect. This technique may lead to the rapid control of pain and allow the patient to maintain adequate oral hydration and nutrition and avoid hospitalization.

Chapter 9

Temporomandibular Joint Dysfunction

ICD-9 CODE **524.60**

THE CLINICAL SYNDROME

Temporomandibular joint (TMJ) dysfunction (also known as myofascial pain dysfunction of the muscles of mastication) is characterized by pain in the joint itself that radiates into the mandible, ear, neck, and tonsillar pillars. The TMJ is a true joint that is divided into upper and lower synovial cavities by a fibrous articular disk. Internal derangement of this disk may result in pain and TMJ dysfunction, but extracapsular causes of TMJ pain are much more common. The TMJ is innervated by branches of the mandibular nerve. The muscles involved in TMJ dysfunction often include the temporalis, masseter, and external and internal pterygoids; the trapezius and sternocleidomastoid may be involved as well.

SIGNS AND SYMPTOMS

Headache often accompanies the pain of TMJ dysfunction and is clinically indistinguishable from tension-type headache. Stress is often the precipitating or an exacerbating factor in the development of TMJ dysfunction (Fig. 9-1). Dental malocclusion may also play a role in its evolution. Internal derangement and arthritis of the TMJ may present as clicking or grating when the mouth is opened and closed. If untreated, the patient may experience increasing pain in the aforementioned areas, as well as limitation of jaw movement and mouth opening.

Trigger points may be identified when palpating the muscles involved in TMJ dysfunction. Crepitus on range of motion of the joint is suggestive of arthritis rather than of dysfunction of myofascial origin. A history of bruxism or jaw clenching is often present.

TESTING

Radiographs of the TMJ are usually within normal limits in patients suffering from TMJ dysfunction, but they may

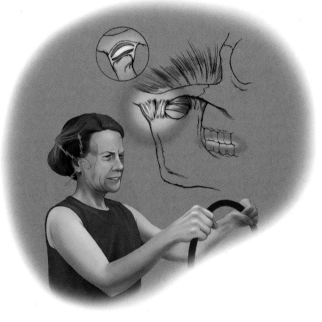

Figure 9–1. Stress is often a trigger for temporomandibular joint dysfunction.

be useful to help identify inflammatory or degenerative arthritis of the joint. Imaging of the joint can help the clinician identify derangement of the disk as well as other abnormalities of the joint itself (Fig. 9-2). A complete blood count, erythrocyte sedimentation rate, and antinuclear antibody testing are indicated if inflammatory arthritis or temporal arteritis is suspected. Injection of the joint with small amounts of local anesthetic can serve as a diagnostic maneuver to determine whether the TMJ is in fact the source of the patient's pain (Fig. 9-3).

DIFFERENTIAL DIAGNOSIS

The clinical symptoms of TMJ dysfunction may be confused with pain of dental or sinus origin or may be characterized as atypical facial pain. However, with

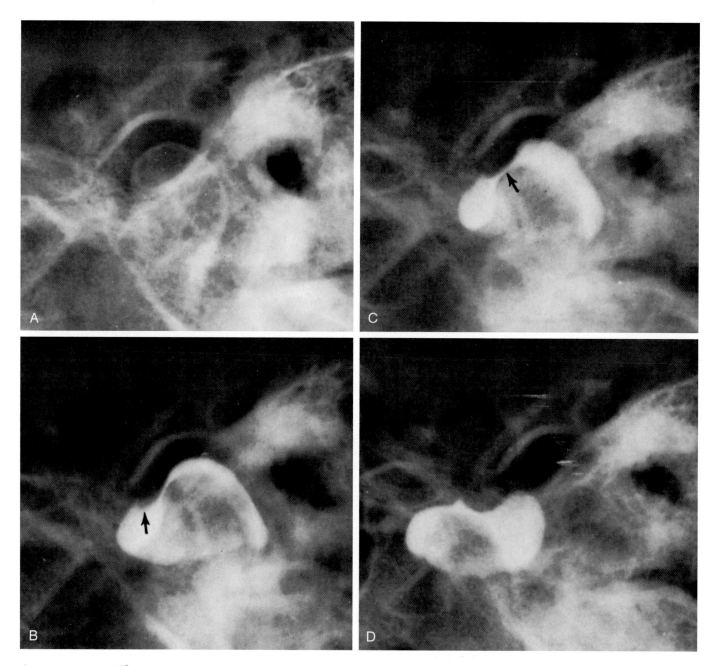

Figure 9–2. Arthrography of an abnormal temporomandibular joint showing disk dislocation with reduction in a 20-year-old woman with clicking and intermittent pain. **A,** Magnification transcranial radiograph with the mouth closed shows normal osseous anatomy and isocentric condyle position in the mandibular fossa. **B,** With the mouth closed, contrast agent fills the inferior joint space and outlines the undersurface of the disk. Note that the posterior band of the disk is located anterior to the condyle *(arrow)* and bulges prominently in the anterior recess. This appearance is diagnostic of anterior dislocation of the disk. **C,** With the mouth half opened, contrast agent has been redistributed, and the condyle has moved onto the posterior band *(arrow)*, which is now compressed between the condyle and the eminence. **D,** With the mouth fully opened, the condyle has translated anterior to the eminence; in so doing, it has crossed the prominent, thick posterior band and is causing a click. The posterior band is now in a normal position posterior to the condyle. (From Resnick D: Diagnosis of Bone and Joint Disorders, 4th ed. Philadelphia, Saunders, 2002, p 1723.)

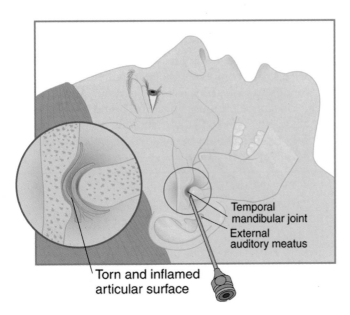

Figure 9–3. Correct needle placement for injections of the temporomandibular joint. (From Waldman SD: Atlas of Pain Management Injection Techniques. Philadelphia, Saunders, 2000, p 5.)

careful questioning and physical examination, the clinician can usually distinguish these overlapping pain syndromes. Tumors of the zygoma and mandible, as well as retropharyngeal tumors, may produce ill-defined pain attributed to the TMJ, and these potentially life-threatening diseases must be excluded in any patient with facial pain. Reflex sympathetic dystrophy of the face should also be considered in any patient presenting with ill-defined facial pain after trauma, infection, or central nervous system injury. The pain of TMJ dysfunction is dull and aching in character, whereas the pain of reflex sympathetic dystrophy of the face is burning, with significant allodynia often present. Stellate ganglion block may help distinguish the two pain syndromes, because the pain of reflex sympathetic dystrophy of the face readily responds to this sympathetic nerve block, whereas the pain of TMJ dysfunction does not. In addition, the pain of TMJ dysfunction must be distinguished from the pain of jaw claudication associated with temporal arteritis.

TREATMENT

The mainstay of therapy is a combination of drug treatment with tricyclic antidepressants, physical modalities such as oral orthotic devices and physical therapy, and intra-articular injection of the joint with small amounts of local anesthetic and steroid. Antidepressant compounds such as nortriptyline at a single bedtime dose of 25 mg can help alleviate sleep disturbance and treat any

underlying myofascial pain syndrome. Orthotic devices help the patient avoid jaw clenching and bruxism, which may exacerbate the clinical syndrome. Intra-articular injection is useful to palliate acute pain to allow physical therapy, as well as to treat joint arthritis that may contribute to the patient's pain and joint dysfunction. Rarely, surgical treatment of the displaced intra-articular disk is required to restore the joint to normal function and reduce pain.

For intra-articular injection of the TMJ, the patient is placed in the supine position with the cervical spine in the neutral position. The TMJ is identified by asking the patient to open and close the mouth several times and palpating the area just anterior and slightly inferior to the acoustic auditory meatus. After the joint is identified, the patient is asked to hold his or her mouth in the neutral position. A total of 0.5 mL of local anesthetic is drawn up in a 3-mL sterile syringe. When treating TMJ dysfunction, internal derangement of the TMJ, or arthritis or other painful conditions involving the TMJ, a total of 20 mg methylprednisolone is added to the local anesthetic with the first block; 10 mg methylprednisolone is added to the local anesthetic with subsequent blocks. After the skin overlying the TMJ is prepared with antiseptic solution, a 1-inch, 25-gauge styleted needle is inserted just below the zygomatic arch directly in the middle of the joint space. The needle is advanced approximately $\frac{1}{4}$ to $\frac{3}{4}$ inch in a plane perpendicular to the skull until a pop is felt, indicating that the joint space has been entered (see Fig. 9-3). After careful aspiration, 1 mL of solution is slowly injected. Injection of the joint may be repeated at 5- to 7-day intervals if symptoms persist.

COMPLICATIONS AND PITFALLS

The vascularity of the region and the proximity to major blood vessels lead to an increased incidence of postblock ecchymosis and hematoma formation, and the patient should be warned of this potential complication. Despite the region's vascularity, intra-articular injection can be performed safely (albeit with an increased risk of hematoma formation) in the presence of anticoagulation by using a 25- or 27-gauge needle, if the clinical situation indicates a favorable risk-benefit ratio. These complications can be decreased if manual pressure is applied to the area of the block immediately after injection. Application of cold packs for 20 minutes after the block also decreases the amount of postprocedural pain and bleeding. Another complication that occurs with some frequency is inadvertent block of the facial nerve, with associated facial weakness. When this occurs, protection of the cornea with sterile ophthalmic lubricant and patching is mandatory.

Clinical Pearls

Pain from TMJ dysfunction requires careful evaluation to design an appropriate treatment plan. Infection and inflammatory causes, including collagen vascular diseases, must be ruled out. When TMJ pain occurs in older patients, it must be distinguished from the jaw claudication associated with temporal arteritis. Stress and anxiety often accompany TMJ dysfunction, and these factors must be addressed and managed. The myofascial pain component is best treated with tricyclic antidepressants, such as amitriptyline. Dental malocclusion and nighttime bruxism should be treated with an acrylic bite appliance. Narcotic analgesics and benzodiazepines should be avoided in patients suffering from TMJ dysfunction.

Chapter 10

Atypical Facial Pain

ICD-9 CODE 350.2

THE CLINICAL SYNDROME

Atypical facial pain (also known as atypical facial neuralgia) describes a heterogeneous group of pain syndromes that share in common the fact that the facial pain cannot be classified as trigeminal neuralgia. The pain is continuous but may vary in intensity. It is almost always unilateral and may be characterized as aching or cramping rather than the shocklike neuritic pain typical of trigeminal neuralgia. The vast majority of patients suffering from atypical facial pain are female. The pain is felt in the distribution of the trigeminal nerve but invariably overlaps the divisions of the nerve (Fig. 10-1).

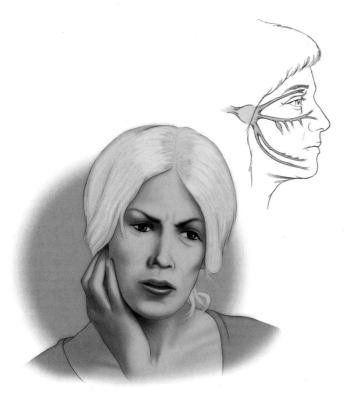

Figure 10–1. Patients with atypical facial pain often rub the affected area; those with trigeminal neuralgia do not.

Table 10–1. Comparison of Trigeminal Neuralgia and Atypical Facial Pain

	Trigeminal Neuralgia	Atypical Facial Pain
Temporal pattern of pain	Sudden and intermittent	Constant
Character of pain	Shocklike and neuritic	Dull, cramping, aching
Pain-free intervals	Usual	Rare
Distribution of pain	One division of trigeminal nerve	Overlapping divisions of trigeminal nerve
Trigger areas	Present	Absent
Underlying psychopathology	Rare	Common

Headache often accompanies atypical facial pain and is clinically indistinguishable from tension-type headache. Stress is often the precipitating or an exacerbating factor in the development of atypical facial pain. Depression and sleep disturbance are also present in a significant number of patients. A history of facial trauma, infection, or tumor of the head and neck may be elicited in some patients with atypical facial pain, but in most cases, no precipitating event can be identified.

SIGNS AND SYMPTOMS

Table 10-1 compares atypical facial pain with trigeminal neuralgia. Unlike trigeminal neuralgia, which is characterized by sudden paroxysms of neuritic shocklike pain, atypical facial pain is constant and has a dull, aching quality, but it may vary in intensity. The pain of trigeminal neuralgia is always within the distribution of one division of the trigeminal nerve, whereas atypical facial pain invariably overlaps these divisional boundaries. The trigger areas characteristic of trigeminal neuralgia are absent in patients suffering from atypical facial pain.

TESTING

Radiographs of the head are usually within normal limits in patients suffering from atypical facial pain, but they may be useful to identify a tumor or bony abnormality (Fig. 10-2). Magnetic resonance imaging (MRI) of the

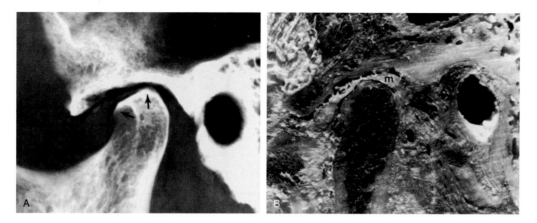

Figure 10-2. Osteoarthritis compared in a specimen radiograph **(A)** and photograph **(B)** of a sagittally sectioned specimen. (From Resnick D: Diagnosis of Bone and Joint Disorders, 4th ed. Philadelphia, Saunders, 2002, p 1739.)

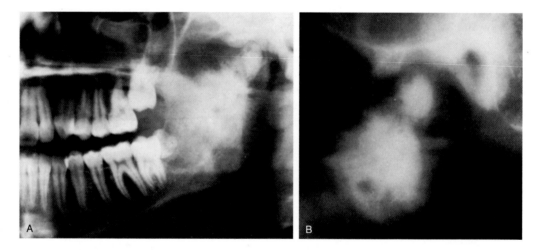

Figure 10-3. Osteosarcoma of the mandible **(A)** and the condylar head and neck **(B)** in a 12-year-old girl. (From Resnick D: Diagnosis of Bone and Joint Disorders, 4th ed. Philadelphia, Saunders, 2002, p 1726.)

brain and sinuses can help the clinician identify intracranial pathology such as tumor, sinus disease, and infection. A complete blood count, erythrocyte sedimentation rate, and antinuclear antibody testing are indicated if inflammatory arthritis or temporal arteritis is suspected. Injection of the temporomandibular joint with small amounts of local anesthetic can serve as a diagnostic maneuver to determine whether the temporomandibular joint is the source of the patient's pain. MRI of the cervical spine is also indicated if the patient is experiencing significant occipital or nuchal pain.

DIFFERENTIAL DIAGNOSIS

The clinical symptoms of atypical facial pain may be confused with pain of dental or sinus origin or may be erroneously characterized as trigeminal neuralgia. Careful questioning and physical examination usually allow the clinician to distinguish these overlapping pain syndromes. Tumors of the zygoma and mandible, as well as posterior fossa and retropharyngeal tumors, may produce ill-defined pain that is attributed to atypical facial pain, and these potentially life-threatening diseases must be excluded in any patient with facial pain (Fig. 10-3). Reflex sympathetic dystrophy of the face should also be considered in any patient presenting with ill-defined facial pain after trauma, infection, or central nervous system injury. As noted, atypical facial pain is dull and aching, whereas reflex sympathetic dystrophy of the face causes burning pain, and significant allodynia is often present. Stellate ganglion block may help distinguish these two pain syndromes; the pain of reflex sympathetic dystrophy of the face readily responds to this sympathetic nerve block, whereas atypical facial pain does not. Atypical facial pain must also be distinguished from the pain of jaw claudication associated with temporal arteritis.

TREATMENT

The mainstay of therapy is a combination of drug treatment with tricyclic antidepressants and physical modalities such as oral orthotic devices and physical therapy. Trigeminal nerve block and intra-articular injection of the temporomandibular joint with small amounts of local anesthetic and steroid may also be of value. Antidepressants such as nortriptyline at a single bedtime dose of 25 mg can help alleviate sleep disturbance and treat any underlying myofascial pain syndrome. Orthotic devices help the patient avoid jaw clenching and bruxism, which may exacerbate the clinical syndrome. Management of underlying depression and anxiety is also mandatory.

COMPLICATIONS AND PITFALLS

The major pitfall when caring for patients thought to be suffering from atypical facial pain is the failure to diagnose underlying pathology that may be responsible for the patient's pain. Atypical facial pain is essentially a diagnosis of exclusion. If trigeminal nerve block or intra-articular injection of the temporomandibular joint is being considered as part of the treatment plan, it must be remembered that the region's vascularity and proximity to major blood vessels can lead to an increased incidence of postblock ecchymosis and hematoma formation, and the patient should be warned of this potential complication.

Clinical Pearls

Atypical facial pain requires careful evaluation to design an appropriate treatment plan. Infection and inflammatory causes, including collagen vascular diseases, must be ruled out. Stress and anxiety often accompany atypical facial pain, and these factors must be addressed and treated. The myofascial pain component of atypical facial pain is best treated with tricyclic antidepressants such as amitriptyline. Dental malocclusion and nighttime bruxism should be treated with an acrylic bite appliance. Narcotic analgesics and benzodiazepines should be avoided in patients suffering from atypical facial pain.

Chapter 11

Hyoid Syndrome

IDC-9 Code **727.82**

THE CLINICAL SYNDROME

Hyoid syndrome is caused by calcification and inflammation of the attachment of the stylohyoid ligament to the hyoid bone. The styloid process extends in a caudal and ventral direction from the temporal bone from its origin just below the auditory meatus. The stylohyoid ligament's cephalad attachment is to the styloid process, and its caudad attachment is to the hyoid bone. In hyoid syndrome, the stylohyoid ligament becomes calcified at its caudad attachment to the hyoid bone (Fig. 11-1). Tendinitis of the other muscular attachments to the hyoid bone may contribute to this painful condition. Hyoid syndrome also may be seen in conjunction with Eagle's syndrome. Patient's suffering from diffuse idiopathic skeletal hyperostosis are thought to be prone to the development of hyoid syndrome because of the propensity for calcification of the stylohyoid ligament in this disease (Fig. 11-2).

SIGNS AND SYMPTOMS

The pain of hyoid syndrome is sharp and stabbing in nature and occurs with movement of the mandible, turning of the neck, or swallowing. The pain starts below the angle of the mandible and radiates into the anterolateral neck (Fig. 11-3); it is often referred to the ipsilateral ear. Some patients complain of a foreign body sensation in the pharynx. Injection of local anesthetic and steroid into the attachment of the stylohyoid ligament to the greater cornu of the hyoid bone is both a diagnostic and a therapeutic maneuver.

TESTING

There is no specific test for hyoid syndrome. Plain radiography, computed tomography, or magnetic resonance imaging of the neck may reveal calcification of the

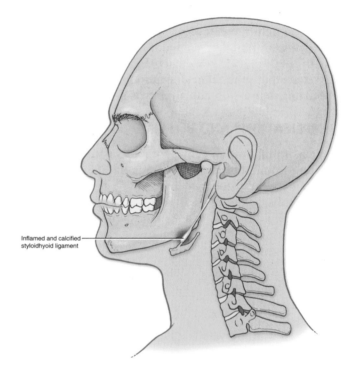

Inflamed and calcified styloidhyoid ligament

Figure 11–1. In hyoid syndrome, the stylohyoid ligament becomes calcified at its caudad attachment to the hyoid bone.

caudad attachment of the stylohyoid ligament at the hyoid bone, which is highly suggestive of hyoid syndrome in patients suffering from the previously described constellation of symptoms. A complete blood count, erythrocyte sedimentation rate, and antinuclear antibody testing are indicated if inflammatory arthritis or temporal arteritis is suspected. As noted earlier, injection of small amounts of anesthetic into the attachment of the stylohyoid ligament to the hyoid bone can help determine whether this is the source of the patient's pain. If difficulty swallowing is a prominent feature of the clinical presentation, endoscopy of the esophagus, with special attention to the gastroesophageal junction, is mandatory to identify esophageal tumors or strictures due to gastric reflux.

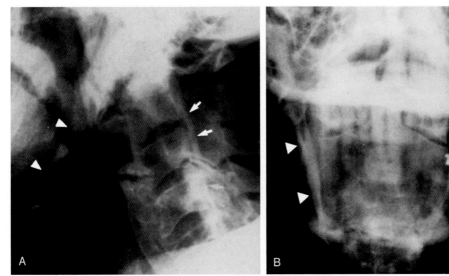

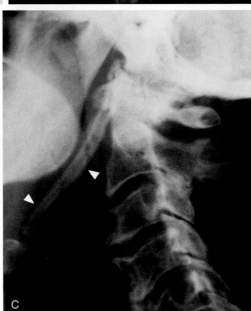

Figure 11–2. Cervical spine abnormalities in diffuse idiopathic skeletal hyperostosis (DISH). **A** and **B,** Radiographic abnormalities in this patient with DISH include extensive anterior bone formation, ossification of the posterior longitudinal ligament *(arrows),* and ossification of both stylohyoid ligaments *(arrowheads).* **C,** In another patient, note the extensive ossification of the stylohyoid ligament *(arrowheads)* and the changes caused by spinal DISH. (From Resnick D: Diagnosis of Bone and Joint Disorders, 4th ed. Philadelphia, Saunders, 2002, 9 1483.)

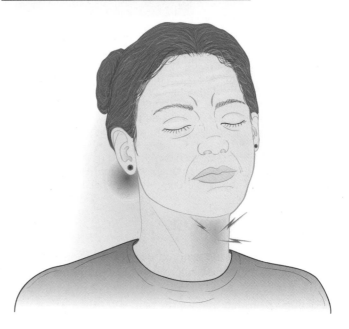

Figure 11–3. The pain of hyoid syndrome is sharp and stabbing and occurs with movement of the mandible, turning of the neck, or swallowing. The pain starts below the angle of the mandible and radiates to the anterolateral neck.

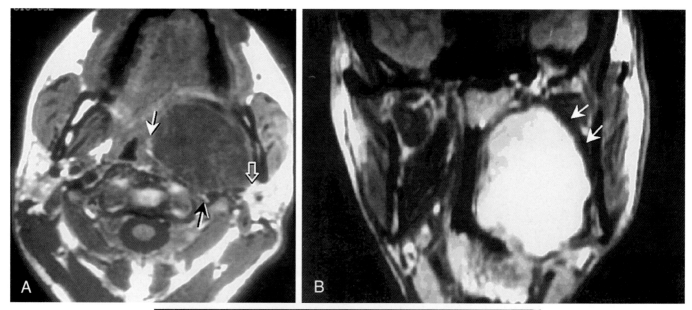

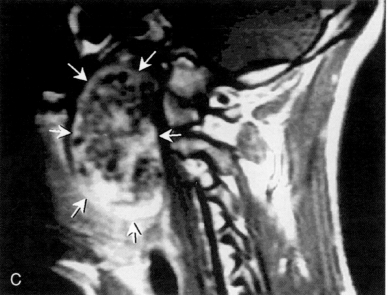

Figure 11–4. Pleomorphic adenoma. **A,** Nonenhanced, T1-weighted axial image demonstrates a well-defined mass of lower signal intensity than adjacent muscle. The mass is displacing the prestyloid parapharyngeal fat medially *(solid white arrow)* and the internal carotid artery posteriorly *(solid black arrow)*. No intact fat plane can be demonstrated between the lesion and the deep lobe of the parotid gland *(open arrow)*. **B,** Intermediate-weighted coronal image demonstrates a relatively homogeneous, well-defined mass of increased signal intensity relative to adjacent muscle and lymphoid tissue. The oropharyngeal mucosa is displaced medially. The left medial pterygoid muscle is compressed and displaced superolaterally *(arrows)*. **C,** Contrast-enhanced, T1-weighted sagittal image demonstrates a markedly heterogeneous mass, with multiple low-signal-intensity regions that may represent areas of calcification or fibrosis. (From Haaga JR, Lanzieri CF, Gilkeson RC [eds]: CT and MR Imaging of the Whole Body, 4th ed. Philadelphia, Mosby, 2003, p 653.)

DIFFERENTIAL DIAGNOSIS

The diagnosis of hyoid syndrome is one of exclusion, and the clinician must first rule out other conditions (Table 11-1). Retropharyngeal infection and tumor may produce ill-defined pain that mimics the pain and other symptoms of hyoid syndrome, and these potentially life-threatening diseases must be excluded (Fig. 11-4). Glossopharyngeal neuralgia is another painful condition that can be mistaken for hyoid syndrome. However, the pain of glossopharyngeal neuralgia is similar to the paroxysms of shocklike pain in trigeminal neuralgia rather than the sharp, shooting pain

Table 11-1. Conditions That Can Mimic Hyoid Syndrome

Glossopharyngeal neuralgia
Retropharyngeal tumor
Retropharyngeal abscess
Atypical facial pain
Mandibular tumor
Esophageal disease
Jaw claudication of temporal arteritis

with movement associated with hyoid syndrome. Because glossopharyngeal neuralgia may be associated with serious cardiac bradyarrhythmias and syncope, it is important to distinguish the two syndromes.

TREATMENT

The pain of hyoid syndrome is best treated with local anesthetic and steroid injection of the attachment of the stylohyoid ligament. Owing to the vascularity of this area and the proximity to neural structures, this technique should be performed only by those familiar with the regional anatomy. Antidepressants such as nortriptyline at a single bedtime dose of 25 mg can help alleviate sleep disturbance and treat any underlying myofascial pain syndrome.

COMPLICATIONS AND PITFALLS

The major pitfall when caring for patients thought to be suffering from hyoid syndrome is the failure to diagnose some other underlying pathology that may be responsible for the pain. If injection of the caudad attachment of the stylohyoid ligament is being considered as part of the treatment plan, it should be remembered that the area's vascularity and proximity to major blood vessels can lead to an increased incidence of postblock ecchymosis and hematoma formation, and the patient should be warned of this potential complication.

Clinical Pearls

The clinician should always look for occult malignancy in patients suffering from pain in this region. Tumors of the larynx, hypopharynx, and anterior triangle of the neck may present with clinical symptoms identical to those of hyoid syndrome. Given the low incidence of hyoid syndrome compared with pain secondary to malignancy, hyoid syndrome must be considered a diagnosis of exclusion.

Chapter 12

Reflex Sympathetic Dystrophy of the Face

ICD-9 CODE 337.29

THE CLINICAL SYNDROME

Reflex sympathetic dystrophy (RSD) is an infrequent cause of face and neck pain. Although the symptom complex in this disorder is relatively constant from patient to patient, and although RSD of the face and neck closely parallels its presentation in the upper or lower extremity, the diagnosis is often missed. As a result, extensive diagnostic and therapeutic procedures may be performed in an effort to palliate the patient's pain. The common denominator in all patients suffering from RSD of the face is trauma (Fig. 12-1), which may take the form of actual injury to the soft tissues, dentition, or bones of the face; infection; cancer; arthritis; or insults to the central nervous system or cranial nerves.

SIGNS AND SYMPTOMS

The hallmark of RSD of the face is burning pain. The pain is frequently associated with cutaneous or mucosal allodynia and does not follow the path of either the cranial or the peripheral nerves. Trigger areas, especially in the oral mucosa, are common, as are trophic skin and mucosal changes in the area affected by RSD. Sudomotor and vasomotor changes may also be identified, but these are often less obvious than in patients suffering from RSD of the extremities. Often, patients with RSD of the face have evidence of previous dental extractions performed in an effort to achieve pain relief. They frequently experience significant sleep disturbance and depression as well.

TESTING

Although there is no specific test for RSD, a presumptive diagnosis can be made if the patient experiences significant pain relief after stellate ganglion block with local anesthetic. Given the diverse nature of the tissue injury

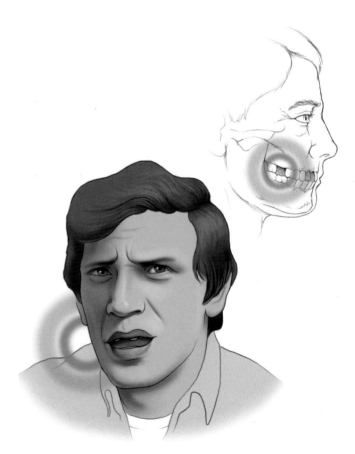

Figure 12–1. Reflex sympathetic dystrophy of the face frequently occurs following trauma, such as dental extractions.

that can cause RSD of the face, however, the clinician must assiduously search for occult pathology that may mimic or coexist with RSD (see Differential Diagnosis). All patients with a presumptive diagnosis of RSD of the face should undergo magnetic resonance imaging of the brain and, if significant occipital or nuchal symptoms are present, of the cervical spine. Screening laboratory tests consisting of a complete blood count, erythrocyte sedimentation rate, and automated blood chemistry should be performed to rule out infection or other inflammatory

Table 12–1. Differential Diagnosis of Reflex Sympathetic Dystrophy (RSD) of the Face

	Trigeminal Neuralgia	Atypical Facial Pain	RSD of the Face
Temporal pattern of pain	Sudden and intermittent	Constant	Constant
Character of pain	Shocklike and neuritic	Dull, cramping, aching	Burning with allodynia
Pain-free intervals	Usual	Rare	Rare
Distribution of pain	One division of trigeminal nerve	Overlapping divisions of trigeminal nerve	Overlapping divisions of trigeminal nerve
Trigger areas	Present	Absent	Present
Underlying psychopathology	Rare	Common	Common
Trophic skin changes	Absent	Absent	Present
Sudomotor and vasomotor changes	Absent	Absent	Often present

causes of tissue injury that may serve as a nidus for RSD.

DIFFERENTIAL DIAGNOSIS

The clinical symptoms of RSD of the face may be confused with pain of dental or sinus origin or may be erroneously characterized as atypical facial pain or trigeminal neuralgia (Table 12-1). Careful questioning and physical examination usually allow the clinician to distinguish these overlapping pain syndromes. Stellate ganglion block may help distinguish RSD from atypical facial pain, because the former readily responds to sympathetic nerve block, whereas the latter does not. Tumors of the zygoma and mandible, as well as posterior fossa and retropharyngeal tumors, may produce ill-defined pain attributed to RSD of the face, and these potentially life-threatening diseases must be excluded in any patient with facial pain. RSD of the face must also be distinguished from the pain of jaw claudication associated with temporal arteritis.

TREATMENT

The successful treatment of RSD of the face requires two phases. First, any nidus of tissue trauma that is contributing to the ongoing sympathetic dysfunction responsible for the symptoms must be identified and removed. Second, interruption of the sympathetic innervation of the face via stellate ganglion block with local anesthetic must be implemented. This may require daily stellate ganglion block for a significant period. Occupational therapy consisting of tactile desensitization of the affected skin may also be of value. Underlying depression and sleep disturbance are best treated with a tricyclic antidepressant such as nortriptyline, given as a single 25-mg dose at bedtime. Gabapentin may help palliate any neuritic pain component. Opioid analgesics and benzodiazepines should be avoided to prevent iatrogenic chemical dependence.

COMPLICATIONS AND PITFALLS

The main complications of RSD of the face are those associated with its misdiagnosis. In this case, chemical dependence, depression, and multiple failed therapeutic procedures are the rule rather than the exception. Stellate ganglion block is a safe and effective technique for pain management, but it is not without side effects and risks.

Clinical Pearls

The key to recognizing RSD of the face is a high index of clinical suspicion. RSD should be suspected in any patient who has burning pain or allodynia associated with antecedent trauma. Once the syndrome is recognized, blockade of the sympathetic nerves subserving the painful area confirms the diagnosis. Repeated sympathetic blockade, combined with adjunctive therapies, results in pain relief in most cases. The frequency and number of sympathetic blocks recommended to treat RSD vary among pain practitioners; however, it is believed that early, aggressive neural blockade provides more rapid resolution of pain and disability.

Section 3

Pain Syndromes of the Neck and Brachial Plexus

Chapter 13

Cervical Facet Syndrome

ICD-9 CODE 724.5

THE CLINICAL SYNDROME

Cervical facet syndrome is a constellation of symptoms consisting of neck, head, shoulder, and proximal upper extremity pain that radiates in a nondermatomal pattern. The pain is ill defined and dull in character. It may be unilateral or bilateral and is thought to be the result of pathology of the facet joint. The pain of cervical facet syndrome is exacerbated by flexion, extension, and lateral bending of the cervical spine. It is often worse in the morning after physical activity. Each facet joint receives innervation from two spinal levels; it receives fibers from the dorsal ramus at the corresponding vertebral level and from the vertebra above. This explains the ill-defined nature of facet-mediated pain and explains why the dorsal nerve from the vertebra above the offending level must often be blocked to provide complete pain relief.

SIGNS AND SYMPTOMS

Most patients with cervical facet syndrome have tenderness to deep palpation of the cervical paraspinous musculature; muscle spasm may also be present. Patients exhibit decreased range of motion of the cervical spine and usually complain of pain on flexion, extension, rotation, and lateral bending of the cervical spine (Fig. 13-1). There is no motor or sensory deficit unless there is coexisting radiculopathy, plexopathy, or entrapment neuropathy.

If the C1-2 facet joints are involved, the pain is referred to the posterior auricular and occipital region. If the C2-3 facet joints are involved, the pain may radiate to the forehead and eyes. Pain emanating from the C3-4 facet joints is referred superiorly to the suboccipital region and inferiorly to the posterolateral neck, and pain from the C4-5 facet joints radiates to the base of the neck. Pain from the C5-6 joints is referred to the shoulders and interscapular region, and pain from the C6-7 facet joints radiates to the supraspinous and infraspinous fossae.

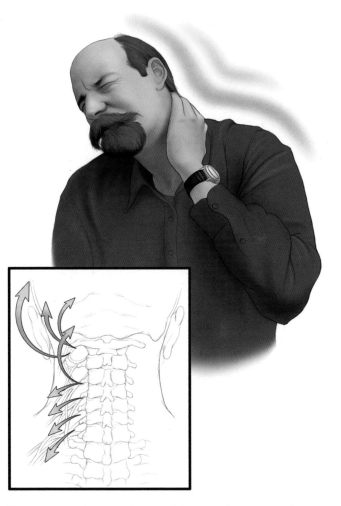

Figure 13–1. The pain of cervical facet syndrome is made worse by flexion, extension, and lateral bending of the cervical spine.

TESTING

By the fifth decade of life, almost all individuals exhibit some abnormality of the facet joints of the cervical spine on plain radiographs (Fig. 13-2). The clinical significance of these findings has long been debated by pain specialists, but it was not until the advent of computed tomography scanning and magnetic resonance imaging (MRI)

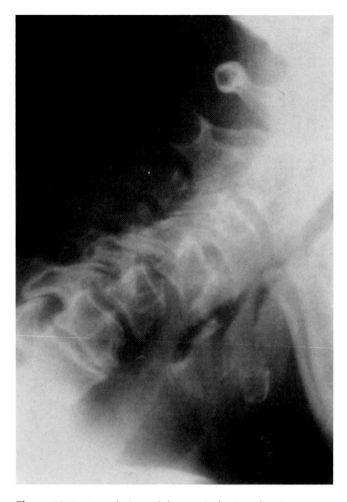

Figure 13–2. Lateral view of the cervical spine showing osteoarthritis of the apophyseal joints of the upper cervical spine, with resultant subluxation of C4 on C5. Additional findings are degenerative disk disease at C5-6 and C6-7, associated osteophyte formation at C6-7, and subluxation of C5 on C6. (From Brower AC, Flemming DJ: Arthritis in Black and White, 2nd ed. Philadelphia, Saunders, 1997, p 290.)

that the relationship between these abnormal facet joints and the cervical nerve roots and other surrounding structures was clearly understood. MRI of the cervical spine should be performed in all patients suspected of suffering from cervical facet syndrome. However, any data gleaned from this sophisticated imaging technique can provide only a presumptive diagnosis. To prove that a specific facet joint is contributing to the patient's pain, a diagnostic intra-articular injection of that joint with local anesthetic is required. If the diagnosis of cervical facet syndrome is in doubt, screening laboratory tests consisting of a complete blood count, erythrocyte sedi-

mentation rate, antinuclear antibody testing, HLA B-27 antigen screening, and automated blood chemistry should be performed to rule out other causes of the patient's pain.

DIFFERENTIAL DIAGNOSIS

Cervical facet syndrome is a diagnosis of exclusion that is supported by a combination of clinical history, physical examination, radiography, MRI, and intra-articular injection of the suspect facet joint. Pain syndromes that may mimic cervical facet syndrome include cervicalgia, cervical bursitis, cervical fibromyositis, inflammatory arthritis, and disorders of the cervical spinal cord, roots, plexus, and nerves.

TREATMENT

Cervical facet syndrome is best treated with a multimodality approach. Physical therapy consisting of heat modalities and deep sedative massage, combined with nonsteroidal anti-inflammatory drugs and skeletal muscle relaxants, is a reasonable starting point. The addition of cervical facet blocks is a logical next step. For symptomatic relief, blockade of the medial branch of the dorsal ramus or intra-articular injection of the facet joint with local anesthetic and steroid is extremely effective. Underlying sleep disturbance and depression are best treated with a tricyclic antidepressant such as nortriptyline, which can be started at a single bedtime dose of 25 mg.

Cervical facet block is often combined with atlanto-occipital block when treating pain in this area. Although the atlanto-occipital joint is not a true facet joint in the anatomic sense, the technique is analogous to the facet joint block commonly used by pain practitioners and may be viewed as such.

COMPLICATIONS AND PITFALLS

The proximity to the spinal cord and exiting nerve roots makes it imperative that cervical facet block be carried out only by those familiar with the regional anatomy and experienced in interventional pain management techniques. The proximity to the vertebral artery, combined with the vascular nature of this region, makes the potential for intravascular injection high, and the injection of even a small amount of local anesthetic into the vertebral artery can result in seizures. Given the proximity of the brain and brainstem, ataxia due to vascular uptake of local anesthetic is not uncommon after cervical facet block. Many patients also complain of a transient increase in headache and cervicalgia after injection of the joint.

Clinical Pearls

Cervical facet syndrome is a common cause of neck, occipital, shoulder, and upper extremity pain. It is often confused with cervicalgia and cervical fibromyositis. Diagnostic intra-articular facet block can confirm the diagnosis. The clinician must take care to rule out diseases of the cervical spinal cord, such as syringomyelia, that may initially present in a similar manner. Ankylosing spondylitis may also present as cervical facet syndrome and must be correctly identified to avoid ongoing joint damage and functional disability.

Many pain specialists believe that cervical facet block and atlanto-occipital block are underused in the treatment of "post-whiplash" cervicalgia and cervicogenic headaches and that they should be considered whenever cervical epidural or occipital nerve blocks fail to provide palliation of headache and neck pain syndromes.

Chapter 14

Cervical Radiculopathy

ICD-9 CODE 724.3

THE CLINICAL SYNDROME

Cervical radiculopathy is a constellation of symptoms consisting of neurogenic neck and upper extremity pain emanating from the cervical nerve roots. In addition to pain, the patient may experience numbness, weakness, and loss of reflexes. The causes of cervical radiculopathy include herniated disk, foraminal stenosis, tumor, osteophyte formation, and, rarely, infection.

SIGNS AND SYMPTOMS

Patients suffering from cervical radiculopathy complain of pain, numbness, tingling, and paresthesias in the distribution of the affected nerve root or roots (Table 14-1). Patients may also note weakness and lack of coordination in the affected extremity. Muscle spasms and neck pain, as well as pain referred to the trapezius and interscapular region, are common. Decreased sensation, weakness, and reflex changes are demonstrated on physical examination. Patients with C7 radiculopathy commonly place the hand of the affected extremity on top of the head to obtain relief (Fig. 14-1). Occasionally, patients suffering from cervical radiculopathy experi-

ence compression of the cervical spinal cord, resulting in myelopathy. Cervical myelopathy is most commonly due to a midline herniated cervical disk, spinal stenosis, tumor, or, rarely, infection. Patients suffering from cervical myelopathy experience lower extremity weakness and bowel and bladder symptoms. This represents a neurosurgical emergency and should be treated as such.

TESTING

Magnetic resonance imaging (MRI) provides the best information regarding the cervical spine and its contents (Fig. 14-2). MRI is highly accurate and can identify abnormalities that may put the patient at risk for cervical myelopathy (Fig. 14-3). In patients who cannot undergo MRI, such as those with pacemakers, computed tomography or myelography is a reasonable alternative. Radionuclide bone scanning and plain radiography are indicated if fractures or bony abnormalities such as metastatic disease are being considered.

Although these tests provide the clinician with useful neuroanatomic information, electromyography and nerve conduction velocity testing provide the clinician with neurophysiologic information that can determine the actual status of each individual nerve root and the brachial plexus. Electromyography can also

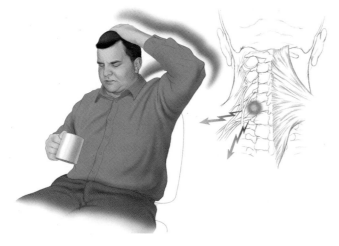

Figure 14–1. Patients with C7 radiculopathy often place the hand of the affected extremity on the head to obtain relief.

Table 14–1. Clinical Features of Cervical Radiculopathy

Cervical Root	Pain	Sensory Changes	Weakness	Reflex Changes
C5	Neck, shoulder, anterolateral arm	Numbness in deltoid area	Deltoid and biceps	Biceps reflex
C6	Neck, shoulder, lateral aspect of arm	Dorsolateral aspect of thumb and index finger	Biceps, wrist extensors, pollicis longus	Brachioradialis reflex
C7	Neck, shoulder, lateral aspect of arm, dorsal forearm	Index and middle fingers and dorsum of hand	Triceps	Triceps reflex

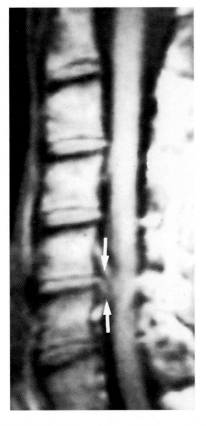

Figure 14–2. Disk herniation at the C5-6 level. Sagittal T1-weighted spin echo image showing a herniated fragment *(arrows)* extending below the disk space level. (From Stark DD, Bradley WG Jr: Magnetic Resonance Imaging, vol 3, 3rd ed. St Louis, Mosby, 1999, p 1848.)

distinguish plexopathy from radiculopathy and can identify a coexistent entrapment neuropathy, such as carpal tunnel syndrome. Screening laboratory tests consisting of a complete blood count, erythrocyte sedimentation rate, antinuclear antibody testing, HLA B-27 antigen screening, and automated blood chemistry should be performed if the diagnosis of cervical radiculopathy is in question.

DIFFERENTIAL DIAGNOSIS

Cervical radiculopathy is a clinical diagnosis supported by a combination of clinical history, physical examination, radiography, and MRI. Pain syndromes that may mimic cervical radiculopathy include cervicalgia, cervical bursitis, cervical fibromyositis, inflammatory arthritis, and disorders of the cervical spinal cord, roots, plexus, and nerves.

TREATMENT

Cervical radiculopathy is best treated with a multimodality approach. Physical therapy, including heat modalities and deep sedative massage, combined with nonsteroidal anti-inflammatory drugs and skeletal muscle relaxants, is a reasonable starting point. The addition of cervical epidural nerve blocks is a logical next step. Cervical epidural blocks with local anesthetic and steroid are extremely effective in the treatment of cervical radiculopathy. Underlying sleep disturbance and depression are best treated with a tricyclic antidepressant such as nortriptyline, which can be started at a single bedtime dose of 25 mg.

COMPLICATIONS AND PITFALLS

Failure to accurately diagnose cervical radiculopathy may put the patient at risk for the development of cervical myelopathy, which, if untreated, may progress to quadriparesis or quadriplegia.

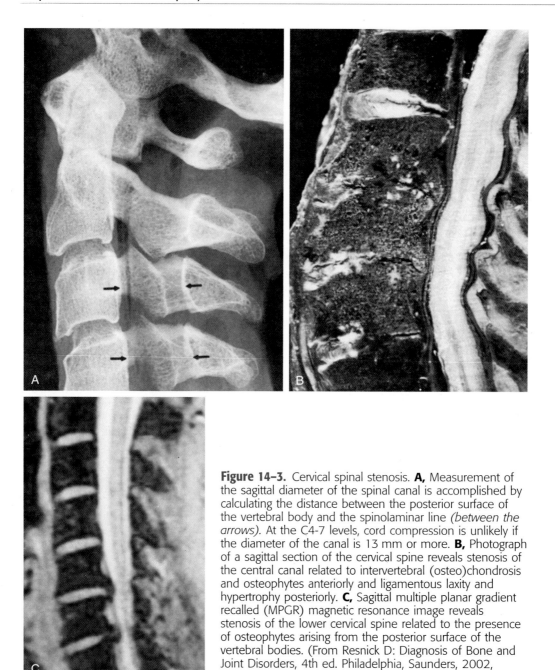

Figure 14–3. Cervical spinal stenosis. **A,** Measurement of the sagittal diameter of the spinal canal is accomplished by calculating the distance between the posterior surface of the vertebral body and the spinolaminar line *(between the arrows)*. At the C4-7 levels, cord compression is unlikely if the diameter of the canal is 13 mm or more. **B,** Photograph of a sagittal section of the cervical spine reveals stenosis of the central canal related to intervertebral (osteo)chondrosis and osteophytes anteriorly and ligamentous laxity and hypertrophy posteriorly. **C,** Sagittal multiple planar gradient recalled (MPGR) magnetic resonance image reveals stenosis of the lower cervical spine related to the presence of osteophytes arising from the posterior surface of the vertebral bodies. (From Resnick D: Diagnosis of Bone and Joint Disorders, 4th ed. Philadelphia, Saunders, 2002, p 1455.)

Clinical Pearls

Carpal tunnel syndrome should be differentiated from cervical radiculopathy involving the cervical nerve roots, which may mimic median nerve compression. Further, it should be remembered that cervical radicu-lopathy and median nerve entrapment may coexist in the "double crush" syndrome, which is seen most commonly with carpal tunnel syndrome.

Chapter 15

Fibromyalgia of the Cervical Musculature

ICD-9 CODE 729.1

THE CLINICAL SYNDROME

Fibromyalgia is a chronic pain syndrome that affects a focal or regional portion of the body. Fibromyalgia of the cervical spine is one of the most common painful conditions encountered in clinical practice. The sine qua non for diagnosis is the finding of myofascial trigger points on physical examination. These trigger points are thought to be the result of microtrauma to the affected muscles. Stimulation of the myofascial trigger points reproduces or exacerbates the patient's pain. Although these trigger points are generally localized to the cervical paraspinous musculature, the trapezius, and other muscles of the neck, the pain is often referred to other areas. This referred pain may be misdiagnosed or attributed to other organ systems, leading to extensive evaluation and ineffective treatment.

The pathophysiology of the myofascial trigger points of fibromyalgia of the cervical spine remains unclear, but tissue trauma seems to be the common denominator. Acute trauma to muscle as a result of overstretching commonly results in fibromyalgia. More subtle muscle injury in the form of repetitive microtrauma, damage to muscle fibers from exposure to extreme heat or cold, overuse, chronic deconditioning of the agonist and antagonist muscle unit, or other coexistent disease processes such as radiculopathy may also result in fibromyalgia of the cervical spine.

A variety of other factors seems to predispose patients to the development of fibromyalgia of the cervical spine. For example, a weekend athlete who subjects his or her body to unaccustomed physical activity may develop fibromyalgia. Poor posture while sitting at a computer or while watching television has also been implicated as a predisposing factor. In addition, previous injuries may result in abnormal muscle function and increase the risk of developing fibromyalgia. All these predisposing factors may be intensified if the patient also suffers from poor nutritional status or coexisting psychological abnormalities.

Often, stiffness and fatigue accompany the pain of fibromyalgia of the cervical spine, increasing the functional disability associated with this disease and complicating its treatment. Fibromyalgia may occur as a primary disease state or in conjunction with other painful conditions, including radiculopathy and chronic regional pain syndromes. Psychological or behavioral abnormalities, including depression, frequently coexist with the muscle abnormalities, and their management must be an integral part of any successful treatment plan.

SIGNS AND SYMPTOMS

As noted earlier, the sine qua non of fibromyalgia of the cervical spine is the myofascial trigger point. This trigger point represents the pathologic lesion and is characterized by a local point of exquisite tenderness in the affected muscle. Mechanical stimulation of the trigger point by palpation or stretching produces not only intense local pain but also referred pain. Taut bands of muscle fibers are often identified when myofascial trigger points are palpated. In addition, there is often involuntary withdrawal of the stimulated muscle, called a "jump sign" (Fig. 15-1). A positive jump sign is characteristic of fibromyalgia of the cervical spine, as is stiffness of the neck, pain on range of motion, and pain referred to the upper extremities in a nondermatomal pattern. Although this referred pain has been well studied and occurs in a characteristic pattern, it often leads to misdiagnosis.

TESTING

Biopsies of clinically identified trigger points have not revealed consistently abnormal histology. The muscle hosting the trigger points has been described either as "moth eaten" or as containing "waxy degeneration." Increased plasma myoglobin has been reported in some patients with fibromyalgia of the cervical spine, but

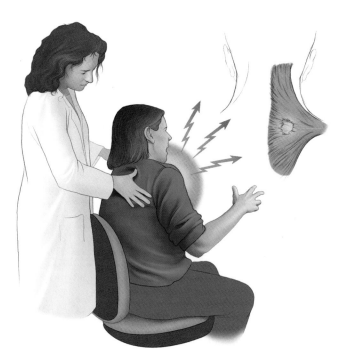

Figure 15–1. Palpation of a trigger point results in a positive jump sign.

other investigators have not corroborated this finding. Electrodiagnostic testing has revealed an increase in muscle tension in some patients, but again, this finding has not been reproducible. Thus, the diagnosis is based on the clinical findings of trigger points in the cervical paraspinous muscles and an associated jump sign, rather than on specific laboratory, electrodiagnostic, or radiographic testing.

DIFFERENTIAL DIAGNOSIS

The clinician must rule out other disease processes that may mimic fibromyalgia of the cervical spine, including primary inflammatory muscle disease, multiple sclerosis, and collagen vascular disease. The judicious use of electrodiagnostic testing and radiography can identify coexisting pathology such as a herniated nucleus pulposus or rotator cuff tear. The clinician must also identify any psychological and behavioral abnormalities that may mask or exacerbate the symptoms associated with fibromyalgia or other pathologic processes.

TREATMENT

Treatment is focused on blocking the myofascial trigger and achieving prolonged relaxation of the affected muscle. Because the mechanism of action is poorly understood, an element of trial and error is often required when developing a treatment plan. Conservative therapy consisting of trigger point injections with local anes-

thetic or saline is the starting point. Because underlying depression and anxiety are present in many patients suffering from fibromyalgia of the cervical spine, the administration of antidepressants is an integral part of most treatment plans.

In addition, a number of adjuvant methods are available for the treatment of fibromyalgia of the cervical spine. The therapeutic use of heat and cold is often combined with trigger point injections and antidepressants to achieve pain relief. Some patients experience decreased pain with the application of transcutaneous nerve stimulation or electrical stimulation to fatigue the affected muscles. Although not currently approved by the Food and Drug Administration for this indication, the injection of minute quantities of botulinum toxin type A directly into trigger points has been used with success in patients who have not responded to traditional treatment modalities.

COMPLICATIONS AND PITFALLS

Trigger point injections are extremely safe if careful attention is paid to the clinically relevant anatomy. Sterile technique is required to prevent infection, as are universal precautions to minimize any risk to the operator. Most side effects of trigger point injection are related to needle-induced trauma at the injection site and in underlying tissues. The incidence of ecchymosis and hematoma formation can be decreased if pressure is applied to the injection site immediately after injection. The avoidance of overly long needles can decrease the incidence of trauma to underlying structures. Special care must be taken to avoid pneumothorax when injecting trigger points in proximity to the underlying pleural space.

Clinical Pearls

Fibromyalgia of the cervical spine is a common disorder that often coexists with a variety of somatic and psychological disorders, yet it is often misdiagnosed. In patients suspected of suffering from fibromyalgia of the cervical spine, a careful evaluation is mandatory to identify any underlying disease processes. Treatment is focused on blocking the myofascial trigger to achieve pain relief. This is accomplished with trigger point injections with local anesthetic or saline, along with antidepressants to treat underlying depression. Physical therapy, therapeutic heat and cold, transcutaneous nerve stimulation, and electrical stimulation may be helpful in some cases. For patients who do not respond to traditional measures, consideration should be given to the use of botulinum toxin type A injection.

Chapter **16**

Cervical Strain

ICD-9 CODE 847.0

THE CLINICAL SYNDROME

Acute cervical strain is a constellation of symptoms consisting of nonradicular neck pain that radiates in a nondermatomal pattern into the shoulders and interscapular region; headache often accompanies these symptoms. The trapezius is commonly affected, with resultant spasm and limited range of motion of the cervical spine. Cervical strain is usually the result of trauma to the cervical spine and associated soft tissues (Fig. 16-1), but it may occur without an obvious inciting incident. The pathologic lesions responsible for this clinical syndrome may emanate from the soft tissues, facet joints, or intervertebral disks.

SIGNS AND SYMPTOMS

Neck pain is the hallmark of cervical strain. It may begin in the occipital region and radiate in a nondermatomal pattern into the shoulders and interscapular region. The pain of cervical strain is often exacerbated by movement of the cervical spine and shoulders. Headaches often occur and may worsen with emotional stress. Sleep disturbance is common, as is difficulty concentrating on simple tasks. Depression may occur with prolonged symptoms.

On physical examination, there is tenderness on palpation; spasm of the paraspinous musculature and trapezius is often present. Decreased range of motion is invariably present, and pain is increased when this maneuver is attempted. The neurologic examination of the upper extremities is within normal limits, despite the frequent complaint of upper extremity pain.

TESTING

There is no specific test for cervical strain. Testing is aimed primarily at identifying occult pathology or other diseases that may mimic cervical strain (see Differential Diagnosis). Plain radiographs can delineate any bony abnormality of the cervical spine, including arthritis,

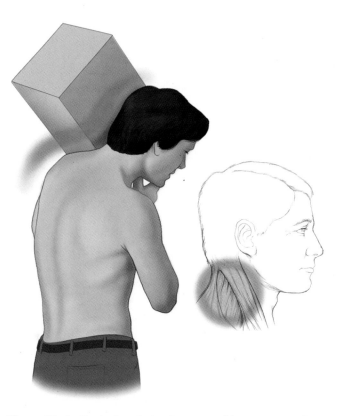

Figure 16–1. Cervical strain is often caused by trauma to the cervical spine and adjacent soft tissues.

fracture, congenital abnormality (e.g., Arnold-Chiari malformation), and tumor. Straightening of the lordotic curve is frequently noted. All patients with the recent onset of cervical strain should undergo magnetic resonance imaging (MRI) of the cervical spine and, if significant occipital or headache symptoms are present, of the brain (Fig. 16-2). Screening laboratory tests consisting of a complete blood count, erythrocyte sedimentation rate, antinuclear antibody testing, HLA B-27 antigen screening, and automated blood chemistry should be performed to rule out occult inflammatory arthritis, infection, and tumor.

DIFFERENTIAL DIAGNOSIS

Cervical strain is a clinical diagnosis supported by a combination of clinical history, physical examination,

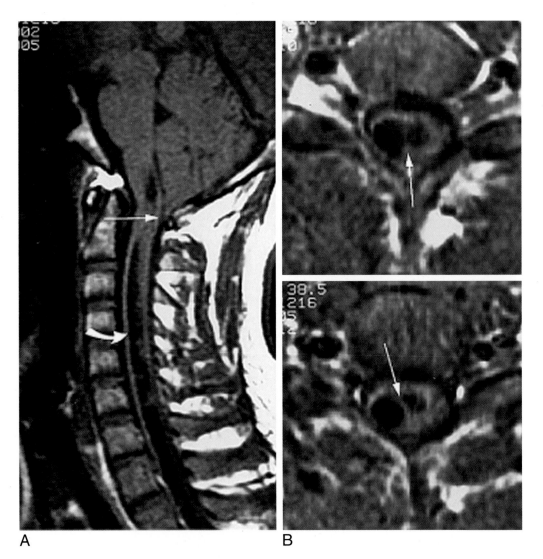

Figure 16–2. Syringohydromyelia. **A,** T1-weighted sagittal MRI of the cervical spine demonstrating a Chiari type I malformation with low-lying cerebellar tonsils *(straight arrow)* and a tight foramen magnum. A syrinx cavity is noted in the cervical spinal cord *(curved arrow).* **B,** T1-weighted axial image demonstrating the eccentric nature of the syrinx cavity, with internal septa or haustrations *(arrows).* (From Edelman RR, Hessellink JR, Zlatkin MB, Crues JV: Clinical Magnetic Resonance Imaging, 3rd ed. Philadelphia, Saunders, 2006, p 2304.)

radiography, and MRI. Pain syndromes that may mimic cervical strain include cervical bursitis, cervical fibromyositis, inflammatory arthritis, and disorders of the cervical spinal cord, roots, plexus, and nerves.

TREATMENT

Cervical strain is best treated with a multimodality approach. Physical therapy, including heat modalities and deep sedative massage, combined with nonsteroidal anti-inflammatory drugs and skeletal muscle relaxants, is a reasonable starting point. For symptomatic relief, cervi-

cal epidural block, blockade of the medial branch of the dorsal ramus, or intra-articular injection of the facet joint with local anesthetic and steroid is extremely effective. Underlying sleep disturbance and depression are best treated with a tricyclic antidepressant such as nortripty-line, which can be started at a single bedtime dose of 25 mg.

Cervical facet block is often combined with atlanto-occipital block when treating pain in this area. Although the atlanto-occipital joint is not a true facet joint in the anatomic sense, the technique is analogous to the facet joint block commonly used by pain practitioners and may be viewed as such.

COMPLICATIONS AND PITFALLS

The proximity to the spinal cord and exiting nerve roots makes it imperative that cervical epidural block and cervical facet block be carried out only by those familiar with the regional anatomy and experienced in interventional pain management techniques. The proximity to the vertebral artery, combined with the vascular nature of this region, makes the potential for intravascular injection high, and the injection of even a small amount of local anesthetic into the vertebral artery can result in seizures. Given the proximity of the brain and brainstem, ataxia due to vascular uptake of local anesthetic is not uncommon after cervical facet block. Many patients also complain of a transient increase in headache and cervicalgia after injection of the cervical facet joints.

Clinical Pearls

Cervical strain is a common cause of neck, occipital, shoulder, and upper extremity pain. It is often confused with cervical radiculopathy and cervical fibromyositis. The clinician must rule out diseases of the cervical spinal cord, such as syringomyelia, that may initially present in a manner similar to cervical strain. Ankylosing spondylitis may also present as cervical strain and must be correctly identified to avoid ongoing joint damage and functional disability.

Many pain specialists believe that cervical facet block and atlanto-occipital block are underused in the treatment of "post-whiplash" cervicalgia and cervicogenic headaches and that they should be considered whenever cervical epidural or occipital nerve blocks fail to provide palliation.

Chapter **17**

Cervicothoracic Interspinous Bursitis

ICD-9 Code **727.3**

THE CLINICAL SYNDROME

The interspinous ligaments of the lower cervical and upper thoracic spine and their associated muscles are susceptible to the development of acute and chronic pain symptoms following overuse. It is thought that bursitis is responsible for this pain. Frequently, the patient presents with midline pain after prolonged activity requiring hyperextension of the neck, such as painting a ceiling, or following prolonged use of a computer monitor with too high a focal point.

SIGNS AND SYMPTOMS

The pain is localized to the interspinous region between C7 and T1 and does not radiate. It is constant, dull, and aching in character. The patient may attempt to relieve the constant ache by assuming a posture of dorsal kyphosis with a thrusting forward of the neck (Fig. 17-1). In contrast to the pain of cervical strain, the pain of cervicothoracic interspinous bursitis often improves with activity and worsens with rest. On physical examination, there is tenderness on deep palpation of the C7-T1 region, often with reflex spasm of the associated paraspinous musculature. Decreased range of motion is invariably present, and pain increases with extension of the lower cervical and upper thoracic spine.

TESTING

There is no specific test for cervicothoracic bursitis. Testing is aimed primarily at identifying occult pathology or other diseases that may mimic cervicothoracic bursitis (see Differential Diagnosis). Plain radiographs can delineate any bony abnormality of the cervical spine, including arthritis, fracture, congenital abnormality (e.g., Arnold-Chiari malformation), and tumor. All patients with the recent onset of cervicothoracic bursitis should undergo

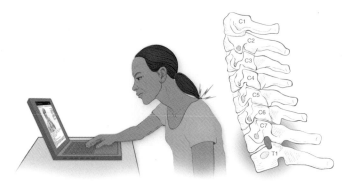

Figure 17–1. A patient with cervicothoracic interspinous bursitis may attempt to relieve the constant ache by assuming a posture of dorsal kyphosis with a thrusting forward of the neck.

magnetic resonance imaging (MRI) of the cervical spine and, if significant occipital or headache symptoms are present, of the brain (Fig. 17-2). Screening laboratory tests consisting of a complete blood count, erythrocyte sedimentation rate, antinuclear antibody testing, and automated blood chemistry should be performed to rule out occult inflammatory arthritis, infection, and tumor.

DIFFERENTIAL DIAGNOSIS

Cervicothoracic bursitis is a clinical diagnosis of exclusion supported by a combination of clinical history, physical examination, radiography, and MRI. Pain syndromes that may mimic cervicothoracic bursitis include cervical strain, cervical fibromyositis, inflammatory arthritis, and disorders of the cervical spinal cord, roots, plexus, and nerves. Congenital abnormalities such as Arnold-Chiari malformation and Klippel-Feil syndrome may also present similarly to cervicothoracic bursitis.

TREATMENT

Cervicothoracic bursitis is best treated with a multimodality approach. Physical therapy consisting of the correction of functional abnormalities (e.g., poor posture,

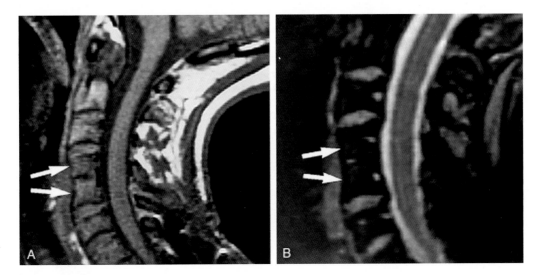

Figure 17–2. Klippel-Feil anomaly. T1-weighted **(A)** and T2-weighted **(B)** sagittal images of the cervical spine demonstrating lack of segmentation of the C4 and C5 vertebrae *(arrows).* (From Edelman RR, Hessellink JR, Zlatkin MB, Crues JV: Clinical Magnetic Resonance Imaging, 3rd ed. Philadelphia, Saunders, 2006, p 2306.)

improper chair or computer height), heat modalities, and deep sedative massage, combined with nonsteroidal anti-inflammatory drugs and skeletal muscle relaxants, is a reasonable starting point. If these treatments fail to provide rapid relief, injection of local anesthetic and steroid into the area between the interspinous ligament and the ligamentum flavum is a reasonable next step. For symptomatic relief, cervical epidural block, blockade of the medial branch of the dorsal ramus, or intra-articular injection of the facet joint with local anesthetic and steroid may also be considered. Antimyotonic agents such as tizanidine may be used if symptoms persist. Underlying sleep disturbance and depression are best treated with a tricyclic antidepressant such as nortriptyline, which can be started at a single bedtime dose of 25 mg.

COMPLICATIONS AND PITFALLS

The proximity to the spinal cord and exiting nerve roots makes it imperative that injections be performed only by those familiar with the regional anatomy and experienced in interventional pain management techniques. The proximity to the vertebral artery, combined with the vascular nature of this region, makes the potential for

intravascular injection high, and the injection of even a small amount of local anesthetic into the vertebral artery can result in seizures. Given the proximity of the brain and brainstem, ataxia due to vascular uptake of local anesthetic is not uncommon after injection in this region. Many patients also complain of a transient increase in headache and cervicalgia after injection of the cervical facet joints.

Clinical Pearls

Correction of the functional abnormalities responsible for the development of cervicothoracic bursitis is mandatory if long-lasting relief is to be achieved. Physical modalities, including local heat, gentle stretching exercises, and deep sedative massage, are beneficial and may be started concurrently with a trial of nonsteroidal anti-inflammatory agents. Injection of local anesthetic and steroid is extremely effective in the treatment of cervicothoracic bursitis pain that fails to respond to more conservative measures. Vigorous exercise should be avoided, because it will exacerbate the patient's symptoms.

Chapter 18

Brachial Plexopathy

ICD-9 CODE 353.0

THE CLINICAL SYNDROME

Brachial plexopathy is a constellation of symptoms consisting of neurogenic pain and associated weakness that radiates from the shoulder into the supraclavicular region and upper extremity (Fig. 18-1). There are many causes of brachial plexopathy, but some of the more common ones include compression of the plexus by cervical ribs or abnormal muscles (e.g., thoracic outlet syndrome), invasion of the plexus by tumor (e.g., Pancoast's tumor syndrome), direct trauma to the plexus (e.g., stretch injuries and avulsions), inflammatory causes (e.g., Parsonage-Turner syndrome), and postradiation plexopathy.

SIGNS AND SYMPTOMS

Patients suffering from brachial plexopathy complain of pain radiating to the supraclavicular region and upper extremity. The pain is neuritic in character and may take on a deep, boring quality as the plexus is invaded by tumor. Movement of the neck and shoulder exacerbates the pain, so patients often try to avoid such movement. Frozen shoulder often results and may confuse the diagnosis. If thoracic outlet syndrome is suspected, the Adson test may be performed (Fig. 18-2). The test is positive if the radial pulse disappears with the neck extended and the head turned toward the affected side. Because the Adson test is nonspecific, treatment decisions should not be based on this finding alone (see Testing). If the patient presents with severe pain that is followed shortly by profound weakness, brachial plexitis should be considered; this can be confirmed with electromyography.

TESTING

All patients presenting with brachial plexopathy, especially those without a clear history of antecedent trauma, must undergo magnetic resonance imaging (MRI) of the cervical spine and the brachial plexus. Computed tomography scanning is a reasonable alternative if MRI is contraindicated. Electromyography and nerve conduction velocity testing are extremely sensitive, and a skilled

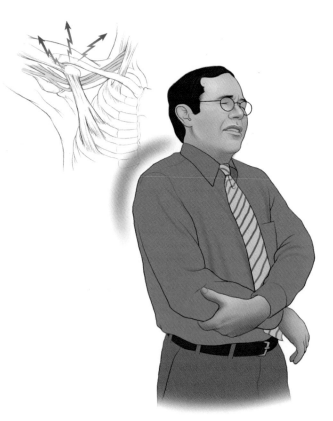

Figure 18–1. The pain of brachial plexopathy radiates from the shoulder and supraclavicular region into the upper extremity.

electromyographer can delineate which portion of the plexus is abnormal. If an inflammatory basis for the plexopathy is suspected, serial electromyography is indicated, and MRI of the shoulder muscles often reveals muscle edema and denervation-induced atrophy (Fig. 18-3). If Pancoast's tumor or some other tumor of the brachial plexus is suspected, chest radiographs with apical lordotic views may be helpful. If the diagnosis is in question, screening laboratory tests consisting of a complete blood count, erythrocyte sedimentation rate, antinuclear antibody testing, and automated blood chemistry should be performed to rule out other causes of the patient's pain.

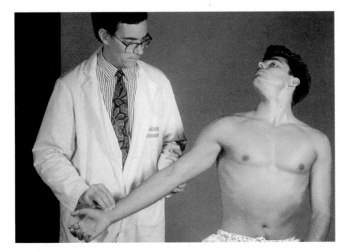

Figure 18–2. Adson test. The patient inhales deeply, extends the neck fully, and turns the head to the affected side. This maneuver tests for compression in the scalene triangle; it is positive if there is a diminution in the radial pulse and reproduction of the patient's symptoms. (From Klippel JH, Dieppe PA: Rheumatology, 2nd ed. London, Mosby, 1998.)

DIFFERENTIAL DIAGNOSIS

Diseases of the cervical spinal cord, bony cervical spine, and disk can mimic brachial plexopathy. Appropriate testing, including MRI and electromyography, can help sort out the myriad possibilities, but the clinician should be aware that more than one pathologic process may be contributing to the patient's symptoms. Syringomyelia, tumor of the cervical spinal cord, and tumor of the cervical nerve root as it exits the spinal cord (e.g., schwannoma)

can have an insidious onset and be quite difficult to diagnosis. Pancoast's tumor should be high on the list of diagnostic possibilities in all patients presenting with brachial plexopathy in the absence of clear antecedent trauma, especially if there is a history of tobacco use. Lateral herniated cervical disk, metastatic tumor, or cervical spondylosis resulting in significant nerve root compression may also present as brachial plexopathy. Rarely, infection involving the apex of the lung may compress and irritate the plexus.

TREATMENT

Drug Therapy

Gabapentin

Gabapentin is first-line treatment for the neuritic pain of brachial plexopathy. Start with 300 mg gabapentin at bedtime for 2 nights, and caution the patient about potential side effects, including dizziness, sedation, confusion, and rash. The drug is then increased in 300-mg increments given in equally divided doses over 2 days, as side effects allow, until pain relief is obtained or a total dose of 2400 mg/day is reached. At this point, if the patient has experienced partial pain relief, blood values are measured, and the drug is carefully titrated upward using 100-mg tablets. Rarely is a dose greater than 3600 mg/day required.

Carbamazepine

Carbamazepine is useful in patients who do not obtain pain relief with gabapentin. Despite the safety and

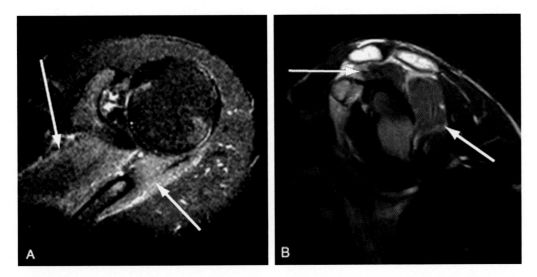

Figure 18–3. Parsonage-Turner syndrome. Axial short tau inversion recovery **(A)** and sagittal oblique T2-weighted **(B)** images. Increased signal intensity consistent with interstitial muscle edema associated with denervation is seen in the supraspinatus and infraspinatus muscles *(arrows)*. (From Edelman RR, Hessellink JR, Zlatkin MB, Crues JV: Clinical Magnetic Resonance Imaging, 3rd ed. Philadelphia, Saunders, 2006, p 3272.)

efficacy of carbamazepine, confusion and anxiety have surrounded its use. It is sometimes discontinued owing to laboratory abnormalities erroneously attributed to it. Therefore, baseline laboratory values consisting of a complete blood count, urinalysis, and automated chemistry profile should be obtained before starting the drug.

Carbamazepine should be initiated slowly if the pain is not out of control at a starting dose of 100 to 200 mg at bedtime for 2 nights. The patient should be cautioned about side effects, including dizziness, sedation, confusion, and rash. The drug is increased in 100- to 200-mg increments given in equally divided doses over 2 days, as side effects allow, until pain relief is obtained or a total dose of 1200 mg/day is reached. Careful monitoring of laboratory parameters is mandatory to avoid the rare possibility of a life-threatening blood dyscrasia, and at the first sign of blood count abnormality or rash, the drug should be discontinued. Failure to monitor patients started on carbamazepine can be disastrous, because aplastic anemia can occur. When pain relief is obtained, the patient should be kept at that dosage of carbamazepine for at least 6 months before tapering of the medication is considered. The patient should be instructed that under no circumstances should the drug dosage be changed or the drug refilled or discontinued without the physician's knowledge.

Baclofen

Baclofen may be of value in some patients who fail to obtain relief from gabapentin or carbamazepine. Baseline laboratory tests should be obtained before starting baclofen, and the patient should be cautioned about potential adverse effects, which are the same as those associated with carbamazepine and gabapentin. Baclofen is started with a 10-mg dose at bedtime for 2 nights; the dosage is then increased in 10-mg increments given in equally divided doses over 7 days, as side effects allow, until pain relief is obtained or a total dose of 80 mg/day is reached. This drug has significant hepatic and central nervous system side effects, including weakness and sedation. As with carbamazepine, careful monitoring of laboratory values is indicated.

When treating individuals with any of these drugs, the physician should make sure that the patient knows that premature tapering or discontinuation of the medication may lead to the recurrence of pain, which will be more difficult to control.

Invasive Therapy

Brachial Plexus Block

Brachial plexus block with local anesthetic and steroid is an excellent adjunct to drug treatment. This technique rapidly relieves pain while medications are being titrated to effective levels. The initial block is carried out with preservative-free bupivacaine combined with methylprednisolone. Subsequent daily nerve blocks are carried out in a similar manner, substituting a lower dose of methylprednisolone. This approach can also be used to control breakthrough pain.

Radiofrequency Destruction of the Brachial Plexus

The brachial plexus can be destroyed by creating a radiofrequency lesion under biplanar fluoroscopic guidance. This procedure is reserved for patients who have failed to respond to all aforementioned treatments and whose pain is secondary to tumor or avulsion of the brachial plexus.

Dorsal Root Entry Zone Lesioning

Dorsal root entry zone lesioning is the neurosurgical procedure of choice for intractable brachial plexopathy in patients who have failed to respond to all aforementioned treatments and whose pain is secondary to tumor or avulsion of the brachial plexus. This is a major neurosurgical procedure and carries significant risks.

Physical Modalities

Physical and occupational therapy to maintain function and palliate pain is a crucial part of the treatment plan for patients suffering from brachial plexopathy. Shoulder abnormalities, including subluxation and adhesive capsulitis, must be treated aggressively. Occupational therapy to assist in activities of daily living is important to avoid further deterioration of function.

COMPLICATIONS AND PITFALLS

The pain of brachial plexopathy is difficult to treat. It responds poorly to opioid analgesics and may respond poorly to the medications discussed. The uncontrolled pain of brachial plexopathy can lead to suicide, and strong consideration should be given to hospitalizing such patients. Correct diagnosis of the underlying cause is crucial to the successful treatment of the pain and dysfunction associated with brachial plexopathy, because stretch injuries and contusions of the plexus may respond with time, but plexopathy secondary to tumor or avulsion of the cervical roots requires aggressive treatment.

Clinical Pearls

Brachial plexus block with local anesthetic and steroid represents an excellent stopgap measure for patients suffering from the uncontrolled pain of brachial plexopathy while waiting for drug treatments to take effect. Correct diagnosis is paramount to allow the clinician to design a logical treatment plan.

Chapter 19

Pancoast's Tumor Syndrome

ICD-9 CODE **162.3**

THE CLINICAL SYNDROME

Pancoast's tumor syndrome is the result of local growth of tumor from the apex of the lung directly into the brachial plexus. Such tumors usually involve the first and second thoracic nerves as well as the eighth cervical nerve, producing a classic clinical syndrome consisting of severe arm pain and, in some patients, Horner's syndrome. Destruction of the first and second ribs is also common. Diagnosis is usually delayed, and patients are often erroneously treated for cervical radiculopathy or primary shoulder pathology until the diagnosis becomes clear.

SIGNS AND SYMPTOMS

Patients suffering from Pancoast's tumor syndrome complain of pain radiating to the supraclavicular region and upper extremity (Fig. 19-1). Initially, the lower portion of the brachial plexus is involved because the tumor growth is from below, causing pain in the upper thoracic and lower cervical dermatomes. The pain is neuritic in character and may take on a deep, boring quality as the tumor invades the brachial plexus. Movement of the neck and shoulder exacerbates the pain, so patients often try to avoid such movement. Frozen shoulder often results and may confuse the diagnosis. As the disease progresses, Horner's syndrome may occur.

TESTING

All patients presenting with brachial plexopathy, especially those without a clear history of antecedent trauma, must undergo magnetic resonance imaging (MRI) of the cervical spine and the brachial plexus (Fig. 19-2). Computed tomography is a reasonable alternative if MRI is contraindicated. Electromyography and nerve conduction velocity testing are extremely sensitive, and a skilled electromyographer can determine which portion of the plexus is abnormal. All patients with a significant smoking

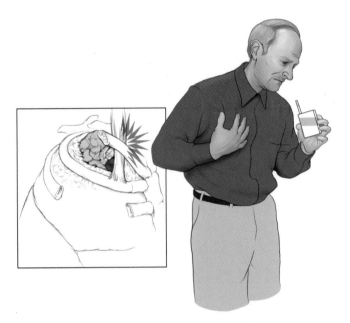

Figure 19–1. Pancoast's tumor should be suspected in patients suffering from shoulder and upper extremity pain who have a history of smoking.

history and suspected Pancoast's tumor or other tumor of the brachial plexus should undergo chest radiography with apical lordotic views or computed tomography scanning through the apex of the lung. If the diagnosis is in question, screening laboratory tests consisting of a complete blood count, erythrocyte sedimentation rate, antinuclear antibody testing, and automated blood chemistry should be performed to rule out other causes of the patient's pain.

DIFFERENTIAL DIAGNOSIS

Diseases of the cervical spinal cord, bony cervical spine, and disk can mimic the brachial plexopathy associated with Pancoast's tumor syndrome. Appropriate testing, including MRI and electromyography, can help sort out the myriad possibilities, but the clinician should be aware that more than one pathologic process may be contributing to the patient's symptoms. Syringomyelia,

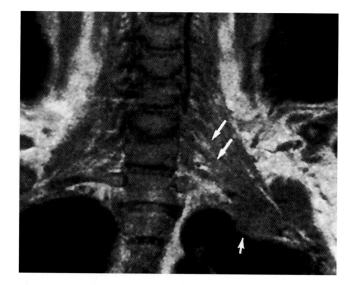

Figure 19–2. Pancoast's tumor (adenocarcinoma) with infiltration of the brachial plexus. A 65-year-old man complained of severe pain in the shoulder radiating to the elbow, medial side of the forearm, and fourth and fifth fingers in an ulnar nerve distribution. Screening coronal T1-weighted image shows the brachial plexus from the region of the roots *(long arrows)* to the region of the trunks and divisions, where there is tumor invasion *(short arrow)* and loss of fat planes on the left. (From Stark DD, Bradley WG Jr: Magnetic Resonance Imaging, 3rd ed. St Louis, Mosby, 1999.)

tumor of the cervical spinal cord, and tumor of the cervical nerve root as it exits the spinal cord (e.g., schwannoma) can have an insidious onset and be quite difficult to diagnose. Pancoast's tumor should be high on the list of diagnostic possibilities in all patients presenting with brachial plexopathy in the absence of clear antecedent trauma, especially if there is a history of tobacco use. Lateral herniated cervical disk, metastatic tumor, or cervical spondylosis that results in significant nerve root compression may also present as brachial plexopathy. Rarely, infection involving the apex of the lung may compress and irritate the plexus.

TREATMENT

The primary treatment of Pancoast's tumor syndrome is aimed at the tumor itself. Based on the cell type and extent of involvement, chemotherapy and radiation therapy may be indicated. Primary surgical treatment of tumors involving the brachial plexus is difficult, and the results are disappointing.

Drug Therapy

Opioid Analgesics

Opioid analgesics are the mainstay of treatment for the pain associated with Pancoast's tumor syndrome.

Although neuropathic pain generally responds poorly to opioid analgesics, given the severity of the pain and the lack of other options, a trial of opioid analgesics is warranted. Administration of a short-acting, potent opioid such as oxycodone is a reasonable starting point. Immediate-release morphine or methadone can also be considered. These drugs can be used in combination with nonsteroidal anti-inflammatory drugs and the adjuvant analgesics described here.

Gabapentin

Gabapentin is used to treat the neuritic pain of Pancoast's tumor syndrome. Start with 300 mg gabapentin at bedtime for 2 nights, and caution the patient about potential side effects, including dizziness, sedation, confusion, and rash. The drug is then increased in 300-mg increments given in equally divided doses over 2 days, as side effects allow, until pain relief is obtained or a total dose of 2400 mg/day is reached. At this point, if the patient has experienced partial pain relief, blood values are measured, and the drug is carefully titrated upward using 100-mg tablets. Rarely is a dose greater than 3600 mg/day required.

Carbamazepine

Carbamazepine is useful in patients who do not obtain pain relief with gabapentin. Despite the safety and efficacy of carbamazepine, confusion and anxiety have surrounded its use. It is sometimes discontinued owing to laboratory abnormalities erroneously attributed to it. Therefore, baseline laboratory values consisting of a complete blood count, urinalysis, and automated chemistry profile should be obtained before starting the drug.

Carbamazepine should be initiated slowly if the pain is not out of control at a starting dose of 100 to 200 mg at bedtime for 2 nights. The patient should be cautioned about side effects, including dizziness, sedation, confusion, and rash. The drug is increased in 100- to 200-mg increments given in equally divided doses over 2 days, as side effects allow, until pain relief is obtained or a total dose of 1200 mg/day is reached. Careful monitoring of laboratory parameters is mandatory to avoid the rare possibility of a life-threatening blood dyscrasia, and at the first sign of blood count abnormality or rash, the drug should be discontinued. Failure to monitor patients started on carbamazepine can be disastrous, because aplastic anemia can occur. When pain relief is obtained, the patient should be kept at that dosage of carbamazepine for at least 6 months before tapering of the medication is considered. The patient should be instructed that under no circumstances should the drug dosage be changed or the drug refilled or discontinued without the physician's knowledge.

Baclofen

Baclofen may be of value in some patients who fail to obtain relief from the previously mentioned medications. Baseline laboratory tests should be obtained before starting baclofen, and the patient should be cautioned about potential adverse effects, which are the same as those associated with carbamazepine and gabapentin. Baclofen is started with a 10-mg dose at bedtime for 2 nights; the drug is then increased in 10-mg increments given in equally divided doses over 7 days, as side effects allow, until pain relief is obtained or a total dose of 80 mg/day is reached. This drug has significant hepatic and central nervous system side effects, including weakness and sedation. As with carbamazepine, careful monitoring of laboratory values is indicated.

Invasive Therapy

Brachial Plexus Block

Brachial plexus block with local anesthetic and steroid is an excellent adjunct to drug treatment of Pancoast's tumor syndrome. This technique rapidly relieves pain while medications are being titrated to effective levels. The initial block is carried out with preservative-free bupivacaine combined with methylprednisolone. Subsequent daily nerve blocks are carried out in a similar manner, substituting a lower dose of methylprednisolone. This approach can also be used to control breakthrough pain.

Radiofrequency Destruction of the Brachial Plexus

The brachial plexus can be destroyed by creating a radiofrequency lesion under biplanar fluoroscopic guidance. This procedure is reserved for patients for whom all aforementioned treatments have failed.

Dorsal Root Entry Zone Lesioning

Dorsal root entry zone lesioning is the neurosurgical procedure of choice for intractable brachial plexopathy associated with Pancoast's tumor in patients who have failed all aforementioned treatment options. This is a major neurosurgical procedure and carries significant risks.

Other Neurosurgical Options

Cordotomy, deep brain stimulation, and thalamotomy have all been tried, with varying degrees of success.

Physical Modalities

Physical and occupational therapy to maintain function and palliate pain is a crucial part of the treatment plan for patients suffering from Pancoast's tumor syndrome. Shoulder abnormalities, including subluxation and adhesive capsulitis, must be aggressively treated. Occupational therapy to assist in activities of daily living is important to avoid further deterioration of function.

COMPLICATIONS AND PITFALLS

The pain of Pancoast's tumor syndrome is difficult to treat. It may respond poorly to any or all of the recommended medications. The uncontrolled pain of Pancoast's tumor syndrome can lead to suicide, and strong consideration should be given to hospitalizing such patients. Correct diagnosis of the underlying cause is crucial, because the pain and dysfunction associated with brachial plexopathy secondary to Pancoast's tumor require aggressive treatment.

Clinical Pearls

Brachial plexus block with local anesthetic and steroid is an excellent stopgap measure for patients suffering from the uncontrolled pain of brachial plexopathy while waiting for drug treatments to take effect. Correct diagnosis is paramount to allow the clinician to design a logical treatment plan.

Chapter **20**

Thoracic Outlet Syndrome

ICD-9 CODE **353.0**

THE CLINICAL SYNDROME

Thoracic outlet syndrome consists of a constellation of signs and symptoms, including paresthesias and aching pain of the neck, shoulder, and arm. The cause is thought to be compression of the brachial plexus and subclavian artery and vein as they exit the space between the shoulder girdle and the first rib (Fig. 20-1) or compression from congenitally abnormal structures such as cervical ribs. One or all the structures may be compressed, giving the syndrome a varied clinical expression. Thoracic outlet syndrome is seen most commonly in women between 25 and 50 years of age. It has been the subject of significant debate, and the diagnosis and treatment of thoracic outlet syndrome remain controversial.

SIGNS AND SYMPTOMS

Although the symptoms of thoracic outlet syndrome vary, compression of neural structures accounts for most of them. Paresthesias of the upper extremity radiating into the distribution of the ulnar nerve may be misdiagnosed as tardy ulnar palsy. Aching and incoordination of the affected extremity are also common findings. If vascular compression exists, edema or discoloration of the arm may be noted; in rare instances, venous or arterial thrombosis may occur. Rarely, the symptoms of thoracic outlet syndrome are caused by arterial aneurysm, and auscultation of the supraclavicular region reveals a bruit.

The symptoms of thoracic outlet syndrome may be elicited by a variety of maneuvers, including the Adson test and the elevated arm stress test. The Adson test is carried out by palpating the radial pulse on the affected side with the patient's neck extended and the head turned toward the affected side. A diminished pulse is suggestive of thoracic outlet syndrome. The elevated arm stress test is performed by having the patient hold his or her arms over the head and open and close the hands. Normally, patients without thoracic outlet syn-

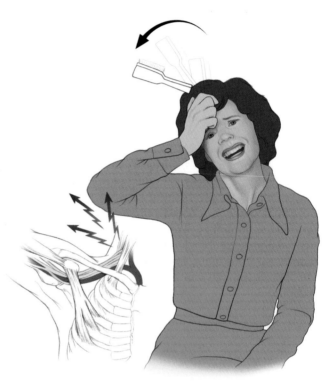

Figure 20–1. Compression of the brachial plexus results in pain and weakness in the affected upper extremity.

drome can perform this maneuver for approximately 3 minutes, whereas those suffering from thoracic outlet syndrome experience the onset of symptoms within 30 seconds.

TESTING

Plain radiographs of the cervical spine should be performed in all patients suspected of having thoracic outlet syndrome. These films should be carefully reviewed for congenital abnormalities such as cervical ribs or overly elongated transverse processes. Patients should also undergo chest radiography with apical lordotic views to rule out Pancoast's tumor. Magnetic resonance imaging (MRI) of the cervical spine is indicated to identify lesions of the cervical spinal cord and exiting nerve roots, as

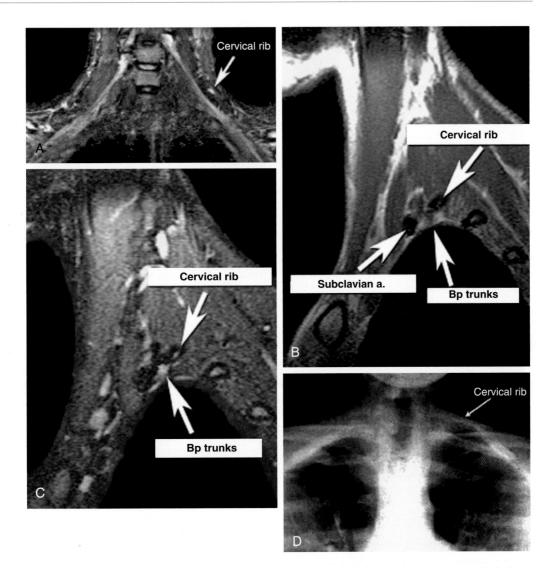

Figure 20–2. Patient with thoracic outlet syndrome on the left side secondary to a cervical rib. **A,** Coronal T2-weighted image shows the subtle deviation of the brachial plexus as it crosses the area of the cervical rib. **B** and **C,** Sagittal T1- and T2-weighted images at the level of the interscalene triangle show the close proximity of the cervical rib to the lower trunk of the brachial plexus (Bp). **D,** Plain chest film shows the left cervical rib. The patient underwent surgical removal of the cervical rib, resulting in relief of symptoms. (From Edelman RR, Hessellink JR, Zlatkin MB, Crues JV: Clinical Magnetic Resonance Imaging, 3rd ed. Philadelphia, Saunders, 2006, p 2382.)

well as cervical ribs (Fig. 20-2). If the diagnosis is still in doubt, MRI of the brachial plexus is indicated to search for occult pathology, including primary tumors of the plexus. Screening laboratory tests consisting of a complete blood count, erythrocyte sedimentation rate, antinuclear antibody testing, and automated blood chemistry may be performed to rule out other causes of the patient's pain.

DIFFERENTIAL DIAGNOSIS

Diseases of the cervical spinal cord, bony cervical spine, and disk can mimic thoracic outlet syndrome. Appropri-

ate testing, including MRI and electromyography, can help sort out the myriad possibilities, but the clinician should be aware that more than one pathologic process may be contributing to the patient's symptoms. Syringomyelia, tumor of the cervical spinal cord, and tumor of the cervical nerve root as it exits the spinal cord (e.g., schwannoma) can have an insidious onset and be quite difficult to diagnose. Pancoast's tumor should be high on the list of diagnostic possibilities in the absence of clear antecedent trauma, especially if there is a history of tobacco use. Lateral herniated cervical disk, metastatic tumor, or cervical spondylosis that results in significant nerve root compression should also be considered.

Rarely, infection involving the apex of the lung may compress and irritate the plexus.

TREATMENT

Physical Modalities

The primary treatment for patients suffering from thoracic outlet syndrome is the rational use of physical therapy to maintain function and palliate pain. Shoulder abnormalities, including subluxation and adhesive capsulitis, must be aggressively treated. Occupational therapy to assist in activities of daily living is important to avoid further deterioration of function.

Drug Therapy

Gabapentin

Gabapentin is first-line pharmacologic treatment for the neuritic pain of thoracic outlet syndrome. Start with 300 mg gabapentin at bedtime for 2 nights, and caution the patient about potential side effects, including dizziness, sedation, confusion, and rash. The drug is then increased in 300-mg increments given in equally divided doses over 2 days, as side effects allow, until pain relief is obtained or a total dosage of 2400 mg/day is reached. At this point, if the patient has experienced partial pain relief, blood values are measured, and the drug is carefully titrated upward using 100-mg tablets. Rarely is a dosage greater than 3600 mg/day required.

Carbamazepine

Carbamazepine is useful in patients who do not obtain pain relief with gabapentin. Despite the safety and efficacy of carbamazepine, confusion and anxiety have surrounded its use. It is sometimes discontinued owing to laboratory abnormalities erroneously attributed to it. Therefore, baseline laboratory values consisting of a complete blood count, urinalysis, and automated chemistry profile should be obtained before starting the drug.

Carbamazepine should be initiated slowly if the pain is not out of control at a starting dose of 100 to 200 mg at bedtime for 2 nights. The patient should be cautioned about side effects, including dizziness, sedation, confusion, and rash. The drug is increased in 100- to 200-mg increments given in equally divided doses over 2 days, as side effects allow, until pain relief is obtained or a total dosage of 1200 mg/day is reached. Careful monitoring of laboratory parameters is mandatory to avoid the rare possibility of a life-threatening blood dyscrasia, and at the first sign of blood count abnormality or rash, the drug should be discontinued. Failure to monitor patients started on carbamazepine can be disastrous, because aplastic anemia can occur. When pain relief is obtained, the patient should be kept at that dosage of carbamazepine for at least 6 months before considering tapering of the medication. The patient should be instructed that under no circumstances should the drug dosage be changed or the drug refilled or discontinued without the physician's knowledge.

Baclofen

Baclofen may be of value in some patients who fail to obtain relief with gabapentin and carbamazepine. Baseline laboratory tests should be obtained before starting baclofen, and the patient should be cautioned about potential adverse effects, which are the same as those associated with carbamazepine and gabapentin. Baclofen is started with a 10-mg dose at bedtime for 2 nights; the drug is then increased in 10-mg increments given in equally divided doses over 7 days, as side effects allow, until pain relief is obtained or a total dosage of 80 mg/day is reached. This drug has significant hepatic and central nervous system side effects, including weakness and sedation. As with carbamazepine, careful monitoring of laboratory values is indicated.

When treating individuals with any of these drugs, the physician should make sure that the patient knows that premature tapering or discontinuation of the medication may lead to the recurrence of pain, which will be more difficult to control.

Invasive Therapy

Brachial Plexus Block

Brachial plexus block with local anesthetic and steroid is an excellent adjunct to drug treatment of thoracic outlet syndrome. This technique rapidly relieves pain while medications are being titrated to effective levels. The initial block is carried out with preservative-free bupivacaine combined with methylprednisolone. Subsequent daily nerve blocks are carried out in a similar manner, substituting a lower dose of methylprednisolone. This approach can also be used to control breakthrough pain.

Surgery

In the absence of demonstrable pathology (e.g., a cervical rib), the outcome of surgical treatment for thoracic outlet syndrome is dismal, regardless of the technique chosen. However, in patients with a clear cause of their symptoms who have failed to achieve relief from more conservative therapies, the judicious use of surgical treatment may be a reasonable last step.

COMPLICATIONS AND PITFALLS

The pain and dysfunction of thoracic outlet syndrome are difficult to treat. Physical therapy should be the primary modality in any well thought out treatment plan. In general, the pain of thoracic outlet syndrome responds poorly to opioid analgesics, and these drugs should be avoided. The careful use of adjuvant analgesics may help palliate the pain and allow the patient to participate in physical therapy. Correct diagnosis is crucial, because stretch injuries and contusions of the plexus may respond with time, but plexopathy secondary to tumor or avulsion of the cervical roots requires aggressive treatment.

Clinical Pearls

Brachial plexus block with local anesthetic and steroid represents an excellent stopgap measure while waiting for drug treatments to take effect. Correct diagnosis is paramount to allow the clinician to design a logical treatment plan.

Section 4

Pain Syndromes of the Shoulder

Chapter 21

Arthritis Pain of the Shoulder

ICD-9 CODE 715.91

THE CLINICAL SYNDROME

The shoulder joint is susceptible to the development of arthritis from a variety of conditions that cause damage to the joint cartilage. Osteoarthritis is the most common cause of shoulder pain and functional disability (Fig. 21-1). It may occur after seemingly minor trauma or may be the result of repeated microtrauma. Pain around the shoulder and upper arm that is worse with activity is present in most patients suffering from osteoarthritis of the shoulder. Difficulty sleeping is also common, as is progressive loss of motion.

SIGNS AND SYMPTOMS

The majority of patients presenting with shoulder pain secondary to osteoarthritis, rotator cuff arthropathy, or post-traumatic arthritis complain of pain that is localized around the shoulder and upper arm. Activity makes the pain worse, whereas rest and heat provide some relief. The pain is constant and is characterized as aching in nature; it may interfere with sleep. Some patients complain of a grating or popping sensation with use of the joint, and crepitus may be present on physical examination.

In addition to pain, patients suffering from arthritis of the shoulder joint often experience a gradual reduction in functional ability because of decreasing shoulder range of motion, making simple everyday tasks such as combing one's hair, fastening a brassiere, or reaching overhead quite difficult. With continued disuse, muscle wasting may occur, and a frozen shoulder may develop.

TESTING

Plain radiographs are indicated in all patients who present with shoulder pain (Fig. 21-2). Based on the patient's clinical presentation, additional testing may be indicated, including a complete blood count, erythrocyte sedimentation rate, and antinuclear antibody testing. Magnetic resonance imaging of the shoulder is indicated if a rotator

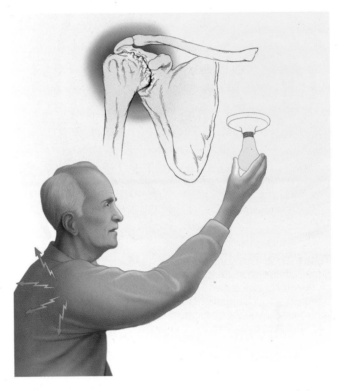

Figure 21–1. Range of motion of the shoulder can precipitate the pain of osteoarthritis.

cuff tear is suspected. Radionuclide bone scanning is indicated if metastatic disease or primary tumor involving the shoulder is a possibility.

DIFFERENTIAL DIAGNOSIS

Osteoarthritis of the joint is the most common form of arthritis that results in shoulder pain; however, rheumatoid arthritis, post-traumatic arthritis, and rotator cuff arthropathy are also common causes of shoulder pain. Less common causes of arthritis-induced shoulder pain include collagen vascular diseases, infection, villonodular synovitis, and Lyme disease. Acute infectious arthritis is usually accompanied by significant systemic symptoms, including fever and malaise, and should be easily recognized; it is diagnosed with culture and treated with

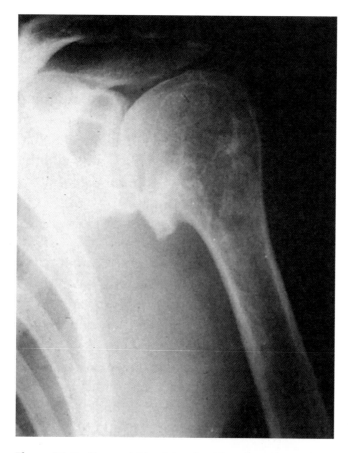

Figure 21–2. Osteoarthritis of the shoulder. The radiograph shows all the characteristic features of a "hypertrophic" form of osteoarthritis of the glenohumeral joint, with joint space narrowing, subchondral sclerosis, large cysts in the glenoid, and massive inferior osteophytosis. (From Klippel JH, Dieppe PA: Rheumatology, 2nd ed. London, Mosby, 1998.)

antibiotics rather than injection therapy. Collagen vascular diseases generally present as a polyarthropathy rather than a monoarthropathy limited to the shoulder joint; however, shoulder pain secondary to collagen vascular disease responds exceedingly well to the intra-articular injection technique described here.

TREATMENT

Initial treatment of the pain and functional disability associated with osteoarthritis of the shoulder includes a combination of nonsteroidal anti-inflammatory drugs or cyclooxygenase-2 inhibitors and physical therapy. Local application of heat and cold may also be beneficial. For patients who do not respond to these treatment modalities, intra-articular injection of local anesthetic and steroid is a reasonable next step.

Intra-articular injection of the shoulder is performed by placing the patient in the supine position and preparing the skin overlying the shoulder, subacromial region, and joint space with antiseptic solution. A sterile syringe containing 2 mL of 0.25% preservative-free bupivacaine and 40 mg methylprednisolone is attached to a 1½-inch, 25-gauge needle using strict aseptic technique. The midpoint of the acromion is identified, and at a point approximately 1 inch below the midpoint, the shoulder joint space is identified. The needle is carefully advanced through the skin and subcutaneous tissues, through the joint capsule, and into the joint. If bone is encountered, the needle is withdrawn into the subcutaneous tissues and redirected superiorly and slightly more medially. After entering the joint space, the contents of the syringe is gently injected. There should be little resistance to injection; if resistance is encountered, the needle is probably in a ligament or tendon and should be advanced slightly into the joint space until the injection can proceed without significant resistance. The needle is then removed, and a sterile pressure dressing and ice pack are applied to the injection site.

Physical modalities, including local heat and gentle range-of-motion exercises, should be introduced several days after the patient undergoes injection for shoulder pain. Vigorous exercises should be avoided, because they will exacerbate the patient's symptoms.

COMPLICATIONS AND PITFALLS

This injection technique is safe if careful attention is paid to the clinically relevant anatomy. Sterile technique must be used to avoid infection, along with universal precautions to minimize any risk to the operator. The incidence of ecchymosis and hematoma formation can be decreased if pressure is applied to the injection site immediately after injection. The major complication of intra-articular injection of the shoulder is infection, although it should be exceedingly rare if strict aseptic technique is followed. Approximately 25% of patients complain of a transient increase in pain after intra-articular injection of the shoulder joint, and they should be warned of this possibility.

> ### Clinical Pearls
>
> Osteoarthritis of the shoulder is a common complaint encountered in clinical practice. It must be distinguished from other causes of shoulder pain, including rotator cuff tears. Intra-articular injection is extremely effective in the treatment of pain secondary to arthritis of the shoulder joint. Coexistent bursitis and tendinitis may contribute to shoulder pain and necessitate additional treatment with more localized injection of local anesthetic and methylprednisolone. Simple analgesics and nonsteroidal anti-inflammatory drugs or cyclooxygenase-2 inhibitors can be used concurrently with this injection technique.

Chapter 22

Acromioclavicular Joint Pain

ICD-9 CODE 719.41

THE CLINICAL SYNDROME

The acromioclavicular joint is vulnerable to injury from both acute trauma and repeated microtrauma (Fig. 22-1). Acute injuries are frequently the result of falling directly onto the shoulder when playing sports or riding a bicycle. Repeated strain from throwing or working with the arm raised across the body may also result in trauma to the joint. After trauma, the joint may become acutely inflamed, and if the condition becomes chronic, arthritis of the acromioclavicular joint may develop.

SIGNS AND SYMPTOMS

Patients suffering from acromioclavicular joint dysfunction frequently complain of pain when reaching across the chest (Fig. 22-2). Often, patients are unable to sleep on the affected shoulder and may complain of a grinding sensation in the joint, especially on first awakening. Physical examination may reveal enlargement or swelling of the joint, with tenderness to palpation. Downward traction or passive adduction of the affected shoulder

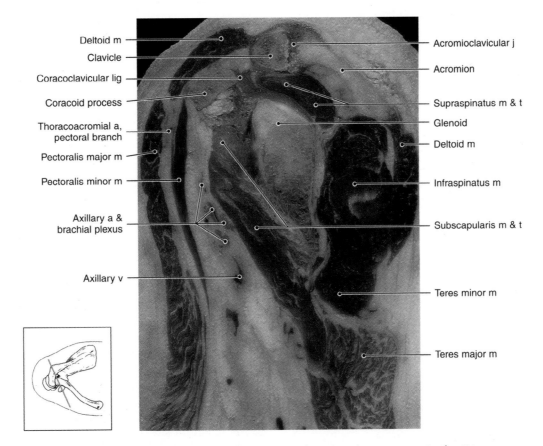

Figure 22–1. Acromioclavicular joint viewed in sagittal section. (From Kang HS, Ahn JM, Resnick D: MRI of the Extremities: An Anatomic Atlas, 2nd ed. Philadelphia, Saunders, 2002, p 29.)

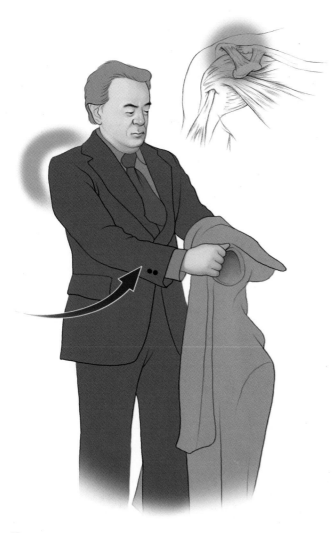

Figure 22–2. Acromioclavicular joint pain is made worse by reaching across the chest.

may cause increased pain. If there is disruption of the ligaments of the acromioclavicular joint, these maneuvers may reveal joint instability.

TESTING

Plain radiographs of the joint may reveal narrowing or sclerosis, consistent with osteoarthritis. Magnetic resonance imaging is indicated if disruption of the ligaments is suspected. The injection technique described later serves as both a diagnostic and a therapeutic maneuver. If polyarthritis is present, screening laboratory tests consisting of a complete blood count, erythrocyte sedimentation rate, and antinuclear antibody testing should be performed.

DIFFERENTIAL DIAGNOSIS

Osteoarthritis of the acromioclavicular joint is a frequent cause of shoulder pain, and it is usually the result of

trauma. However, rheumatoid arthritis and rotator cuff arthropathy are also common causes of shoulder pain that may mimic acromioclavicular joint pain and confuse the diagnosis. Less common causes of arthritis-induced shoulder pain include the collagen vascular diseases, infection, and Lyme disease. Acute infectious arthritis is usually accompanied by significant systemic symptoms, including fever and malaise, and should be easily recognized; it is treated with culture and antibiotics rather than injection therapy. Collagen vascular diseases generally present as a polyarthropathy rather than a monoarthropathy limited to the shoulder joint; however, shoulder pain secondary to collagen vascular disease responds exceedingly well to the intra-articular injection technique described here.

TREATMENT

Initial treatment of the pain and functional disability associated with acromioclavicular joint pain includes a combination of nonsteroidal anti-inflammatory drugs or cyclooxygenase-2 inhibitors and physical therapy. Local application of heat and cold may also be beneficial. For patients who do not respond to these treatment modalities, intra-articular injection of local anesthetic and steroid is a reasonable next step.

Intra-articular injection of the acromioclavicular joint is performed by placing the patient in the supine position and preparing the skin overlying the superior shoulder and distal clavicle with antiseptic solution. A sterile syringe containing 1 mL of 0.25% preservative-free bupivacaine and 40 mg methylprednisolone is attached to a 1½-inch, 25-gauge needle using strict aseptic technique. The top of the acromion is identified, and at a point approximately 1 inch medially, the acromioclavicular joint space is identified. The needle is carefully advanced through the skin and subcutaneous tissues, through the joint capsule, and into the joint (Fig. 22-3). If bone is encountered, the needle is withdrawn into the subcutaneous tissues and redirected slightly more medially. After the joint space is entered, the contents of the syringe are gently injected. There should be some resistance to injection, because the joint space is small and the joint capsule is dense. If significant resistance is encountered, however, the needle is probably in a ligament and should be advanced slightly into the joint space until the injection can proceed with only limited resistance. If no resistance is encountered on injection, the joint space is probably not intact, and magnetic resonance imaging is recommended. After injection the needle is removed, and a sterile pressure dressing and ice pack are applied to the injection site.

Physical modalities, including local heat and gentle range-of-motion exercises, should be introduced several days after the patient undergoes injection for shoulder

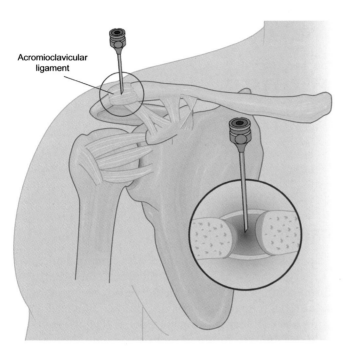

Figure 22–3. Proper needle placement for acromioclavicular joint injection. (From Waldman SD: Atlas of Pain Management Injection Techniques. Philadelphia, Saunders, 2000, p 41.)

pain. Vigorous exercises should be avoided, because they will exacerbate the patient's symptoms.

COMPLICATIONS AND PITFALLS

This injection technique is safe if careful attention is paid to the clinically relevant anatomy. Sterile technique must be used to avoid infection, along with universal precautions to minimize any risk to the operator. The incidence of ecchymosis and hematoma formation can be decreased if pressure is applied to the injection site immediately after injection. The major complication of intra-articular injection of the acromioclavicular joint is infection, although it should be exceedingly rare if strict aseptic technique is followed. Approximately 25% of patients complain of a transient increase in pain after intra-articular injection of the acromioclavicular joint, and they should be warned of this possibility.

Clinical Pearls

Intra-articular injection is extremely effective in the treatment of pain secondary to arthritis of the acromioclavicular joint. Coexistent bursitis and tendinitis may contribute to shoulder pain and necessitate additional treatment with more localized injection of local anesthetic and methylprednisolone. Simple analgesics and nonsteroidal anti-inflammatory drugs or cyclooxygenase-2 inhibitors can be used concurrently with this injection technique.

Chapter 23

Subdeltoid Bursitis

ICD-9 CODE 726.19

THE CLINICAL SYNDROME

The subdeltoid bursa lies primarily under the acromion, extending laterally between the deltoid muscle and the joint capsule under the deltoid muscle (Fig. 23-1). It may exist as a single bursal sac or, in some patients, as a multisegmented series of loculated sacs. The subdeltoid bursa is vulnerable to injury from both acute trauma and repeated microtrauma. Acute injuries frequently take the form of direct trauma to the shoulder when playing sports or falling off a bicycle. Repeated strain from throwing, bowling, carrying a heavy briefcase, working with the arm raised across the body, rotator cuff injuries, or repetitive motion associated with assembly-line work may result in inflammation of the subdeltoid bursa. If the inflammation becomes chronic, calcification of the bursa may occur.

Patients suffering from subdeltoid bursitis frequently complain of pain with any movement of the shoulder, but especially with abduction (Fig. 23-2). The pain is localized to the subdeltoid area, with referred pain often noted at the insertion of the deltoid at the deltoid tuberosity on the upper third of the humerus. Patients are often unable to sleep on the affected shoulder and may complain of a sharp, catching sensation when abducting the shoulder, especially on first awakening.

SIGNS AND SYMPTOMS

Physical examination may reveal point tenderness over the acromion; occasionally, swelling of the bursa gives the affected deltoid muscle an edematous feel. Passive elevation and medial rotation of the affected shoulder reproduce the pain, as do resisted abduction and lateral rotation. Sudden release of resistance during this maneuver markedly increases the pain. Rotator cuff tear may mimic or coexist with subdeltoid bursitis and may confuse the diagnosis (see Differential Diagnosis).

TESTING

Plain radiographs of the shoulder may reveal calcification of the bursa and associated structures, consistent with chronic inflammation. Magnetic resonance imaging is indicated if tendinitis, partial disruption of the ligaments, or rotator cuff tear is being considered (Fig. 23-3). Based on the patient's clinical presentation, additional testing may be indicated, including a complete blood count, erythrocyte sedimentation rate, and antinuclear antibody testing. Radionuclide bone scanning is indicated if metastatic disease or primary tumor involving the shoulder is a possibility. The injection technique described later serves as both a diagnostic and a therapeutic maneuver.

DIFFERENTIAL DIAGNOSIS

Subdeltoid bursitis is one of the most common causes of shoulder joint pain. Osteoarthritis, rheumatoid arthritis, post-traumatic arthritis, and rotator cuff arthropathy are also common causes of shoulder pain that may coexist with subdeltoid bursitis. Less common causes of arthritis-induced shoulder pain include collagen vascular diseases, infection, villonodular synovitis, and Lyme disease. Acute infectious arthritis is usually accompanied by significant systemic symptoms, including fever and malaise, and should be easily recognized; it is treated with culture and antibiotics rather than injection therapy. Collagen vascular diseases generally present as a polyarthropathy rather than a monoarthropathy limited to the shoulder joint; however, shoulder pain secondary to collagen vascular disease responds exceedingly well to the injection technique described here.

TREATMENT

Initial treatment of the pain and functional disability associated with subdeltoid bursitis includes a combination of nonsteroidal anti-inflammatory drugs or cyclooxygenase-2 inhibitors and physical therapy. Local application of heat and cold may also be beneficial. For patients who do not respond to these treatment

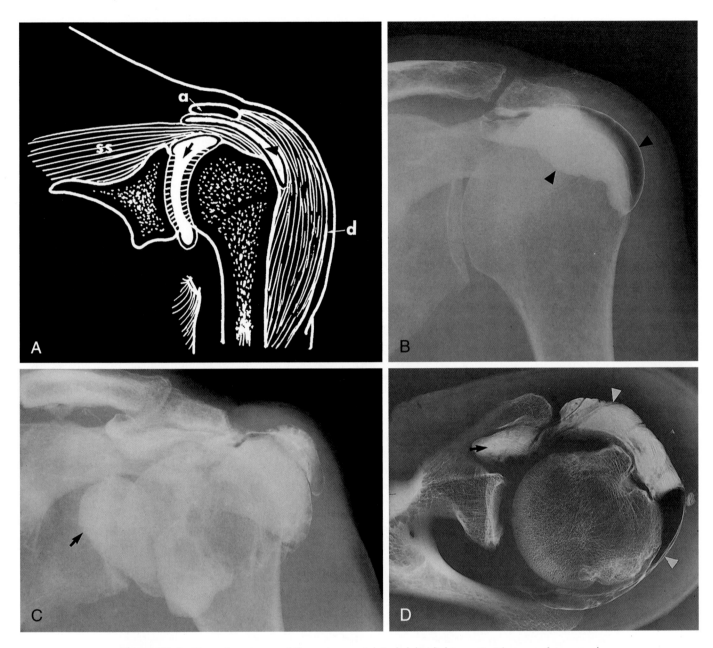

Figure 23–1. Normal anatomy of the subacromial (subdeltoid) bursa. **A,** Diagram of a coronal section of the shoulder shows the glenohumeral joint *(arrow)* and subacromial (subdeltoid) bursa *(arrowhead)*, separated by a portion of the rotator cuff (i.e., supraspinatus tendon). The supraspinatus (ss) and deltoid (d) muscles and the acromion (a) are indicated.
B, Subdeltoid-subacromial bursogram, accomplished with the injection of both radiopaque contrast material and air, shows the bursa *(arrowheads)* sitting like a cap on the humeral head and greater tuberosity of the humerus. Note that the joint is not opacified, indicative of an intact rotator cuff. **C,** In a different cadaver, a subacromial-subdeltoid bursogram shows much more extensive structure as a result of opacification of the subacromial, subdeltoid, and subcoracoid *(arrow)* portions of the bursa. **D,** Radiograph of a transverse section of the specimen illustrated in **C** shows both the subdeltoid *(arrowheads)* and subcoracoid *(arrow)* portions of the bursa. The glenohumeral joint is not opacified. (From Resnick D: Diagnosis of Bone and Joint Disorders, 4th ed. Philadelphia, Saunders, 2002, p 3072.)

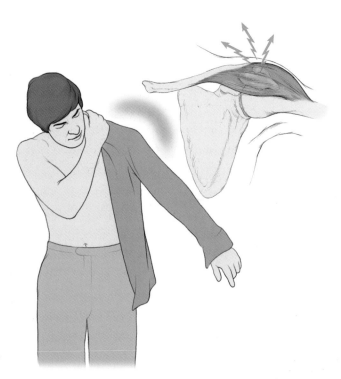

Figure 23–2. Abduction of the shoulder exacerbates the pain of subdeltoid bursitis.

modalities, injection of local anesthetic and steroid into the subdeltoid bursa is a reasonable next step.

Injection into the subdeltoid bursa is performed by placing the patient in the supine position and preparing the skin overlying the superior shoulder, acromion, and distal clavicle with antiseptic solution. A sterile syringe containing 4 mL of 0.25% preservative-free bupivacaine and 40 mg methylprednisolone is attached to a 1½-inch, 25-gauge needle using strict aseptic technique. The lateral edge of the acromion is identified, and at the midpoint of the lateral edge, the injection site is identified. At this point, the needle is carefully advanced with a slightly cephalad trajectory through the skin and subcutaneous tissues beneath the acromion capsule and into the bursa (Fig. 23-4). If bone is encountered, the needle is withdrawn into the subcutaneous tissues and redirected slightly more inferiorly. After entering the bursa, the contents of the syringe are gently injected while the needle is slowly withdrawn. There should be minimal resistance to injection unless calcification of the bursal sac is present, in which case resistance to needle advancement is associated with a gritty feel. Significant calcific bursitis may ultimately require surgical excision to achieve complete relief of symptoms. After injection the needle is removed, and a sterile pressure dressing and ice pack are applied to the injection site.

Physical modalities, including local heat and gentle range-of-motion exercises, should be introduced several days after the patient undergoes injection for shoulder pain. Vigorous exercises should be avoided, because they will exacerbate the patient's symptoms.

COMPLICATIONS AND PITFALLS

This injection technique is safe if careful attention is paid to the clinically relevant anatomy. Sterile technique must

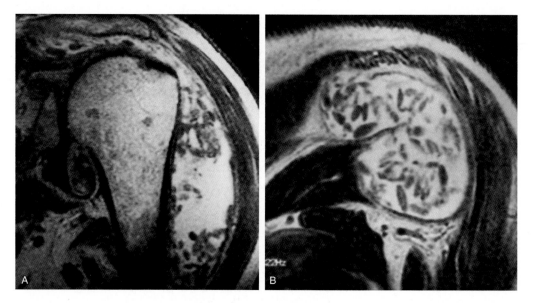

Figure 23–3. Subacromial-subdeltoid bursitis. **A** and **B,** Oblique, coronal, fast spin echo (TR 300, TE 99) magnetic resonance images (**B** is posterior to **A**) show massive distention of the bursa with fluid of high signal intensity, and synovial proliferative tissue and rice bodies of low signal intensity, in a patient with probable rheumatoid arthritis. The rotator cuff is torn and retracted, and the glenohumeral joint is also involved. (From Resnick D: Diagnosis of Bone and Joint Disorders, 4th ed. Philadelphia, Saunders, 2002, p 4256.)

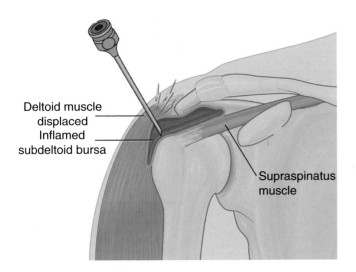

Figure 23–4. Proper needle placement for injection of the subdeltoid bursa. (From Waldman SD: Atlas of Pain Management Injection Techniques. Philadelphia, Saunders, 2000.)

be used to avoid infection, along with universal precautions to minimize any risk to the operator. The incidence of ecchymosis and hematoma formation can be decreased if pressure is applied to the injection site immediately after injection. The major complication of injection of the subdeltoid bursa is infection, although it should be exceedingly rare if strict aseptic technique is followed. Approximately 25% of patients complain of a transient increase in pain after injection of the subdeltoid bursa, and they should be warned of this possibility.

Clinical Pearls

This injection technique is extremely effective in the treatment of pain secondary to subdeltoid bursitis. Coexistent arthritis and tendinitis may contribute to shoulder pain, necessitating additional treatment with more localized injection of local anesthetic and methylprednisolone. Simple analgesics and nonsteroidal anti-inflammatory agents can be used concurrently with this injection technique.

Chapter 24

Bicipital Tendinitis

ICD-9 CODE 726.12

THE CLINICAL SYNDROME

The tendons of the long and short heads of the biceps are particularly prone to the development of tendinitis. Bicipital tendinitis is usually caused at least partially by impingement on the tendons of the biceps at the coracoacromial arch. The onset of bicipital tendinitis is generally acute, occurring after overuse or misuse of the shoulder joint, such as trying to start a recalcitrant lawn mower, practicing an overhead tennis serve, or overaggressive follow-through when driving golf balls. The biceps muscle and tendons are susceptible to trauma and to wear and tear, and if the damage is severe enough, the tendon of the long head of the biceps can rupture, leaving the patient with a telltale "Popeye" biceps (named after the cartoon character). This deformity can be accentuated by having the patient perform Luningston's maneuver: placing his or her hands behind the head and flexing the biceps muscle.

SIGNS AND SYMPTOMS

The pain of bicipital tendinitis is constant and severe and is localized in the anterior shoulder over the bicipital groove (Fig. 24-1). A catching sensation may accompany the pain. Significant sleep disturbance is often reported. The patient may attempt to splint the inflamed tendons by internal rotation of the humerus, which moves the biceps tendon from beneath the coracoacromial arch. Patients with bicipital tendinitis have a positive Yergason's test—that is, production of pain on active supination of the forearm against resistance with the elbow flexed at a right angle (Fig. 24-2). Bursitis often accompanies bicipital tendinitis.

In addition to pain, patients suffering from bicipital tendinitis often experience a gradual reduction in functional ability because of decreasing shoulder range of motion, making simple everyday tasks such as combing one's hair, fastening a brassiere, and reaching overhead quite difficult. With continued disuse, muscle wasting may occur, and a frozen shoulder may develop.

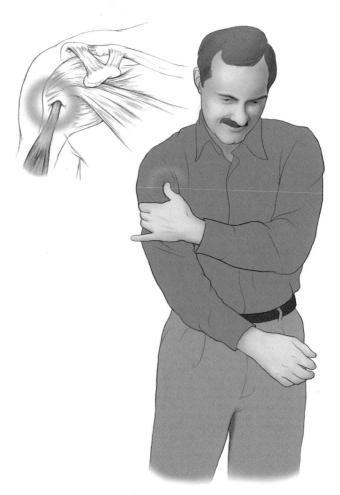

Figure 24–1. Palpation of the bicipital groove exacerbates the pain of bicipital tendinitis.

TESTING

Plain radiographs are indicated for all patients who present with shoulder pain. Based on the patient's clinical presentation, additional testing may be indicated, including a complete blood count, erythrocyte sedimentation rate, and antinuclear antibody testing. Magnetic resonance imaging of the shoulder is indicated if rotator cuff tear is suspected (Fig. 24-3). The injection technique described later serves as both a diagnostic and a therapeutic maneuver.

with local anesthetic and steroid is a reasonable next step.

Injection for bicipital tendinitis is carried out by placing the patient in the supine position with the arm externally rotated approximately 45 degrees. The coracoid process is identified anteriorly. Just lateral to the coracoid process is the lesser tuberosity, which can be more easily palpated as the arm is passively rotated. The point overlying the tuberosity is marked with a sterile marker. The skin overlying the anterior shoulder is prepared with antiseptic solution. A sterile syringe containing 1 mL of 0.25% preservative-free bupivacaine and 40 mg methylprednisolone is attached to a 1½-inch, 25-gauge needle using strict aseptic technique. The previously marked point is palpated, and the insertion of the biceps tendon is reidentified with the gloved finger. The needle is carefully advanced at this point through the skin, subcutaneous tissues, and underlying tendon until

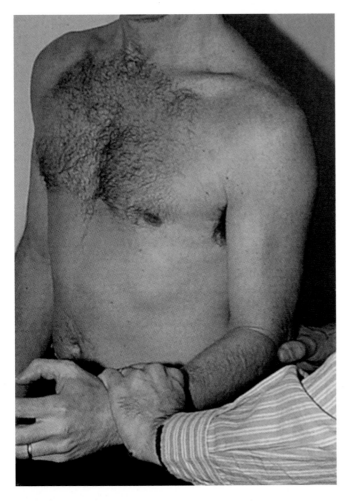

Figure 24–2. Yergason's test for bicipital tendinitis. (From Klippel JH, Dieppe PA: Rheumatology, 2nd ed. London, Mosby, 1998.)

DIFFERENTIAL DIAGNOSIS

Bicipital tendinitis is usually a straightforward clinical diagnosis. However, coexisting bursitis or tendinitis of the shoulder from overuse or misuse may confuse the diagnosis. Occasionally, partial rotator cuff tear can be mistaken for bicipital tendinitis. In some clinical situations, consideration should be given to primary or secondary tumors involving the shoulder, superior sulcus of the lung, or proximal humerus. The pain of acute herpes zoster, which occurs before eruption of a vesicular rash, can also mimic bicipital tendinitis.

TREATMENT

Initial treatment of the pain and functional disability associated with bicipital tendinitis includes a combination of nonsteroidal anti-inflammatory drugs or cyclooxygenase-2 inhibitors and physical therapy. Local application of heat and cold may also be beneficial. For patients who do not respond to these treatment modalities, injection

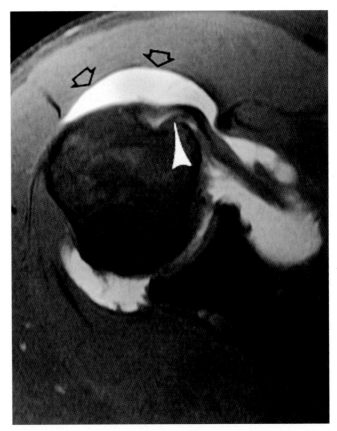

Figure 24–3. "Perched" biceps tendon. Fat-suppressed, T1-weighted, axial magnetic resonance arthrogram reveals a flattened biceps tendon (large arrowhead) draped over the lesser tuberosity in the presence of a normally configured bicipital groove. The presence of contrast material in the subacromial-subdeltoid bursa (open arrowheads) indicates a coexisting full-thickness tear of the rotator cuff. (From Edelman RR, Hessellink JR, Zlatkin MB, Crues JV: Clinical Magnetic Resonance Imaging, 3rd ed. Philadelphia, Saunders, 2006, p 3161.)

it impinges on bone. The needle is then withdrawn 1 to 2 mm out of the periosteum of the humerus, and the contents of the syringe is gently injected. There should be slight resistance to injection. If no resistance is encountered, either the needle tip is in the joint space itself or the tendon is ruptured. If there is significant resistance, the needle tip is probably in the substance of a ligament or tendon and should be advanced or withdrawn slightly until the injection can proceed without significant resistance. The needle is then removed, and a sterile pressure dressing and ice pack are applied to the injection site.

Physical modalities, including local heat and gentle range-of-motion exercises, should be introduced several days after the patient undergoes injection. Vigorous exercises should be avoided, because they will exacerbate the patient's symptoms.

COMPLICATIONS AND PITFALLS

This injection technique is safe if careful attention is paid to the clinically relevant anatomy. Sterile technique must be used to avoid infection, along with universal precautions to minimize any risk to the operator. The incidence of ecchymosis and hematoma formation can be decreased if pressure is applied to the injection site immediately after injection. The major complication of this injection technique is infection, although it should be exceedingly rare if strict aseptic technique is followed. Trauma to the biceps tendon from the injection itself is also a possibility. Tendons that are highly inflamed or previously damaged are subject to rupture if they are injected directly. This complication can often be avoided if the clinician uses a gentle technique and stops injecting immediately if significant resistance is encountered. Approximately 25% of patients complain of a transient increase in pain after injection, and they should be warned of this possibility.

Clinical Pearls

The musculotendinous unit of the shoulder joint is susceptible to the development of tendinitis for several reasons. First, the joint is subjected to a wide range of repetitive motions. Second, the space in which the musculotendinous unit functions is restricted by the coracoacromial arch, making impingement likely with extreme movements of the joint. Third, the blood supply to the musculotendinous unit is poor, making the healing of microtrauma difficult. All these factors can contribute to tendinitis. Calcium deposition around the tendon may occur if the inflammation continues, making subsequent treatment more difficult.

The injection technique described is extremely effective in the treatment of pain secondary to bicipital tendinitis. Coexistent bursitis and arthritis may contribute to shoulder pain, necessitating additional treatment with more localized injection of local anesthetic and methylprednisolone. Simple analgesics and nonsteroidal anti-inflammatory drugs or cyclooxygenase-2 inhibitors can be used concurrently with this injection technique.

Chapter 25

Supraspinatus Syndrome

ICD-9 CODE 729.1

THE CLINICAL SYNDROME

The supraspinatus muscle is susceptible to the development of myofascial pain syndrome. Flexion-extension and lateral motion stretch injuries to the neck, shoulder, and upper back or repeated microtrauma secondary to activities that require working overhead or repeatedly reaching across one's body, such as painting ceilings, assembly-line work, or even watching television while reclining on a couch, may result in the development of myofascial pain in the supraspinatus muscle.

Myofascial pain syndrome is a chronic pain syndrome that affects a focal or regional portion of the body. The sine qua non of myofascial pain syndrome is the finding of myofascial trigger points on physical examination. Although these trigger points are generally localized to the part of the body affected, the pain is often referred to other areas. This referred pain may be misdiagnosed or attributed to other organ systems, leading to extensive evaluation and ineffective treatment. Patients with myofascial pain syndrome involving the supraspinatus muscle often have referred pain in the shoulder radiating down into the upper extremity.

The trigger point is pathognomonic of myofascial pain syndrome and is characterized by a local point of exquisite tenderness in the affected muscle. Mechanical stimulation of the trigger point by palpation or stretching produces not only intense local pain but referred pain as well. In addition, there is often an involuntary withdrawal of the stimulated muscle, called a "jump sign," which is also characteristic of myofascial pain syndrome. In patients with supraspinatus syndrome, the trigger point overlies the superior border of the scapula (Fig. 25-1).

Taut bands of muscle fibers are often identified when myofascial trigger points are palpated. In spite of this consistent physical finding, the pathophysiology of the myofascial trigger point remains elusive, but it is thought that trigger points are the result of microtrauma to the affected muscle. This may occur from a single injury,

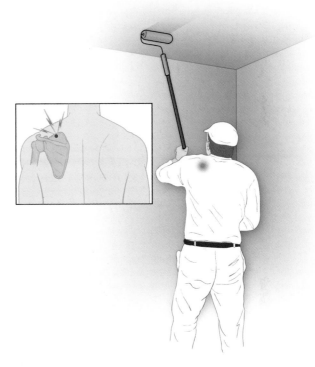

Figure 25–1. In patients with supraspinatus syndrome, the trigger point overlies the superior border of the scapula.

repetitive microtrauma, or chronic deconditioning of the agonist and antagonist muscle unit.

In addition to muscle trauma, a variety of other factors seems to predispose patients to the development of myofascial pain syndrome. For instance, a weekend athlete who subjects his or her body to unaccustomed physical activity may develop myofascial pain syndrome. Poor posture while sitting at a computer or while watching television has also been implicated as a predisposing factor. Previous injuries may result in abnormal muscle function and lead to the development of myofascial pain syndrome. All these factors may be intensified if the patient also suffers from poor nutritional status or coexisting psychological or behavioral abnormalities, including chronic stress and depression. The supraspinatus muscle

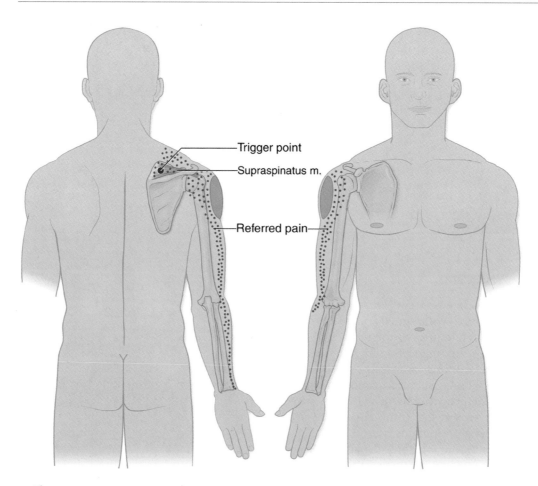

Figure 25–2. Pain on range of motion and pain referred to the shoulder and upper extremities in a nondermatomal pattern are characteristic of supraspinatus syndrome. (From Waldman SD: Atlas of Pain Management Injection Techniques, 2nd ed. Philadelphia, Saunders, 2007.)

seems to be particularly susceptible to stress-induced myofascial pain syndrome.

Stiffness and fatigue often coexist with pain, increasing the functional disability associated with this disease and complicating its treatment. Myofascial pain syndrome may occur as a primary disease state or in conjunction with other painful conditions, including radiculopathy and chronic regional pain syndromes. Psychological or behavioral abnormalities, including depression, frequently coexist with the muscle abnormalities, and management of these psychological disorders is an integral part of any successful treatment plan.

SIGNS AND SYMPTOMS

The sine qua non of supraspinatus syndrome is the identification of a myofascial trigger point—a local point of exquisite tenderness—overlying the superior border of the scapula. Mechanical stimulation of the trigger point by palpation or stretching produces intense local pain as

well as referred pain, and the jump sign may be present. Other findings characteristic of supraspinatus syndrome are pain on range of motion of the affected scapula and shoulder and pain referred to the shoulder and upper extremities in a nondermatomal pattern (Fig. 25-2).

TESTING

Biopsies of clinically identified trigger points have not revealed consistently abnormal histology. The muscle hosting the trigger points has been described either as "moth-eaten" or as containing "waxy degeneration." Increased plasma myoglobin has been reported in some patients with supraspinatus syndrome, but this finding has not been corroborated by other investigators. Electrodiagnostic testing of patients suffering from supraspinatus syndrome has revealed an increase in muscle tension in some patients, but again, this finding has not been reproducible. Because of the lack of objective testing, the clinician must use electrodiagnostic and radiographic means to rule out other disease processes that may mimic supraspinatus syndrome (see Differential Diagnosis).

DIFFERENTIAL DIAGNOSIS

The diagnosis of supraspinatus syndrome is made on the basis of clinical findings rather than specific laboratory, electrodiagnostic, or radiographic testing. For this reason, a targeted history and physical examination, with a systematic search for trigger points and identification of a positive jump sign, must be carried out in every patient suspected of having supraspinatus syndrome. It is incumbent on the clinician to rule out other coexisting disease processes that may mimic supraspinatus syndrome, including primary inflammatory muscle disease, multiple sclerosis, and collagen vascular disease. Electrodiagnostic and radiographic testing can help identify coexisting pathology such as shoulder bursitis, tendinitis, and rotator cuff tears. The clinician must also identify coexisting psychological and behavioral abnormalities that may mask or exacerbate the symptoms associated with supraspinatus syndrome.

TREATMENT

Treatment is focused on blocking the myofascial trigger and achieving prolonged relaxation of the affected muscle. It is hoped that interrupting the pain cycle in this way will allow the patient to obtain long-term pain relief. Because the mechanism of action of the treatment modalities used is poorly understood, an element of trial and error is involved in developing a treatment plan.

Conservative therapy consisting of trigger point injection with local anesthetic or saline is the initial treatment of supraspinatus syndrome. Adjunct therapies, including physical therapy, therapeutic heat and cold, transcutaneous nerve stimulation, and electrical stimulation, can be used on a case-by-case basis. For patients who do not respond to these traditional measures, consideration should be given to the use of botulinum toxin type A; although not currently approved by the Food and Drug Administration for this indication, the injection of minute quantities of botulinum toxin type A directly into trigger points has been successful. Because underlying depression and anxiety are present in many patients suffering from supraspinatus syndrome, the administration of antidepressants is an integral part of most treatment plans.

COMPLICATIONS AND PITFALLS

Trigger point injection is extremely safe if careful attention is paid to the clinically relevant anatomy. Sterile technique must be used to avoid infection, along with universal precautions to minimize any risk to the operator. Most complications of trigger point injection are related to needle-induced trauma at the injection site and in underlying tissues. The incidence of ecchymosis and hematoma formation can be decreased if pressure is applied to the injection site immediately after injection. The avoidance of overly long needles can decrease the trauma to underlying structures. Special care must be taken to avoid pneumothorax when injecting trigger points in proximity to the underlying pleural space.

Clinical Pearls

Although supraspinatus syndrome is a common disorder, it is often misdiagnosed. Therefore, in patients suspected of suffering from supraspinatus syndrome, a careful evaluation is mandatory to identify any underlying disease processes. Supraspinatus syndrome often coexists with a variety of somatic and psychological disorders.

Chapter 26

Rotator Cuff Tear

ICD-9 CODE 840.4 (traumatic) or 726.10 (degenerative)

THE CLINICAL SYNDROME

Rotator cuff tears are a common cause of shoulder pain and dysfunction. A rotator cuff tear frequently occurs after seemingly minor trauma to the musculotendinous unit of the shoulder. However, in most cases, the pathology responsible for the tear has been a long time in the making and is the result of ongoing tendinitis. The rotator cuff is made up of the subscapularis, supraspinatus, infraspinatus, and teres minor muscles and the associated tendons (Fig. 26-1). The function of the rotator cuff is to rotate the arm and help provide shoulder joint stability along with the other muscles, tendons, and ligaments of the shoulder.

The supraspinatus and infraspinatus muscle tendons are particularly susceptible to the development of tendinitis, for several reasons. First, the joint is subjected to a wide variety of repetitive motions. Second, the space in which the musculotendinous unit functions is restricted by the coracoacromial arch, making impingement likely with extreme movements of the joint. Third, the blood supply to the musculotendinous unit is poor, making the healing of microtrauma difficult. All these factors can contribute to tendinitis of one or more tendons of the shoulder joint. Calcium deposition around the tendon may occur if the inflammation continues, making subsequent treatment more difficult. Bursitis often accompanies rotator cuff tears and may require specific treatment.

In addition to pain, patients suffering from rotator cuff tear often experience a gradual reduction in functional ability because of decreasing shoulder range of motion, making simple everyday tasks such as combing one's hair, fastening a brassiere, or reaching overhead quite difficult. With continued disuse, muscle wasting may occur, and a frozen shoulder may develop.

SIGNS AND SYMPTOMS

Patients presenting with rotator cuff tear frequently complain that they cannot raise the affected arm above the level of the shoulder without using the other arm to lift it (Fig. 26-2). On physical examination, there is weakness on external rotation if the infraspinatus is involved, and weakness on abduction above the level of the shoulder if the supraspinatus is involved. Tenderness to palpation in the subacromial region is often present. Patients with partial rotator cuff tears lose the ability to reach overhead smoothly. Patients with complete tears exhibit anterior migration of the humeral head, as well as a complete inability to reach above the level of the shoulder. A positive drop arm test—the inability to hold the arm abducted at the level of the shoulder after the supported arm is released—is often seen with complete tears of the rotator cuff (Figs. 26-3 and 26-4). Moseley's test for rotator cuff tear is also positive; this is performed by having the patient actively abduct the arm to 80 degrees and then adding gentle resistance, which forces the arm to drop if complete rotator cuff tear is present. Passive range of motion of the shoulder is normal, but active range of motion is limited.

The pain of rotator cuff tear is constant and severe and is made worse with abduction and external rotation of the shoulder. Significant sleep disturbance is often reported. Patients may attempt to splint the inflamed subscapularis tendon by limiting medial rotation of the humerus.

TESTING

Plain radiographs are indicated in all patients who present with shoulder pain. Based on the patient's clinical presentation, additional testing may be indicated, including a complete blood count, erythrocyte sedimentation rate, and antinuclear antibody testing. Magnetic resonance imaging (MRI) of the shoulder is indicated if rotator cuff tear is suspected (Fig. 26-5).

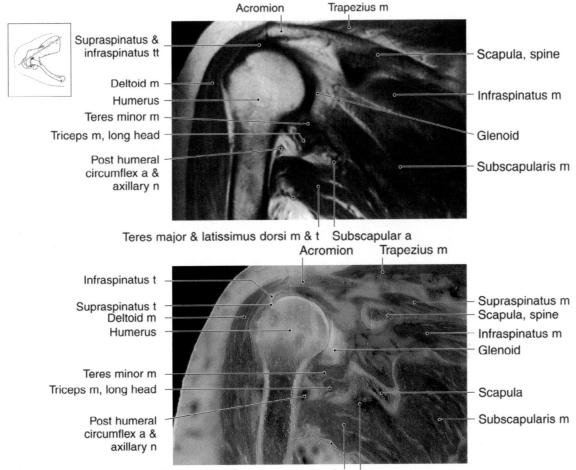

Acromion

Trapezius m

Supraspinatus & infraspinatus tt

Scapula, spine

Deltoid m

Infraspinatus m

Humerus

Teres minor m

Glenoid

Triceps m, long head

Post humeral circumflex a & axillary n

Subscapularis m

Teres major & latissimus dorsi m & t   Subscapular a

Acromion   Trapezius m

Infraspinatus t

Supraspinatus t
Deltoid m
Humerus

Supraspinatus m
Scapula, spine
Infraspinatus m
Glenoid

Teres minor m
Triceps m, long head

Scapula

Post humeral circumflex a & axillary n

Subscapularis m

Teres major & latissimus dorsi m & t   Subscapular a

Figure 26–1. Muscles and tendons of the rotator cuff. (From Kang HS, Ahn JM, Resnick D: MRI of the Extremities: An Anatomic Atlas, 2nd ed. Philadelphia, Saunders, 2002, p 5.)

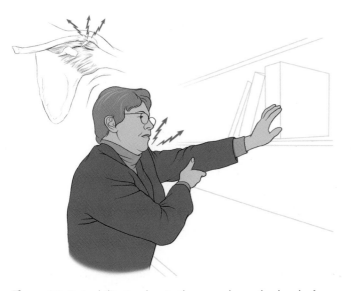

Figure 26–2. Inability to elevate the arm above the level of the shoulder is the hallmark of rotator cuff dysfunction.

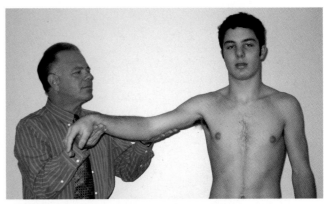

Figure 26–3. The drop arm test for complete rotator cuff tear. (From Waldman SD: Physical Diagnosis of Pain: An Atlas of Signs and Symptoms. Philadelphia, Saunders, 2006, p 91.)

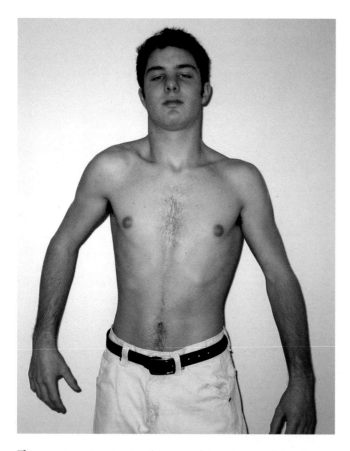

Figure 26–4. A patient with a complete rotator cuff tear is unable to hold the arm in the abducted position, and it falls to the patient's side. The patient often shrugs or hitches the shoulder forward to use the intact muscles of the rotator cuff and the deltoid to keep the arm in the abducted position. (From Waldman SD: Physical Diagnosis of Pain: An Atlas of Signs and Symptoms. Philadelphia, Saunders, 2006, p 92.)

DIFFERENTIAL DIAGNOSIS

Because rotator cuff tears may occur after seemingly minor trauma, the diagnosis is often delayed. The tear may be either partial or complete, further confusing the diagnosis, although a careful physical examination can distinguish the two. Tendinitis of the musculotendinous unit of the shoulder frequently coexists with bursitis of the associated bursae of the shoulder joint, creating additional pain and functional disability. This pain can cause the patient to splint the shoulder group, resulting in abnormal movement of the shoulder, which puts additional stress on the rotator cuff and can lead to further trauma. With rotator cuff tears, passive range of motion is normal, but active range of motion is limited; with frozen shoulder, both passive and active range of motion are limited. Rotator cuff tear rarely occurs before age 40 years, except in cases of severe acute trauma to the shoulder.

TREATMENT

Initial treatment of the pain and functional disability associated with rotator cuff tear includes a combination of nonsteroidal anti-inflammatory drugs or cyclooxygenase-2 inhibitors and physical therapy. Local application of heat and cold may also be beneficial. For patients who do not respond to these treatment modalities, the injection technique described here is a reasonable next step before surgical intervention.

Injection for rotator cuff tear is carried out by placing the patient in the supine position and preparing the skin overlying the superior shoulder, acromion, and distal

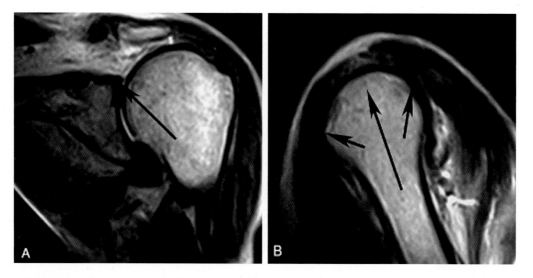

Figure 26–5. Massive tear of the rotator cuff. **A,** Coronal oblique T2-weighted image. The supraspinatus tendon is retracted to the medial glenoid margin *(arrow)*. There is severe atrophy. **B,** Sagittal oblique T2-weighted image. Note the "bald" humeral head. The tear extends from the subscapularis to the infraspinatus tendon *(arrows)*. (From Edelman RR, Hessellink JR, Zlatkin MB, Crues JV: Clinical Magnetic Resonance Imaging, 3rd ed. Philadelphia, Saunders, 2006, p 3225.)

clavicle with antiseptic solution. A sterile syringe containing 4 mL of 0.25% preservative-free bupivacaine and 40 mg methylprednisolone is attached to a $1^1/_2$-inch, 25-gauge needle using strict aseptic technique. The lateral edge of the acromion is identified, and at the midpoint of the lateral edge, the injection site is identified. With a slightly cephalad trajectory, the needle is carefully advanced through the skin, subcutaneous tissues, and deltoid muscle beneath the acromion process. If bone is encountered, the needle is withdrawn into the subcutaneous tissues and redirected slightly more inferiorly. After the needle is in place, the contents of the syringe are gently injected. There should be minimal resistance to injection unless calcification of the subacromial bursal sac is present. This calcification can be recognized as resistance to needle advancement, with an associated gritty feel. Significant calcific bursitis may ultimately require surgical excision to obtain complete relief of symptoms. After injection the needle is removed, and a sterile pressure dressing and ice pack are applied to the injection site.

Physical modalities, including local heat and gentle range-of-motion exercises, should be introduced several days after the patient undergoes injection. Vigorous exercises should be avoided, because they will exacerbate the patient's symptoms and may lead to complete tendon rupture.

COMPLICATIONS AND PITFALLS

One major complication is failure to correctly identify a partial rotator cuff tear and treat it before it becomes complete. This usually occurs because MRI of the shoulder is not performed and the diagnosis is made on clinical grounds alone.

The injection technique described is safe if careful attention is paid to the clinically relevant anatomy. Sterile technique must be used to avoid infection, along with universal precautions to minimize any risk to the operator. The incidence of ecchymosis and hematoma formation can be decreased if pressure is applied to the injection site immediately after injection. The major complication of the injection technique is infection, although it should be exceedingly rare if strict aseptic technique is followed. Trauma to the rotator cuff from the injection itself is also a possibility. Tendons that are highly inflamed or previously damaged are subject to rupture if they are injected directly, which could convert a partial tear into a complete one. This complication can be avoided if the clinician uses gentle technique and stops injecting immediately if significant resistance is encountered. Approximately 25% of patients complain of a transient increase in pain after injection, and they should be warned of this possibility.

Clinical Pearls

Injection is extremely effective in the treatment of pain secondary to rotator cuff tear. This technique is not a substitute for surgery, but it can be used to palliate the pain of partial tears or when surgery for complete tears is not being contemplated. Coexistent bursitis and arthritis may contribute to shoulder pain, necessitating more localized injection of local anesthetic and methylprednisolone. Simple analgesics and nonsteroidal anti-inflammatory drugs can be used concurrently with this injection technique. It should be noted that partial tears may be amenable to arthroscopic or minimal-incision surgery, and the clinician should not wait until the tear is complete before obtaining orthopedic consultation.

Chapter 27

Deltoid Syndrome

ICD-9 CODE 729.1

THE CLINICAL SYNDROME

The deltoid muscle is susceptible to the development of myofascial pain syndrome. Flexion-extension and lateral motion stretch injuries or impact injuries to the deltoid muscle during football or repeated microtrauma secondary to jobs that require prolonged lifting may result in the development of myofascial pain in the deltoid muscle (Fig. 27-1).

Myofascial pain syndrome is a chronic pain syndrome that affects a focal or regional portion of the body. The sine qua non of myofascial pain syndrome is the finding of myofascial trigger points on physical examination. Although these trigger points are generally localized to the part of the body affected, the pain is often referred to other areas. This referred pain may be misdiagnosed or attributed to other organ systems, leading to extensive evaluation and ineffective treatment. Patients with myofascial pain syndrome involving the deltoid muscle often have referred pain in the shoulder radiating down into the upper extremity.

The trigger point is pathognomonic of myofascial pain syndrome and is characterized by a local point of exquisite tenderness in the affected muscle. Mechanical stimulation of the trigger point by palpation or stretching produces not only intense local pain but referred pain as well. In addition, there is often an involuntary withdrawal of the stimulated muscle, called a "jump sign," which is also characteristic of myofascial pain syndrome. Patients with deltoid syndrome exhibit trigger points in both the anterior and posterior fibers of the muscle (Fig. 27-2).

Taunt bands of muscle fibers are often identified when myofascial trigger points are palpated. In spite of this consistent physical finding, the pathophysiology of the myofascial trigger point remains elusive, although it is believed that trigger points are the result of microtrauma to the affected muscle. This may occur from a single injury, repetitive microtrauma, or chronic deconditioning of the agonist and antagonist muscle unit.

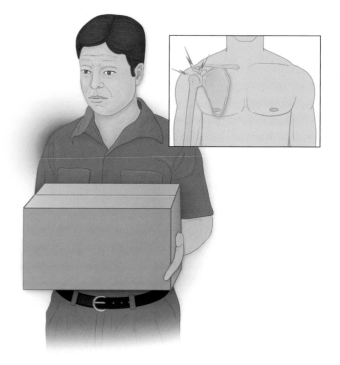

Figure 27–1. Jobs that require prolonged lifting may lead to the development of myofascial pain in the deltoid muscle.

In addition to muscle trauma, a variety of other factors seems to predispose patients to develop myofascial pain syndrome. For instance, a weekend athlete who subjects his or her body to unaccustomed physical activity may develop myofascial pain syndrome. Poor posture while sitting at a computer or while watching television has also been implicated as a predisposing factor. Previous injuries may result in abnormal muscle function and lead to the development of myofascial pain syndrome. All these factors may be intensified if the patient also suffers from poor nutritional status or coexisting psychological or behavioral abnormalities, including chronic stress and depression. The deltoid muscle seems to be particularly susceptible to stress-induced myofascial pain syndrome.

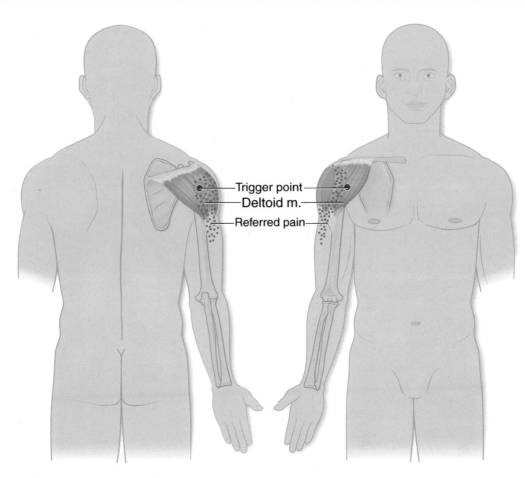

Figure 27–2. Patients with deltoid syndrome have trigger points in both the anterior and posterior fibers of the muscle. (From Waldman SD: Atlas of Pain Management Injection Techniques, 2nd ed. Philadelphia, Saunders, 2007 p 83.)

Stiffness and fatigue often coexist with pain, increasing the functional disability associated with this disease and complicating its treatment. Myofascial pain syndrome may occur as a primary disease state or in conjunction with other painful conditions, including radiculopathy and chronic regional pain syndromes. Psychological or behavioral abnormalities, including depression, frequently coexist with the muscle abnormalities, and management of these psychological disorders is an integral part of any successful treatment plan.

SIGNS AND SYMPTOMS

The sine qua non of deltoid syndrome is the identification of a myofascial trigger point—a local point of exquisite tenderness—overlying the superior border of the scapula. Mechanical stimulation of the trigger point by palpation or stretching produces not only intense local pain but also referred pain. The jump sign is also characteristic of deltoid syndrome, as is pain over the deltoid muscle that is referred into the proximal lateral upper extremity (see Fig. 27-2).

TESTING

Biopsies of clinically identified trigger points have not revealed consistently abnormal histology. The muscle hosting the trigger points has been described either as "moth-eaten" or as containing "waxy degeneration." Increased plasma myoglobin has been reported in some patients with deltoid syndrome, but this finding has not been corroborated by other investigators. Electrodiagnostic testing of patients suffering from deltoid syndrome has revealed an increase in muscle tension in some patients, but again, this finding has not been reproducible. Because of the lack of objective diagnostic testing, the clinician must rule out other coexisting disease processes that may mimic deltoid syndrome (see Differential Diagnosis).

DIFFERENTIAL DIAGNOSIS

The diagnosis of deltoid syndrome is made on the basis of clinical findings rather than specific laboratory, electrodiagnostic, or radiographic testing. For this reason, a

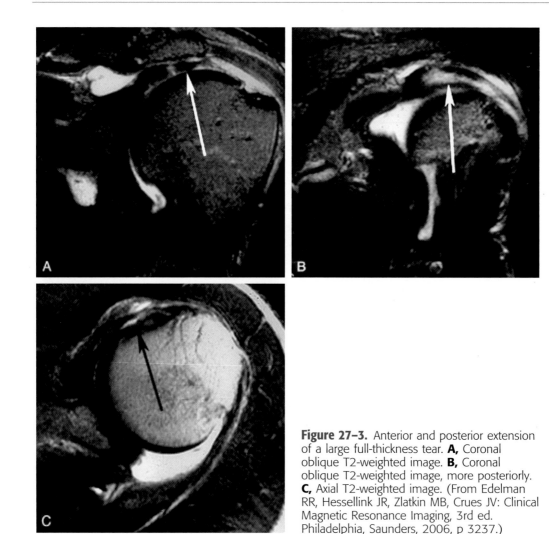

Figure 27–3. Anterior and posterior extension of a large full-thickness tear. **A,** Coronal oblique T2-weighted image. **B,** Coronal oblique T2-weighted image, more posteriorly. **C,** Axial T2-weighted image. (From Edelman RR, Hessellink JR, Zlatkin MB, Crues JV: Clinical Magnetic Resonance Imaging, 3rd ed. Philadelphia, Saunders, 2006, p 3237.)

targeted history and physical examination, with a systematic search for trigger points and identification of a positive jump sign, must be carried out in every patient suspected of suffering from deltoid syndrome. It is incumbent on the clinician to rule out other coexisting disease processes that may mimic deltoid syndrome, including primary inflammatory muscle disease, multiple sclerosis, and collagen vascular disease. Electrodiagnostic and radiographic testing can help identify coexisting pathology such as bursitis, tendinitis, and rotator cuff tears (Fig. 27-3). The clinician must also identify coexisting psychological and behavioral abnormalities that may mask or exacerbate the symptoms associated with deltoid syndrome.

TREATMENT

Treatment is focused on blocking the myofascial trigger and achieving prolonged relaxation of the affected muscle. It is hoped that interrupting the pain cycle in this way will allow the patient to obtain long-term pain relief. Because the mechanism of action of the treatment modalities used is poorly understood, an element of trial and error is involved in developing a treatment plan.

Conservative therapy consisting of trigger point injections with local anesthetic or saline is the initial treatment of deltoid syndrome. Adjunct therapies, including physical therapy, therapeutic heat and cold, transcutaneous nerve stimulation, and electrical stimulation, can be used on a case-by-case basis. For patients who do not respond to these traditional measures, consideration should be given to the use of botulinum toxin type A; although not currently approved by the Food and Drug Administration for this indication, the injection of minute quantities of botulinum toxin type A directly into trigger points has been successful. Because underlying depression and anxiety are present in many patients suffering from deltoid syndrome, the administration of antidepressants is an integral part of most treatment plans.

COMPLICATIONS AND PITFALLS

Trigger point injections are extremely safe if careful attention is paid to the clinically relevant anatomy. Sterile technique must be used to avoid infection, along with universal precautions to minimize any risk to the operator. Most complications of trigger point injection are related to needle-induced trauma at the injection site and in underlying tissues. The incidence of ecchymosis and hematoma formation can be decreased if pressure is applied to the injection site immediately after injection. The avoidance of overly long needles can decrease the incidence of trauma to underlying structures. Special care must be taken to avoid pneumothorax when injecting trigger points in proximity to the underlying pleural space.

Clinical Pearls

Although deltoid syndrome is a common disorder, it is often misdiagnosed. Therefore, in patients suspected of suffering from deltoid syndrome, a careful evaluation to identify underlying disease processes is mandatory. Deltoid syndrome often coexists with a variety of somatic and psychological disorders.

Chapter 28

Teres Major Syndrome

ICD-9 CODE **729.1**

THE CLINICAL SYNDROME

The teres major muscle is susceptible to the development of myofascial pain syndrome. Stretch or impact injuries to the teres major muscle sustained while playing sports or in motor vehicle accidents, as well as falls onto the lateral scapula, have been implicated in the evolution of teres major syndrome. In addition, repeated microtrauma secondary to reaching up and behind, such as when retrieving a briefcase from the backseat of a car, may result in the development of myofascial pain in the teres major muscle (Fig. 28-1).

Myofascial pain syndrome is a chronic pain syndrome that affects a focal or regional portion of the body. The sine qua non of myofascial pain syndrome is the finding of myofascial trigger points on physical examination. Although these trigger points are generally localized to the part of the body affected, the pain is often referred to other areas. This referred pain may be misdiagnosed or attributed to other organ systems, leading to extensive evaluation and ineffective treatment. Patients with myofascial pain syndrome involving the teres major muscle often have referred pain in the shoulder radiating down into the upper extremity.

The trigger point is pathognomonic of myofascial pain syndrome and is characterized by a local point of exquisite tenderness. Mechanical stimulation of the trigger point by palpation or stretching produces not only intense local pain but referred pain as well. In addition, there is often an involuntary withdrawal of the stimulated muscle, called a "jump sign," which is also characteristic of myofascial pain syndrome. Patients with teres major syndrome exhibit trigger points lateral to the scapula in the teres major muscle (Fig. 28-2).

Taut bands of muscle fibers are often identified when myofascial trigger points are palpated. In spite of this consistent physical finding, the pathophysiology of the myofascial trigger point remains elusive, but it is thought that trigger points are the result of microtrauma to the affected muscle. This may occur from a single injury,

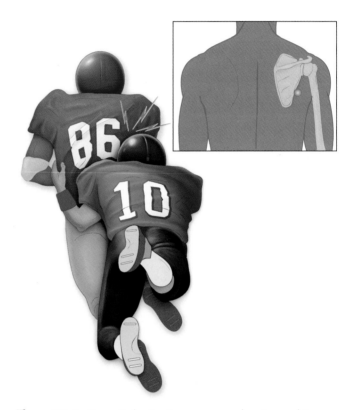

Figure 28–1. Repeated microtrauma secondary to reaching up and behind, as well as playing sports such as football, may result in the development of myofascial pain in the teres major muscle.

repetitive microtrauma, or chronic deconditioning of the agonist and antagonist muscle unit.

In addition to muscle trauma, a variety of other factors seem to predispose patients to the development of myofascial pain syndrome. For instance, a weekend athlete who subjects his or her body to unaccustomed physical activity may develop myofascial pain syndrome. Poor posture while sitting at a computer or while watching television has also been implicated as a predisposing factor. Previous injuries may result in abnormal muscle function and lead to the development of myofascial pain syndrome. All these factors may be intensified if the patient also suffers from poor nutritional status or coexisting psychological or behavioral abnormalities,

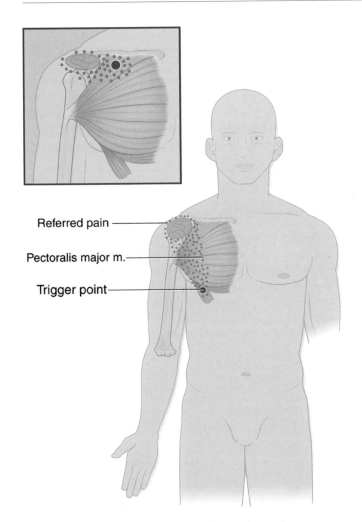

Referred pain

Pectoralis major m.

Trigger point

Figure 28–2. Patients with teres major syndrome have a trigger point lateral to the scapula in the teres major muscle. (From Waldman SD: Atlas of Pain Management Injection Techniques, 2nd ed. Philadelphia, Saunders, 2007, p 86.)

including chronic stress and depression. The teres major muscle seems to be particularly susceptible to stress-induced myofascial pain syndrome.

Stiffness and fatigue often coexist with pain, increasing the functional disability associated with this disease and complicating its treatment. Myofascial pain syndrome may occur as a primary disease state or in conjunction with other painful conditions, including radiculopathy and chronic regional pain syndromes. Psychological or behavioral abnormalities, including depression, frequently coexist with the muscle abnormalities, and management of these psychological disorders is an integral part of any successful treatment plan.

SIGNS AND SYMPTOMS

The trigger point is the pathologic lesion of teres major syndrome and is characterized by a local point of exquisite tenderness in the axillary or posterior portion of the muscle. Mechanical stimulation of the trigger point by palpation or stretching produces both intense local pain and referred pain. In addition, the jump sign is characteristic of teres major syndrome, as is pain over the teres major muscle that is referred to the proximal portion of the posterolateral upper extremity (see Fig. 27-2).

TESTING

Biopsies of clinically identified trigger points have not revealed consistently abnormal histology. The muscle hosting the trigger points has been described either as "moth-eaten" or as containing "waxy degeneration." Increased plasma myoglobin has been reported in some patients with teres major syndrome, but this finding has not been corroborated by other investigators. Electrodiagnostic testing of patients suffering from teres major syndrome has revealed an increase in muscle tension in some patients, but again, this finding has not been reproducible. Because of the lack of objective diagnostic testing, the clinician must rule out other coexisting disease processes that may mimic teres major syndrome (see Differential Diagnosis).

DIFFERENTIAL DIAGNOSIS

The diagnosis of teres major syndrome is made on the basis of clinical findings rather than specific laboratory, electrodiagnostic, or radiographic testing. For this reason, a targeted history and physical examination, with a systematic search for trigger points and identification of a positive jump sign, must be carried out in every patient suspected of suffering from teres major syndrome. It is incumbent on the clinician to rule out other coexisting disease processes that may mimic teres major syndrome, including primary inflammatory muscle disease, multiple sclerosis, and collagen vascular disease. Electrodiagnostic and radiographic testing can help identify coexisting pathology such as shoulder bursitis, tendinitis, and rotator cuff tears. The clinician must also identify coexisting psychological and behavioral abnormalities that may mask or exacerbate the symptoms associated with teres major syndrome.

TREATMENT

Treatment is focused on blocking the myofascial trigger and achieving prolonged relaxation of the affected muscle. It is hoped that interrupting the pain cycle in this way will allow the patient to obtain long-term pain relief. Because the mechanism of action of the treatment modalities used is poorly understood, an element of trial and error is involved in developing a treatment plan.

Conservative therapy consisting of trigger point injections with local anesthetic or saline is the initial treatment of teres major syndrome. Adjunct therapies, including physical therapy, therapeutic heat and cold, transcutaneous nerve stimulation, and electrical stimulation, can be used on a case-by-case basis. For patients who do not respond to these traditional measures, consideration should be given to the use of botulinum toxin type A; although not currently approved by the Food and Drug Administration for this indication, the injection of minute quantities of botulinum toxin type A directly into trigger points has been successful. Because underlying depression and anxiety are present in many patients suffering from teres major syndrome, the administration of antidepressants is an integral part of most treatment plans.

COMPLICATIONS AND PITFALLS

Trigger point injections are extremely safe if careful attention is paid to the clinically relevant anatomy. Sterile technique must be used to avoid infection, along with universal precautions to minimize any risk to the operator. Most complications of trigger point injection are related to needle-induced trauma at the injection site and in underlying tissues. The incidence of ecchymosis and hematoma formation can be decreased if pressure is applied to the injection site immediately after injection. The avoidance of overly long needles can decrease the incidence of trauma to underlying structures. Special care must be taken to avoid pneumothorax when injecting trigger points in proximity to the underlying pleural space.

Clinical Pearls

Although teres major syndrome is a common disorder, it is often misdiagnosed. Therefore, in patients suspected of suffering from teres major syndrome, a careful evaluation to identify underlying disease processes is mandatory. Teres major syndrome commonly coexists with a variety of somatic and psychological disorders.

Chapter 29

Scapulocostal Syndrome

ICD-9 CODE **729.1**

THE CLINICAL SYNDROME

Scapulocostal syndrome consists of a constellation of symptoms including unilateral pain and associated paresthesias at the medial border of the scapula, referred pain radiating from the deltoid region to the dorsum of the hand, and decreased range of motion of the scapula (Fig. 29-1). Scapulocostal syndrome is commonly referred to as "traveling salesman's shoulder," because it is frequently seen in individuals who repeatedly reach backward to get something from the backseat of a car (Fig. 29-2). Scapulocostal syndrome is an overuse syndrome caused by repeated improper use of the muscles of scapular stabilization—the levator scapulae, pectoralis minor, serratus anterior, rhomboids, and, to a lesser extent, infraspinatus and teres minor.

Scapulocostal syndrome is a chronic myofascial pain syndrome, and the sine qua non of myofascial pain syndrome is the finding of myofascial trigger points on physical examination. Although these trigger points are generally localized to the part of the body affected, the pain is often referred to other areas. This referred pain may be misdiagnosed or attributed to other organ systems, leading to extensive evaluation and ineffective treatment. Mechanical stimulation of the trigger point by palpation or stretching produces both intense local pain and referred pain. In addition, there is often an involuntary withdrawal of the stimulated muscle, called a "jump sign," which is also characteristic of myofascial pain syndrome. Almost all patients with scapulocostal syndrome have a prominent infraspinatus trigger point, which is best demonstrated by having the patient place the hand of the affected side over the deltoid of the opposite shoulder (Fig. 29-3). This maneuver laterally rotates the affected scapula and allows palpation and subsequent injection of the infraspinatus trigger point. Other trigger points along the medial border of the scapula may be present and may be amenable to injection therapy.

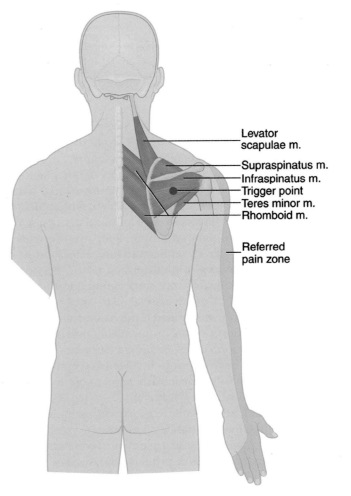

Figure 29–1. Scapulocostal syndrome involves unilateral pain and associated paresthesias at the medial border of the scapula, referred pain radiating from the deltoid region to the dorsum of the hand, and decreased range of motion of the scapula. (From Waldman SD: Atlas of Pain Management Injection Techniques, 2nd ed. Philadelphia, Saunders, 2007.)

Taut bands of muscle fibers are often identified when myofascial trigger points are palpated. In spite of this consistent physical finding, the pathophysiology of the myofascial trigger point remains elusive, although it is believed that trigger points are the result of microtrauma

101

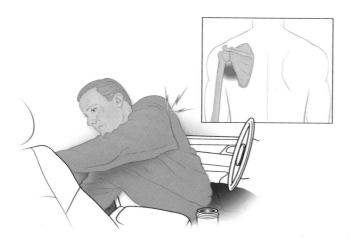

Figure 29-2. Scapulocostal syndrome is also called "traveling salesman's shoulder" because it is frequently seen in individuals who repeatedly reach backward to get something from the backseat of a car.

to the affected muscle. This may occur from a single injury, repetitive microtrauma, or chronic deconditioning of the agonist and antagonist muscle unit.

In addition to muscle trauma, a variety of other factors seem to predispose patients to develop myofascial pain syndrome. For instance, a weekend athlete who subjects his or her body to unaccustomed physical activity may develop myofascial pain syndrome. Poor posture while sitting at a computer or while watching television has also been implicated as a predisposing factor. Previous injuries may result in abnormal muscle function and lead to the development of myofascial pain syndrome. All these factors may be intensified if the patient also suffers from poor nutritional status or coexisting psychological or behavioral abnormalities, including chronic stress and depression. The muscle groups involved in scapulocostal syndrome seem to be particularly susceptible to stress-induced myofascial pain syndrome.

Stiffness and fatigue often coexist with pain, increasing the functional disability associated with this disease and complicating its treatment. Myofascial pain syndrome may occur as a primary disease state or in conjunction with other painful conditions, including radiculopathy and chronic regional pain syndromes. Psychological or behavioral abnormalities, including depression, frequently coexist with the muscle abnormalities, and management of these psychological disorders is an integral part of any successful treatment plan.

SIGNS AND SYMPTOMS

The trigger point is the pathologic lesion of scapulocostal syndrome, and it is characterized by a local point of exquisite tenderness in the infraspinatus muscle. As noted earlier, this infraspinatus trigger point can best be demonstrated by having the patient place the hand of

the affected side over the deltoid of the opposite shoulder. Other trigger points may be present along the medial border of the scapula.

Mechanical stimulation of the trigger point by palpation or stretching produces intense local pain as well as referred pain. The jump sign is characteristic of scapulocostal syndrome, as is pain over the infraspinatus muscle that radiates from the deltoid region to the dorsum of the hand.

TESTING

Biopsies of clinically identified trigger points have not revealed consistently abnormal histology. The muscle hosting the trigger points has been described either as "moth-eaten" or as containing "waxy degeneration." Increased plasma myoglobin has been reported in some patients with scapulocostal syndrome, but this finding has not been corroborated by other investigators. Electrodiagnostic testing of patients suffering from scapulocostal syndrome has revealed an increase in muscle tension in some patients, but again, this finding has not been reproducible. Because of the lack of objective diagnostic testing, the clinician must rule out other coexisting disease processes that may mimic scapulocostal syndrome (see Differential Diagnosis).

DIFFERENTIAL DIAGNOSIS

The diagnosis of scapulocostal syndrome is made on the basis of clinical findings rather than specific laboratory, electrodiagnostic, or radiographic testing. For this reason, a targeted history and physical examination, with a systematic search for trigger points and identification of a positive jump sign, must be carried out in every patient

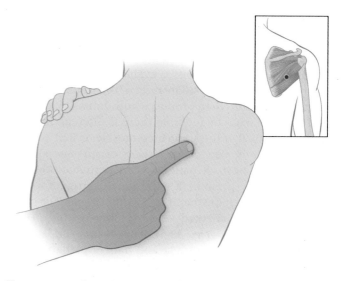

Figure 29-3. The infraspinatus trigger point can be demonstrated by having the patient place the hand of the affected side over the deltoid of the opposite shoulder.

suspected of suffering from scapulocostal syndrome. It is incumbent on the clinician to rule out other coexisting disease processes that may mimic scapulocostal syndrome, including primary inflammatory muscle disease, multiple sclerosis, and collagen vascular disease. Electrodiagnostic and radiographic testing can help identify coexisting pathology such as shoulder bursitis, tendinitis, and rotator cuff tears. The clinician must also identify coexisting psychological and behavioral abnormalities that may mask or exacerbate the symptoms associated with scapulocostal syndrome.

TREATMENT

Treatment is focused on blocking the myofascial trigger and achieving prolonged relaxation of the affected muscle. It is hoped that interrupting the pain cycle in this way will allow the patient to obtain long-term pain relief. Because the mechanism of action of the treatment modalities used is poorly understood, an element of trial and error is involved in developing a treatment plan.

Conservative therapy consisting of trigger point injections with local anesthetic or saline is the initial treatment of scapulocostal syndrome. Adjunct therapies, including physical therapy, therapeutic heat and cold, transcutaneous nerve stimulation, and electrical stimulation, can be used on a case-by-case basis. For patients who do not respond to these traditional measures, consideration should be given to the use of botulinum toxin type A; although not currently approved by the Food and Drug Administration for this indication, the injection of minute quantities of botulinum toxin type A directly into trigger points has been successful. Because underlying depression and anxiety are present in many patients suffering from scapulocostal syndrome, the administration of antidepressants is an integral part of most treatment plans.

COMPLICATIONS AND PITFALLS

Trigger point injections are extremely safe if careful attention is paid to the clinically relevant anatomy. Sterile technique must be used to avoid infection, along with universal precautions to minimize any risk to the operator. Most complications of trigger point injection are related to needle-induced trauma at the injection site and in underlying tissues. The incidence of ecchymosis and hematoma formation can be decreased if pressure is applied to the injection site immediately after injection. The avoidance of overly long needles can decrease the incidence of trauma to underlying structures. Special care must be taken to avoid pneumothorax when injecting trigger points in proximity to the underlying pleural space.

Clinical Pearls

Although scapulocostal syndrome is a common disorder, it is often misdiagnosed. Therefore, in patients suspected of suffering from scapulocostal syndrome, a careful evaluation to identify underlying disease processes is mandatory. Scapulocostal syndrome commonly coexists with a variety of somatic and psychological disorders.

Section 5

Pain Syndromes of the Elbow

Chapter 30

Arthritis Pain of the Elbow

ICD-9 CODE 715.92

THE CLINICAL SYNDROME

Elbow pain secondary to degenerative arthritis is frequently encountered in clinical practice. Osteoarthritis is the most common form of arthritis that results in elbow joint pain. Tendinitis and bursitis may coexist with arthritis pain, making the correct diagnosis more difficult. The olecranon bursa lies in the posterior aspect of the elbow joint and may become inflamed as a result of direct trauma or overuse of the joint. Bursae susceptible to the development of bursitis also exist between the insertion of the biceps and the head of the radius, as well as in the antecubital and cubital areas.

In addition to pain, patients suffering from arthritis of the elbow joint often experience a gradual reduction in functional ability because of decreasing elbow range of motion, making simple everyday tasks such as using a computer keyboard, holding a coffee cup, or turning a doorknob quite difficult (Fig. 30-1). With continued disuse, muscle wasting may occur, and adhesive capsulitis with subsequent ankylosis may develop.

SIGNS AND SYMPTOMS

The majority of patients with elbow pain secondary to osteoarthritis or post-traumatic arthritis complain of pain that is localized around the elbow and forearm. Activity makes the pain worse, whereas rest and heat provide some relief. The pain is constant and is characterized as aching in nature; it may interfere with sleep. Some patients also complain of a grating or popping sensation with use of the joint, and crepitus may be present on physical examination.

TESTING

Plain radiographs should be obtained in all patients who present with elbow pain. Based on the patient's clinical presentation, additional testing may be warranted, including a complete blood count, erythrocyte sedimentation rate, and antinuclear antibody testing. Magnetic

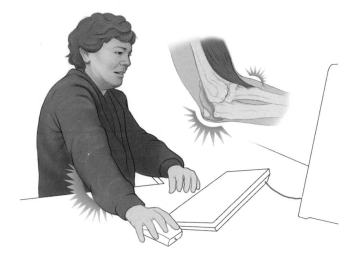

Figure 30–1. Arthritis of the elbow can cause pain and functional disability during common everyday tasks.

resonance imaging of the elbow is indicated if joint instability is suspected (Fig. 30-2).

DIFFERENTIAL DIAGNOSIS

Rheumatoid arthritis, post-traumatic arthritis, and psoriatic arthritis are common causes of elbow pain. Less common causes of arthritis-induced elbow pain include collagen vascular diseases, infection, and Lyme disease. Acute infectious arthritis is usually accompanied by significant systemic symptoms, including fever and malaise, and should be easily recognized; treatment is with culture and antibiotics rather than injection therapy. Collagen vascular diseases generally present as a polyarthropathy rather than a monoarthropathy limited to the elbow joint; however, elbow pain secondary to collagen vascular disease responds exceedingly well to the intra-articular injection technique described later.

TREATMENT

Initial treatment of the pain and functional disability associated with arthritis of the elbow includes a combination of nonsteroidal anti-inflammatory drugs or cyclooxygenase-2 inhibitors and physical therapy. Local

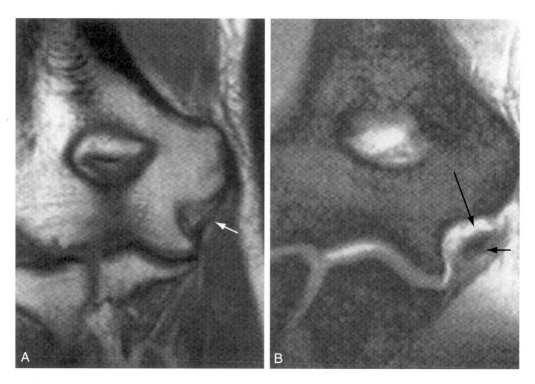

Figure 30–2. Tear of the medial (ulnar) collateral ligament (MCL) of the elbow. **A,** Coronal T1-weighted image of a normal elbow demonstrates an intact MCL as a linear, low-signal structure extending from the medial humeral epicondyle to the proximal ulna *(arrow)*. **B,** Coronal T2-weighted image from a different patient demonstrates disruption of the MCL, with high signal intensity at the expected site of humeral attachment *(long arrow)*. A small focus of low signal is noted at the proximal end of the ligament, which may represent an avulsion fragment *(short arrow)*. The patient was a professional baseball pitcher; these athletes are prone to MCL tears due to the marked valgus stress when throwing a ball. (From Grainger RG, Allison DJ, Adam A, Dixon AK: Grainger & Allison's Diagnostic Radiology: A Textbook of Medical Imaging, 4th ed. Philadelphia, Churchill Livingstone, 2002.)

application of heat and cold may also be beneficial. For patients who do not respond to these treatment modalities, intra-articular injection of local anesthetic and steroid is a reasonable next step.

Intra-articular injection of the elbow is carried out with the patient in the supine position, the arm fully adducted at the patient's side, the elbow flexed, and the dorsum of the hand resting on a folded towel. A total of 5 mL local anesthetic and 40 mg methylprednisolone is drawn up in a 12-mL sterile syringe. After sterile preparation of the skin overlying the posterolateral aspect of the joint, the head of the radius is identified. Just superior to the head of the radius is an indentation that represents the space between the radial head and the humerus. Using strict aseptic technique, a 1-inch, 25-gauge needle is inserted just above the superior aspect of the head of the radius through the skin, subcutaneous tissues, and joint capsule and into the joint (Fig. 30-3). If bone is encountered, the needle is withdrawn into the subcutaneous tissues and redirected superiorly. After entering the joint space, the contents of the syringe are gently injected. There should be little resistance to injection. If

resistance is encountered, the needle is probably in a ligament or tendon and should be advanced slightly into the joint space until the injection can proceed without significant resistance. The needle is then removed, and a sterile pressure dressing and ice pack are applied to the injection site.

Physical modalities, including local heat and gentle range-of-motion exercises, should be introduced several

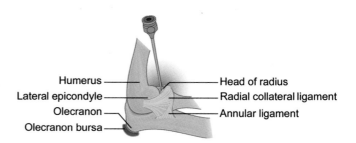

Figure 30–3. Proper needle placement for intra-articular injection of the elbow. (From Waldman SD: Atlas of Pain Management Injection Techniques. Philadelphia, Saunders, 2000.)

days after the patient undergoes injection for elbow pain. Vigorous exercises should be avoided, because they will exacerbate the patient's symptoms.

COMPLICATIONS AND PITFALLS

This injection technique is safe if careful attention is paid to the clinically relevant anatomy. Sterile technique must be used to avoid infection, along with universal precautions to minimize any risk to the operator. The major complication of intra-articular injection of the elbow is infection, although it should be exceedingly rare if strict aseptic technique is followed. The ulnar nerve is especially susceptible to damage at the elbow, and care must be taken to avoid this structure when performing intra-articular injection. Approximately 25% of patients complain of a transient increase in pain after intra-articular injection of the elbow joint, and they should be warned of this possibility.

Clinical Pearls

Pain and functional disability of the elbow are often the result of degenerative arthritis of the joint. Coexistent bursitis and tendinitis may contribute to elbow pain, confusing the diagnosis. Simple analgesics and nonsteroidal anti-inflammatory drugs or cyclooxygenase-2 inhibitors can be used concurrently with the intra-articular injection technique.

Chapter 31

Tennis Elbow

ICD-9 CODE **726.32**

THE CLINICAL SYNDROME

Tennis elbow (also known as lateral epicondylitis) is caused by repetitive microtrauma to the extensor tendons of the forearm. The pathophysiology of tennis elbow is initially caused by microtearing at the origin of the extensor carpi radialis and extensor carpi ulnaris. Secondary inflammation may become chronic as a result of continued overuse or misuse of the extensors of the forearm. Coexistent bursitis, arthritis, or gout may perpetuate the pain and disability of tennis elbow.

The most common nidus of pain from tennis elbow is the bony origin of the extensor tendon of the extensor carpi radialis brevis at the anterior facet of the lateral epicondyle. Less commonly, tennis elbow pain originates from the origin of the extensor carpi radialis longus at the supracondylar crest; rarely, it originates more distally, at the point where the extensor carpi radialis brevis overlies the radial head. The olecranon bursa lies in the posterior aspect of the elbow joint and may also become inflamed (bursitis) as a result of direct trauma to the joint or its overuse. Other bursae susceptible to the development of bursitis lie between the insertion of the biceps and the head of the radius, as well as in the antecubital and cubital areas.

Tennis elbow occurs in individuals engaged in repetitive activities such as hand grasping (e.g., shaking hands) or high-torque wrist turning (e.g., scooping ice cream) (Fig. 31-1). Tennis players develop tennis elbow via two different mechanisms: (1) increased pressure grip strain as a result of playing with too heavy a racket, and (2) making backhand shots with a leading shoulder and elbow rather than keeping the shoulder and elbow parallel to the net (Fig. 31-2). Other racket sports players are also susceptible to the development of tennis elbow.

SIGNS AND SYMPTOMS

The pain of tennis elbow is localized to the region of the lateral epicondyle. It is constant and is made worse with

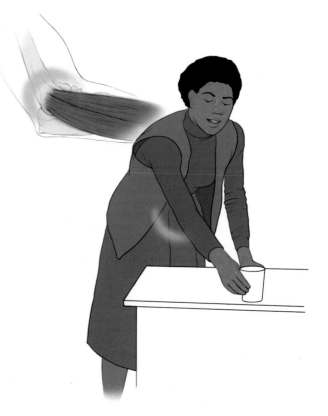

Figure 31–1. The pain of tennis elbow is localized to the lateral epicondyle.

active contraction of the wrist. Patients note the inability to hold a coffee cup or use a hammer. Sleep disturbance is common. On physical examination, there is tenderness along the extensor tendons at or just below the lateral epicondyle. Many patients with tennis elbow exhibit a bandlike thickening within the affected extensor tendons. Elbow range of motion is normal, but grip strength on the affected side is diminished. Patients with tennis elbow demonstrate a positive tennis elbow test, which is performed by stabilizing the patient's forearm and then having the patient clench his or her fist and actively extend the wrist. The examiner then attempts to force the wrist into flexion (Fig. 31-3). Sudden severe pain is highly suggestive of tennis elbow.

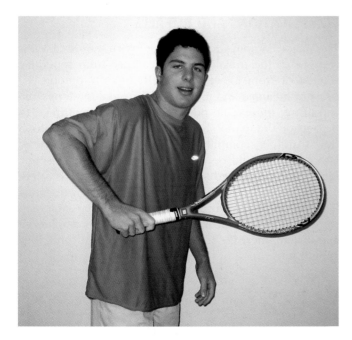

Figure 31–2. Mechanism of elbow injury in tennis players. (From Waldman SD: Physical Diagnosis of Pain: An Atlas of Signs and Symptoms. Philadelphia, Saunders, 2006, p 137.)

TESTING

Electromyography can help distinguish cervical radiculopathy and radial tunnel syndrome from tennis elbow. Plain radiographs should be obtained in all patients who present with elbow pain to rule out joint mice and other occult bony pathology. Based on the patient's clinical presentation, additional testing may be warranted, including a complete blood count, uric acid level, erythrocyte sedimentation rate, and antinuclear antibody testing. Magnetic resonance imaging of the elbow is indicated if joint instability is suspected. The injection technique described later serves as both a diagnostic and a therapeutic maneuver.

DIFFERENTIAL DIAGNOSIS

Radial tunnel syndrome and, occasionally, C6-7 radiculopathy can mimic tennis elbow. Radial tunnel syndrome is caused by entrapment of the radial nerve below the elbow. With radial tunnel syndrome, the maximal tenderness to palpation is distal to the lateral epicondyle over the radial nerve, whereas with tennis elbow, the maximal tenderness to palpation is over the lateral epicondyle.

TREATMENT

Initial treatment of the pain and functional disability associated with tennis elbow includes a combination of nonsteroidal anti-inflammatory drugs or cyclooxygenase-2 inhibitors and physical therapy. Local application of heat and cold may also be beneficial. Any repetitive activity that may exacerbate the patient's symptoms should be avoided. For patients who do not respond to these treatment modalities, injection of local anesthetic and steroid is a reasonable next step.

Injection for tennis elbow is performed by placing the patient in the supine position with the arm fully adducted at the patient's side, the elbow flexed, and the dorsum of the hand resting on a folded towel to relax the affected tendons. A total of 1 mL local anesthetic and 40 mg methylprednisolone is drawn up in a 5-mL sterile syringe. After sterile preparation of the skin overlying the posterolateral aspect of the joint, the lateral epicondyle is identified. Using strict aseptic technique, a 1-inch, 25-gauge needle is inserted perpendicular to the lateral epicondyle through the skin and into the subcutaneous tissue overlying the affected tendon (Fig. 31-4). If bone is encountered, the needle is withdrawn into the subcutaneous tissue. The contents of the syringe are then gently injected. There should be little resistance to injection. If resistance is encountered, the needle is probably in the tendon and should be withdrawn until the injection can proceed without significant resistance. The needle is then removed, and a sterile pressure dressing and ice pack are applied to the injection site.

Physical modalities, including local heat and gentle range-of-motion exercises, should be introduced several days after the patient undergoes injection for tennis elbow. A Velcro band placed around the extensor tendons may also help relieve the symptoms. Vigorous exercises should be avoided, because they will exacerbate the patient's symptoms.

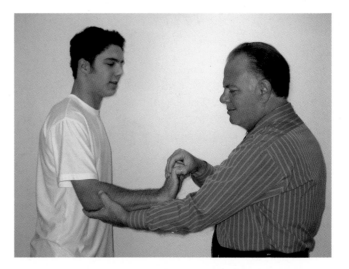

Figure 31–3. Test for tennis elbow. (From Waldman SD: Physical Diagnosis of Pain: An Atlas of Signs and Symptoms. Philadelphia, Saunders, 2006, p 138.)

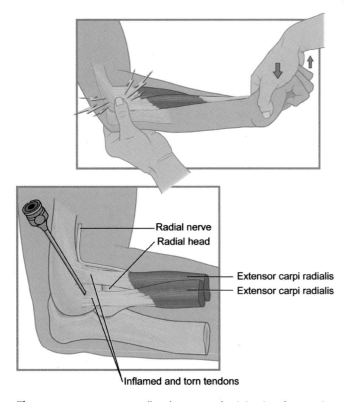

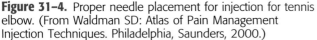

Figure 31–4. Proper needle placement for injection for tennis elbow. (From Waldman SD: Atlas of Pain Management Injection Techniques. Philadelphia, Saunders, 2000.)

COMPLICATIONS AND PITFALLS

The major complication associated with tennis elbow is rupture of the inflamed tendon either from repetitive trauma or from injection directly into the tendon. To prevent inflamed and previously damaged tendons from rupturing, the needle position should be confirmed to be outside the tendon before proceeding with the injection. Another complication of injection is infection, although it should be exceedingly rare if strict aseptic technique is followed. The injection technique is safe if careful attention is paid to the clinically relevant anatomy; in particular, the ulnar nerve is susceptible to damage at the elbow. Approximately 25% of patients complain of a transient increase in pain after injection, and they should be warned of this possibility.

Clinical Pearls

The injection technique described is extremely effective in the treatment of pain secondary to tennis elbow. Coexistent bursitis and tendinitis may contribute to elbow pain, necessitating additional treatment with more localized injection of local anesthetic and methylprednisolone. Simple analgesics and nonsteroidal anti-inflammatory drugs can be used concurrently with the injection technique. Cervical radiculopathy and radial tunnel syndrome may mimic tennis elbow and must be ruled out.

Chapter 32

Golfer's Elbow

ICD-9 CODE 726.31

THE CLINICAL SYNDROME

Golfer's elbow (also known as medial epicondylitis) is caused by repetitive microtrauma to the flexor tendons of the forearm in a manner analogous to tennis elbow. The pathophysiology of golfer's elbow is initially caused by microtearing at the origin of the pronator teres, flexor carpi radialis, flexor carpi ulnaris, and palmaris longus (Fig. 32-1). Secondary inflammation may become chronic as a result of continued overuse or misuse of the flexors of the forearm. The most common nidus of pain from golfer's elbow is the bony origin of the flexor tendon of the flexor carpi radialis and the humeral heads of the flexor carpi ulnaris and pronator teres at the medial epicondyle of the humerus. Less commonly, golfer's elbow pain originates from the ulnar head of the flexor carpi ulnaris at the medial aspect of the olecranon process. Coexistent bursitis, arthritis, or gout may perpetuate the pain and disability of golfer's elbow.

Golfer's elbow occurs in individuals engaged in repetitive flexion activities, such as throwing baseballs or footballs, carrying heavy suitcases, and driving golf balls. These activities have in common repetitive flexion of the wrist and strain on the flexor tendons due to excessive weight or sudden arrested motion. Interestingly, many of the activities that cause tennis elbow can also cause golfer's elbow.

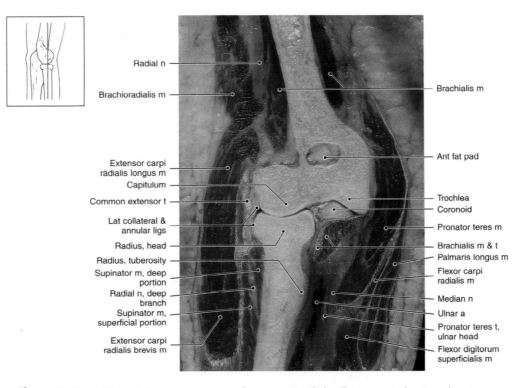

Labels (left): Radial n — Brachioradialis m — Extensor carpi radialis longus m — Capitulum — Common extensor t — Lat collateral & annular ligs — Radius, head — Radius, tuberosity — Supinator m, deep portion — Radial n, deep branch — Supinator m, superficial portion — Extensor carpi radialis brevis m

Labels (right): Brachialis m — Ant fat pad — Trochlea — Coronoid — Pronator teres m — Brachialis m & t — Palmaris longus m — Flexor carpi radialis m — Median n — Ulnar a — Pronator teres t, ulnar head — Flexor digitorum superficialis m

Figure 32–1. Origins of the pronator teres, flexor carpi radialis, flexor carpi ulnaris, palmaris longus, and medial epicondyle. (From Kang HS, Ahn JM, Resnick D: MRI of the Extremities: An Anatomic Atlas, 2nd ed. Philadelphia, Saunders, 2002, p 89.)

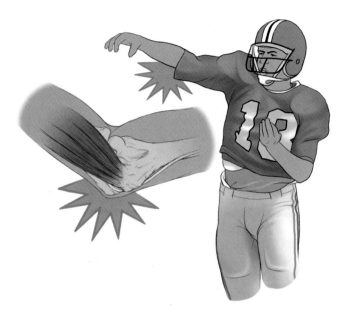

Figure 32–2. The pain of golfer's elbow occurs at the medial epicondyle.

SIGNS AND SYMPTOMS

The pain of golfer's elbow is localized to the region of the medial epicondyle (Fig. 32-2). It is constant and is made worse with active contraction of the wrist. Patients note the inability to hold a coffee cup or use a hammer. Sleep disturbance is common. On physical examination, there is tenderness along the flexor tendons at or just below the medial epicondyle. Many patients with golfer's elbow exhibit a bandlike thickening within the affected flexor tendons. Elbow range of motion is normal, but grip strength on the affected side is diminished. Patients with golfer's elbow demonstrate a positive golfer's elbow test, which is performed by stabilizing the patient's forearm and then having the patient actively flex the wrist. The examiner then attempts to force the wrist into extension (Fig. 32-3). Sudden severe pain is highly suggestive of golfer's elbow.

TESTING

Plain radiographs should be obtained in all patients who present with elbow pain to rule out joint mice and other occult bony pathology. Based on the patient's clinical presentation, additional testing may be warranted, including a complete blood count, uric acid level, erythrocyte sedimentation rate, and antinuclear antibody testing. Magnetic resonance imaging of the elbow is indicated if joint instability is suspected. Electromyography is indicated to diagnosis entrapment neuropathy at the elbow and to distinguish golfer's elbow from cervical radiculopathy. The injection technique described later serves as both a diagnostic and a therapeutic maneuver.

DIFFERENTIAL DIAGNOSIS

Occasionally, C6-7 radiculopathy mimics golfer's elbow; however, patients suffering from cervical radiculopathy usually have neck pain and proximal upper extremity pain in addition to symptoms below the elbow. As noted earlier, electromyography can distinguish radiculopathy from golfer's elbow. Bursitis, arthritis, and gout may also mimic golfer's elbow, confusing the diagnosis. The olecranon bursa lies in the posterior aspect of the elbow joint and may become inflamed as a result of direct trauma to the joint or its overuse. Other bursae susceptible to the development of bursitis are located between the insertion of the biceps and the head of the radius, as well as in the antecubital and cubital areas.

TREATMENT

Initial treatment of the pain and functional disability associated with golfer's elbow includes a combination of nonsteroidal anti-inflammatory drugs or cyclooxygenase-2 inhibitors and physical therapy. Local application of heat and cold may also be beneficial. Any repetitive activity that may exacerbate the patient's symptoms should be avoided. For patients who do not respond to these treatment modalities, injection with local anesthetic and steroid is a reasonable next step.

Injection for golfer's elbow is carried out by placing the patient in the supine position with the arm fully adducted at the patient's side, the elbow fully extended, and the dorsum of the hand resting on a folded towel to relax the affected tendons. A total of 1 mL local anesthetic and 40 mg methylprednisolone is drawn up in a 5-mL sterile syringe. After sterile preparation of the skin overlying the medial aspect of the joint, the medial

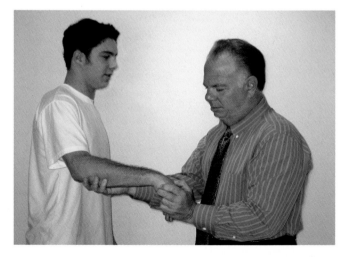

Figure 32–3. Test for golfer's elbow. (From Waldman SD: Physical Diagnosis of Pain: An Atlas of Signs and Symptoms. Philadelphia, Saunders, 2006, p 140.)

epicondyle is identified. Using strict aseptic technique, a 1-inch, 25-gauge needle is inserted perpendicular to the medial epicondyle through the skin and into the subcutaneous tissue overlying the affected tendon. If bone is encountered, the needle is withdrawn into the subcutaneous tissue. The contents of the syringe are then gently injected. There should be little resistance to injection. If significant resistance is encountered, the needle is probably in the tendon and should be withdrawn until the injection can proceed with less resistance. The needle is then removed, and a sterile pressure dressing and ice pack are applied to the injection site.

Physical modalities, including local heat and gentle range-of-motion exercises, should be introduced several days after the patient undergoes injection for elbow pain. A Velcro band placed around the flexor tendons may also help relieve the symptoms. Vigorous exercises should be avoided, because they will exacerbate the patient's symptoms.

COMPLICATIONS AND PITFALLS

The major complications associated with this injection technique are related to trauma to the inflamed and previously damaged tendon, which may rupture if injected directly. Therefore, the needle position should be confirmed to be outside the tendon before proceeding with the injection. Another complication of the injection technique is infection, although it should be exceedingly rare if strict aseptic technique is followed. Injection is safe if careful attention is paid to the clinically relevant anatomy; in particular, the ulnar nerve is susceptible to damage at the elbow. Approximately 25% of patients complain of a transient increase in pain after intra-articular injection of the elbow joint, and they should be warned of this possibility.

Clinical Pearls

The injection technique described is extremely effective in the treatment of pain secondary to golfer's elbow. Coexistent bursitis and tendinitis may contribute to elbow pain, necessitating additional treatment with more localized injection of local anesthetic and methylprednisolone. Simple analgesics and nonsteroidal anti-inflammatory drugs can be used concurrently with this injection technique. Cervical radiculopathy may mimic golfer's elbow and must be ruled out.

Chapter 33

Anconeus Syndrome

ICD-9 CODE **729.1**

THE CLINICAL SYNDROME

The anconeus muscle is susceptible to the development of myofascial pain syndrome. Such pain is most often the result of repetitive microtrauma to the muscle caused by such activities as prolonged ironing, handshaking, or digging (Fig. 33-1). Tennis injuries caused by an improper one-handed backhand technique have also been implicated as an inciting factor in myofascial pain syndrome, as has blunt trauma to the muscle.

Myofascial pain syndrome is a chronic pain syndrome that affects a focal or regional portion of the body. The sine qua non of myofascial pain syndrome is the finding of myofascial trigger points on physical examination. Although these trigger points are generally localized to the part of the body affected, the pain is often referred to other areas. This referred pain may be misdiagnosed or attributed to other organ systems, leading to extensive evaluation and ineffective treatment. Patients with myofascial pain syndrome involving the anconeus often have referred pain in the ipsilateral forearm.

The trigger point is pathognomonic of myofascial pain syndrome and is characterized by a local point of exquisite tenderness in the affected muscle. Mechanical stimulation of the trigger point by palpation or stretching produces not only intense local pain but referred pain as well. In addition, there is often an involuntary withdrawal of the stimulated muscle, called a "jump sign," which is also characteristic of myofascial pain syndrome. Patients with anconeus syndrome have a trigger point over the superior insertion of the muscle (Fig. 33-2).

Taunt bands of muscle fibers are often identified when myofascial trigger points are palpated. In spite of this consistent physical finding, the pathophysiology of the myofascial trigger point remains elusive, although it is believed that trigger points are the result of microtrauma to the affected muscle. This may result from a single injury, repetitive microtrauma, or chronic

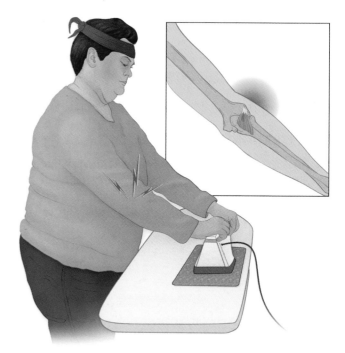

Figure 33–1. Myofascial pain syndrome affecting the anconeus muscle usually occurs as a result of repetitive microtrauma from activities such as prolonged ironing.

deconditioning of the agonist and antagonist muscle unit.

In addition to muscle trauma, a variety of other factors seems to predispose patients to develop myofascial pain syndrome. For instance, a weekend athlete who subjects his or her body to unaccustomed physical activity may develop myofascial pain syndrome. Poor posture while sitting at a computer or while watching television has also been implicated as a predisposing factor. Previous injuries may result in abnormal muscle function and lead to the development of myofascial pain syndrome. All these predisposing factors may be intensified if the patient also suffers from poor nutritional status or coexisting psychological or behavioral abnormalities, including chronic stress and depression. The anconeus muscle

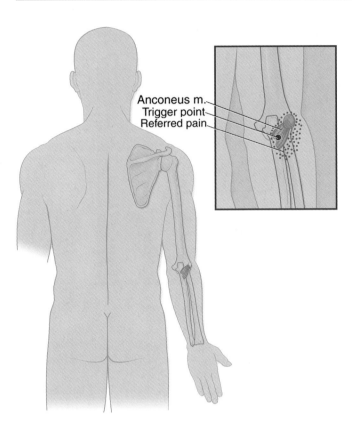

Figure 33-2. Patients with anconeus syndrome have a trigger point over the superior insertion of the muscle. (From Waldman SD: Atlas of Pain Management Injection Techniques, 2nd ed. Philadelphia, Saunders, 2007, p 134.)

seems to be particularly susceptible to stress-induced myofascial pain syndrome.

Stiffness and fatigue often coexist with pain, increasing the functional disability associated with this disease and complicating its treatment. Myofascial pain syndrome may occur as a primary disease state or in conjunction with other painful conditions, including radiculopathy and chronic regional pain syndromes. Psychological or behavioral abnormalities, including depression, frequently coexist with the muscle abnormalities, and management of these psychological disorders is an integral part of any successful treatment plan.

SIGNS AND SYMPTOMS

The trigger point is the pathologic lesion of anconeus syndrome, and it is characterized by a local point of exquisite tenderness over the superior insertion of the muscle (see Fig. 33-2). Mechanical stimulation of the trigger point by palpation or stretching produces both intense local pain and referred pain. The jump sign is also characteristic of anconeus syndrome, as is pain over the anconeus muscle that is referred to the ipsilateral forearm.

TESTING

Biopsies of clinically identified trigger points have not revealed consistently abnormal histology. The muscle hosting the trigger points has been described either as "moth eaten" or as containing "waxy degeneration." Increased plasma myoglobin has been reported in some patients with anconeus syndrome, but this finding has not been corroborated by other investigators. Electrodiagnostic testing of patients suffering from anconeus syndrome has revealed an increase in muscle tension in some patients, but again, this finding has not been reproducible. Because of the lack of objective diagnostic testing, the clinician must rule out other coexisting disease processes that may mimic anconeus syndrome (see Differential Diagnosis).

DIFFERENTIAL DIAGNOSIS

The diagnosis of anconeus syndrome is made on the basis of clinical findings rather than specific laboratory, electrodiagnostic, or radiographic testing. For this reason, a targeted history and physical examination, with a systematic search for trigger points and identification of a positive jump sign, must be carried out in every patient suspected of suffering from anconeus syndrome. It is incumbent on the clinician to rule out other coexisting disease processes that may mimic anconeus syndrome, including primary inflammatory muscle disease, multiple sclerosis, and collagen vascular disease. Electrodiagnostic and radiographic testing can help identify coexisting pathology such as bursitis, tendinitis, and epicondylitis (Fig. 33-3). The clinician must also identify coexisting psychological and behavioral abnormalities that may mask or exacerbate the symptoms associated with anconeus syndrome.

TREATMENT

Treatment is focused on eliminating the myofascial trigger. It is hoped that interrupting the pain cycle in this way will allow the patient to obtain prolonged pain relief. Because the mechanism of action of the treatment modalities used is poorly understood, an element of trial and error is involved in developing a treatment plan.

Conservative therapy consisting of trigger point injections with local anesthetic or saline is the initial treatment of anconeus syndrome. Adjunct therapies, including physical therapy, therapeutic heat and cold, transcutaneous nerve stimulation, and electrical stimulation, can be used on a case-by-case basis. For patients who do not respond to these traditional measures, consideration should be given to the use of botulinum toxin type A; although not currently approved by the Food and Drug Administration for this indication, the injection of minute quantities of botulinum toxin type A directly into trigger

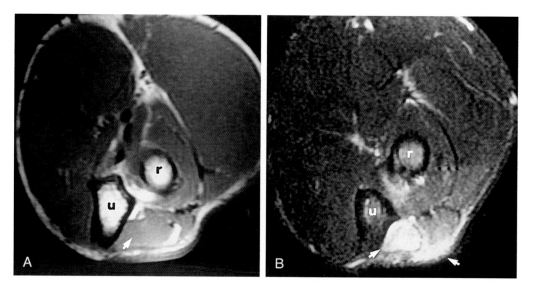

Figure 33–3. Anconeus muscle tear with edema in a 30-year-old male bodybuilder who experienced acute pain during weightlifting. Transaxial T1-weighted **(A)** and T2-weighted **(B)** spin echo magnetic resonance images, the latter obtained with fat suppression, show altered morphology. In **B,** increased signal intensity is evident in the anconeus muscle and surrounding tissues *(arrows).* Inflammatory changes about the biceps tendon are also seen. The radius (r) and ulna (u) are indicated. (From Resnick D: Diagnosis of Bone and Joint Disorders, 4th ed. Philadelphia, Saunders, 2002, p 3065.)

points has been successful. Because underlying depression and anxiety are present in many patients suffering from anconeus syndrome, the administration of antidepressants is an integral part of most treatment plans.

COMPLICATIONS AND PITFALLS

Trigger point injections are extremely safe if careful attention is paid to the clinically relevant anatomy. Sterile technique must be used to avoid infection, along with universal precautions to minimize any risk to the operator. Most complications of trigger point injection are related to needle-induced trauma at the injection site and in underlying tissues. The incidence of ecchymosis and hematoma formation can be decreased if pressure is

applied to the injection site immediately after injection. The avoidance of overly long needles can decrease the incidence of trauma to underlying structures.

Clinical Pearls

Although anconeus syndrome is a common disorder, it is often misdiagnosed. Therefore, in patients suspected of suffering from anconeus syndrome, a careful evaluation to identify underlying disease processes is mandatory. Anconeus syndrome commonly coexists with a variety of somatic and psychological disorders.

Chapter 34

Supinator Syndrome

ICD-9 CODE 729.1

THE CLINICAL SYNDROME

As its name implies, the supinator muscle supinates the forearm. Curving around the upper third of the radius, the supinator muscle is composed of a superficial and a deep layer. The superficial layer originates in a tendinous insertion from the lateral epicondyle of the humerus, the radial collateral ligament of the elbow, and the annular ligament of the supinator crest of the ulna.

The supinator muscle is susceptible to the development of myofascial pain syndrome. Such pain is most often the result of repetitive microtrauma to the muscle caused by such activities as turning a screwdriver, prolonged ironing, handshaking, or digging with a trowel (Fig. 34-1). Tennis injuries caused by an improper one-handed backhand technique have also been implicated as an inciting factor in myofascial pain syndrome, as has blunt trauma to the muscle.

Myofascial pain syndrome is a chronic pain syndrome that affects a focal or regional portion of the body. The sine qua non of myofascial pain syndrome is the finding of myofascial trigger points on physical examination. Although these trigger points are generally localized to the part of the body affected, the pain is often referred to other areas. This referred pain may be misdiagnosed or attributed to other organ systems, leading to extensive evaluation and ineffective treatment. Patients with myofascial pain syndrome involving the supinator muscle often have referred pain in the ipsilateral forearm.

The trigger point is pathognomonic of myofascial pain syndrome and is characterized by a local point of exquisite tenderness in the affected muscle. Mechanical stimulation of the trigger point by palpation or stretching produces not only intense local pain but referred pain as well. In addition, there is often an involuntary withdrawal of the stimulated muscle, called a "jump sign," which is also characteristic of myofascial pain syndrome. Patients with supinator syndrome have a trigger point over the superior portion of the muscle (Fig. 34-2).

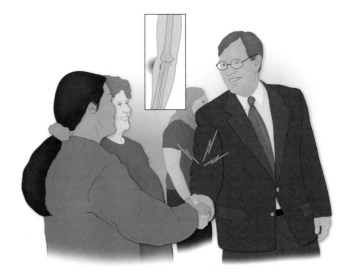

Figure 34-1. Myofascial pain syndrome affecting the supinator muscle is usually the result of repetitive microtrauma caused by activities such as turning a screwdriver, prolonged ironing, handshaking, or digging.

Taunt bands of muscle fibers are often identified when myofascial trigger points are palpated. In spite of this consistent physical finding, the pathophysiology of the myofascial trigger point remains elusive, although it is believed that trigger points are the result of microtrauma to the affected muscle. This may result from a single injury, repetitive microtrauma, or chronic deconditioning of the agonist and antagonist muscle unit.

In addition to muscle trauma, a variety of other factors seems to predispose patients to develop myofascial pain syndrome. For instance, a weekend athlete who subjects his or her body to unaccustomed physical activity may develop myofascial pain syndrome. Poor posture while sitting at a computer or while watching television has also been implicated as a predisposing factor. Previous injuries may result in abnormal muscle function and lead to the development of myofascial pain syndrome. All these predisposing factors may be intensified if the patient also suffers from poor nutritional status or coexisting psychological or behavioral abnormalities, including chronic stress and depression. The supinator muscle

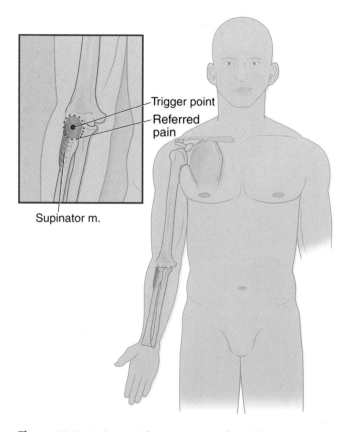

Supinator m.

Figure 34–2. Patients with supinator syndrome have a trigger point over the superior portion of the muscle. (From Waldman SD: Atlas of Pain Management Injection Techniques, 2nd ed. Philadelphia, Saunders, 2007, p 155.)

seems to be particularly susceptible to stress-induced myofascial pain syndrome.

Stiffness and fatigue often coexist with pain, increasing the functional disability associated with this disease and complicating its treatment. Myofascial pain syndrome may occur as a primary disease state or in conjunction with other painful conditions, including radiculopathy and chronic regional pain syndromes. Psychological or behavioral abnormalities, including depression, frequently coexist with the muscle abnormalities, and management of these psychological disorders is an integral part of any successful treatment plan.

SIGNS AND SYMPTOMS

The trigger point is the pathologic lesion of supinator syndrome, and it is characterized by a local point of exquisite tenderness in the supinator muscle. This trigger point can best be demonstrated by having the patient supinate the forearm against active resistance. Point tenderness over the lateral epicondyle may also be present and may be amenable to injection therapy.

Mechanical stimulation of the trigger point by palpation or stretching produces both intense local pain and

referred pain. The jump sign is also characteristic of supinator syndrome, as is pain over the supinator muscle that radiates from the lateral epicondyle and superior portion of the muscle into the forearm.

TESTING

Biopsies of clinically identified trigger points have not revealed consistently abnormal histology. The muscle hosting the trigger points has been described either as "moth eaten" or as containing "waxy degeneration." Increased plasma myoglobin has been reported in some patients with supinator syndrome, but this finding has not been corroborated by other investigators. Electrodiagnostic testing of patients suffering from supinator syndrome has revealed an increase in muscle tension in some patients, but again, this finding has not been reproducible. Because of the lack of objective diagnostic testing, the clinician must rule out other coexisting disease processes that may mimic supinator syndrome (see Differential Diagnosis).

DIFFERENTIAL DIAGNOSIS

The diagnosis of supinator syndrome is made on the basis of clinical findings rather than specific laboratory, electrodiagnostic, or radiographic testing. For this reason, a targeted history and physical examination, with a systematic search for trigger points and identification of a positive jump sign, must be carried out in every patient suspected of suffering from supinator syndrome. It is incumbent on the clinician to rule out other coexisting disease processes that may mimic supinator syndrome, including primary inflammatory muscle disease, collagen vascular disease, inflammatory arthritis, tennis elbow, radial tunnel syndrome, tumor, bursitis, tendinitis, and crystal deposition diseases (Fig. 34-3). Radiographic testing, including magnetic resonance imaging of the elbow, can help identify coexisting pathology such as internal derangement of the elbow, tendinitis, and bursitis. Electromyography can rule out cubital and radial tunnel syndromes. The clinician must also identify coexisting psychological and behavioral abnormalities that may mask or exacerbate the symptoms associated with supinator syndrome.

TREATMENT

Treatment is focused on eliminating the myofascial trigger. It is hoped that interrupting the pain cycle in this way will allow the patient to obtain prolonged pain relief. Because the mechanism of action of the treatment modalities used is poorly understood, an element of trial and error is involved in developing a treatment plan.

Conservative therapy consisting of trigger point injections with local anesthetic or saline is the initial treat-

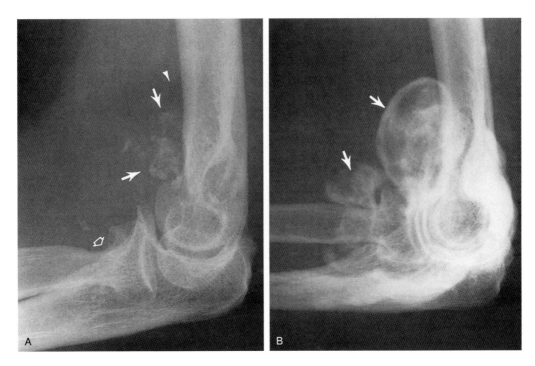

Figure 34–3. Idiopathic synovial osteochondromatosis. This 67-year-old woman reported progressive pain and swelling in her elbow over a 6-month period. **A,** The radiograph outlines irregular ossification in the joint *(solid arrows)*, with displacement of the anterior fat pad *(arrowhead)*, minor osseous erosion *(open arrow)*, and osteophytes. **B,** An arthrogram identifies multiple radiolucent filling defects *(arrows)*. The diagnosis was confirmed histologically. (From Resnick D: Diagnosis of Bone and Joint Disorders, 4th ed. Philadelphia, Saunders, 2002, p 3067.)

ment of supinator syndrome. Adjunct therapies, including physical therapy, therapeutic heat and cold, transcutaneous nerve stimulation, and electrical stimulation, can be used on a case-by-case basis. For patients who do not respond to these traditional measures, consideration should be given to the use of botulinum toxin type A; although not currently approved by the Food and Drug Administration for this indication, the injection of minute quantities of botulinum toxin type A directly into trigger points has been successful. Because underlying depression and anxiety are present in many patients suffering from supinator syndrome, the administration of antidepressants is an integral part of most treatment plans.

COMPLICATIONS AND PITFALLS

Trigger point injections are extremely safe if careful attention is paid to the clinically relevant anatomy. Sterile technique must be used to avoid infection, along with universal precautions to minimize any risk to the operator. Most complications of trigger point injection are related to needle-induced trauma at the injection site and in underlying tissues. The incidence of ecchymosis and hematoma formation can be decreased if pressure is applied to the injection site immediately after injection. The avoidance of overly long needles can decrease the incidence of trauma to underlying structures. Special care must be taken to avoid damage to the underlying neural structures when injecting trigger points in proximity to the elbow and forearm.

Clinical Pearls

Although supinator syndrome is a common disorder, it is often misdiagnosed. Therefore, in patients suspected of suffering from supinator syndrome, a careful evaluation to identify underlying disease processes is mandatory. Supinator syndrome commonly coexists with a variety of somatic and psychological disorders.

Chapter 35

Brachioradialis Syndrome

THE CLINICAL SYNDROME

The brachioradialis muscle flexes the forearm at the elbow, pronates the forearm when supinated, and supinates the forearm when pronated. It originates at the upper lateral supracondylar ridge of the humerus and the lateral intermuscular septum of the humerus. The muscle inserts on the superior aspect of the styloid process of the radius, the lateral side of the distal radius, and the antebrachial fascia. The muscle is innervated by the radial nerve.

The brachioradialis muscle is susceptible to the development of myofascial pain syndrome. Such pain is most often the result of repetitive microtrauma to the muscle from such activities as turning a screwdriver, prolonged ironing, repeated flexing of the forearm at the elbow (e.g., when using exercise equipment), handshaking, or digging with a trowel. Tennis injuries caused by an improper one-handed backhand technique have also been implicated as an inciting factor in myofascial pain syndrome, as has blunt trauma to the muscle (Fig. 35-1).

Myofascial pain syndrome is a chronic pain syndrome that affects a focal or regional portion of the body. The sine qua non of myofascial pain syndrome is the finding of myofascial trigger points on physical examination. Although these trigger points are generally localized to the part of the body affected, the pain is often referred to other areas. This referred pain may be misdiagnosed or attributed to other organ systems, leading to extensive evaluation and ineffective treatment. Patients with myofascial pain syndrome involving the brachioradialis muscle often have referred pain in the ipsilateral forearm and, on occasion, above the elbow.

The trigger point is the pathognomonic lesion of myofascial pain syndrome and is characterized by a local point of exquisite tenderness in the affected muscle. Mechanical stimulation of the trigger point by palpation or stretching produces not only intense local pain but referred pain as well. In addition, there is often an involuntary withdrawal of the stimulated muscle, called a

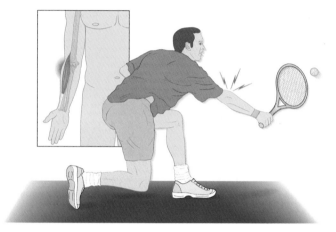

Figure 35–1. Tennis injuries caused by an improper one-handed backhand technique have been implicated in brachioradialis syndrome.

"jump sign," which is also characteristic of myofascial pain syndrome. Patients with brachioradialis syndrome have a trigger point over the superior belly of the muscle (Fig. 35-2).

Taut bands of muscle fibers are often identified when myofascial trigger points are palpated. In spite of this consistent physical finding, the pathophysiology of the myofascial trigger point remains elusive, although it is believed that trigger points are the result of microtrauma to the affected muscle. This may occur from a single injury, repetitive microtrauma, or chronic deconditioning of the agonist and antagonist muscle unit.

In addition to muscle trauma, a variety of other factors seems to predispose patients to develop myofascial pain syndrome. For instance, a weekend athlete who subjects his or her body to unaccustomed physical activity may develop myofascial pain syndrome. Poor posture while sitting at a computer or while watching television has also been implicated as a predisposing factor. Previous injuries may result in abnormal muscle function and lead to the development of myofascial pain syndrome. All these predisposing factors may be intensified if the patient also suffers from poor nutritional status or coexisting psychological or behavioral abnormalities, including chronic stress and depression. The brachioradialis

122

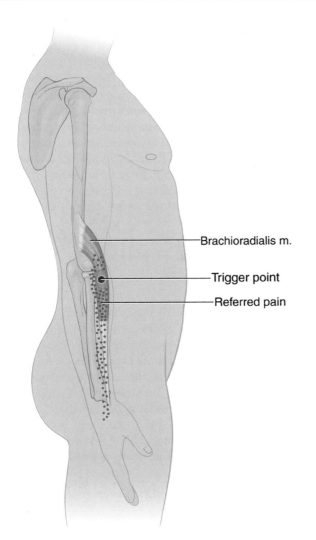

Figure 35-2. Patients with brachioradialis syndrome have a trigger point over the superior belly of the muscle. (From Waldman SD: Atlas of Pain Management Injection Techniques, 2nd ed. Philadelphia, Saunders, 2007.)

muscle seems to be particularly susceptible to stress-induced myofascial pain syndrome.

Stiffness and fatigue often coexist with pain, increasing the functional disability associated with this disease and complicating its treatment. Myofascial pain syndrome may occur as a primary disease state or in conjunction with other painful conditions, including radiculopathy and chronic regional pain syndromes. Psychological or behavioral abnormalities, including depression, frequently coexist with the muscle abnormalities, and management of these psychological disorders is an integral part of any successful treatment plan.

SIGNS AND SYMPTOMS

The trigger point is the pathologic lesion of brachioradialis syndrome, and it is characterized by a local point of exquisite tenderness in the brachioradialis muscle. This trigger point can best be demonstrated by having the patient simultaneously flex and pronate the forearm against active resistance. Point tenderness over the lateral supracondylar ridge of the humerus may also be present and may be amenable to injection therapy.

Mechanical stimulation of the trigger point by palpation or stretching produces both intense local pain and referred pain. The jump sign is also characteristic of brachioradialis syndrome, as is pain over the brachioradialis muscle that radiates from the lateral epicondyle and superior portion of the muscle into the forearm.

TESTING

Biopsies of clinically identified trigger points have not revealed consistently abnormal histology. The muscle hosting the trigger points has been described either as "moth-eaten" or as containing "waxy degeneration." Increased plasma myoglobin has been reported in some patients with brachioradialis syndrome, but this finding has not been corroborated by other investigators. Electrodiagnostic testing of patients suffering from brachioradialis syndrome has revealed an increase in muscle tension in some patients, but again, this finding has not been reproducible. Because of the lack of objective diagnostic testing, the clinician must rule out other coexisting disease processes that may mimic brachioradialis syndrome (see Differential Diagnosis).

DIFFERENTIAL DIAGNOSIS

The diagnosis of brachioradialis syndrome is made on the basis of clinical findings rather than specific laboratory, electrodiagnostic, or radiographic testing. For this reason, a targeted history and physical examination, with a systematic search for trigger points and identification of a positive jump sign, must be carried out in every patient suspected of suffering from brachioradialis syndrome. It is incumbent on the clinician to rule out other coexisting disease processes that may mimic brachioradialis syndrome, including primary inflammatory muscle disease and collagen vascular disease. Radiographic testing, including magnetic resonance imaging, can help identify coexisting pathology such as internal derangement of the elbow, tumor, bursitis, tendinitis, crystal deposition diseases, and tennis elbow (Fig. 35-3). Electromyography can rule out cubital and radial tunnel syndromes. The clinician must also identify coexisting psychological and behavioral abnormalities that may mask or exacerbate the symptoms associated with brachioradialis syndrome.

TREATMENT

Treatment is focused on eliminating the myofascial trigger. It is hoped that interrupting the pain cycle in this

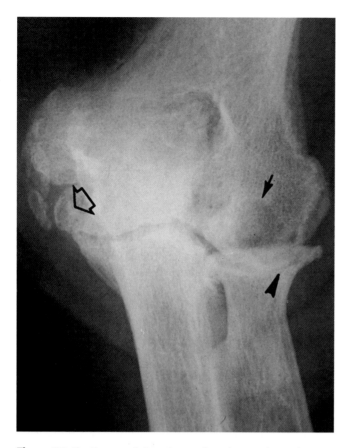

Figure 35–3. Characteristics of pyrophosphate arthropathy, including an unusual articular distribution. Changes in the elbow include joint space narrowing, subchondral cysts *(solid arrow)*, deformity of the radial head *(arrowhead)*, and fragmentation *(open arrow)*. (From Resnick D: Diagnosis of Bone and Joint Disorders, 4th ed. Philadelphia, Saunders, 2002, p 1584.)

way will allow the patient to obtain prolonged pain relief. Because the mechanism of action of the treatment modalities used is poorly understood, an element of trial and error is involved in developing a treatment plan.

Conservative therapy consisting of trigger point injections with local anesthetic or saline is the initial treatment of brachioradialis syndrome. Adjunct therapies, including physical therapy, therapeutic heat and cold, transcutaneous nerve stimulation, and electrical stimulation, can be used on a case-by-case basis. For patients who do not respond to these traditional measures, consideration should be given to the use of botulinum toxin type A; although not currently approved by the Food and Drug Administration for this indication, the injection of minute quantities of botulinum toxin type A directly into trigger points has been successful. Because underlying depression and anxiety are present in many patients suffering from brachioradialis syndrome, the administration of antidepressants is an integral part of most treatment plans.

COMPLICATIONS AND PITFALLS

Trigger point injections are extremely safe if careful attention is paid to the clinically relevant anatomy. Sterile technique must be used to avoid infection, along with universal precautions to minimize any risk to the operator. Most complications of trigger point injection are related to needle-induced trauma at the injection site and in underlying tissues. The incidence of ecchymosis and hematoma formation can be decreased if pressure is applied to the injection site immediately after injection. The avoidance of overly long needles can decrease the incidence of trauma to underlying structures. Special care must be taken to avoid damage to the underlying neural structures when injecting trigger points in proximity to the elbow and forearm.

Clinical Pearls

Although brachioradialis syndrome is a common disorder, it is often misdiagnosed. Therefore, in patients suspected of suffering from brachioradialis syndrome, a careful evaluation to identify underlying disease processes is mandatory. Brachioradialis syndrome commonly coexists with a variety of somatic and psychological disorders.

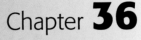

Chapter 36

Ulnar Nerve Entrapment at the Elbow

ICD-9 CODE **354.2**

THE CLINICAL SYNDROME

Ulnar nerve entrapment at the elbow is one of the most common entrapment neuropathies encountered in clinical practice. Causes include compression of the ulnar nerve by an aponeurotic band that runs from the medial epicondyle of the humerus to the medial border of the olecranon, direct trauma to the ulnar nerve at the elbow, and repetitive elbow motion. Ulnar nerve entrapment at the elbow is also called tardy ulnar palsy, cubital tunnel syndrome, and ulnar nerve neuritis. This entrapment neuropathy presents as pain and associated paresthesias in the lateral forearm that radiate to the wrist and to the ring and little fingers. Some patients also notice pain referred to the medial aspect of the scapula on the affected side. Untreated, ulnar nerve entrapment at the elbow can result in a progressive motor deficit and, ultimately, flexion contracture of the affected fingers. Symptoms usually begin after repetitive elbow motion or repeated pressure on the elbow, such as leaning on the elbow while lying on the floor (Fig. 36-1). Direct trauma to the ulnar nerve as it enters the cubital tunnel may result in a similar clinical presentation. Patients with vulnerable nerve syndrome, such as diabetics and alcoholics, are at greater risk for the development of ulnar nerve entrapment at the elbow.

SIGNS AND SYMPTOMS

Physical findings include tenderness over the ulnar nerve at the elbow. A positive Tinel's sign is usually present over the ulnar nerve as it passes beneath the aponeurosis. Weakness of the intrinsic muscles of the forearm and hand that are innervated by the ulnar nerve may be identified with careful manual muscle testing; however, early in the course of cubital tunnel syndrome, the only physical finding other than tenderness over the nerve may be loss of sensation on the ulnar side of the little finger.

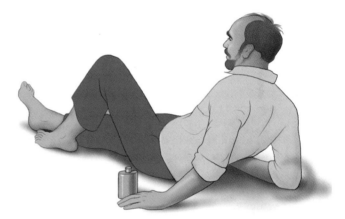

Figure 36–1. The ulnar nerve is susceptible to compression at the elbow.

Muscle wasting of the intrinsic muscles of the hand can best be identified by viewing the hand from above with the palm down. Patients suffering from ulnar nerve entrapment at the elbow often exhibit a positive Froment's sign, which is due to weakness of the adductor pollicis brevis and flexor pollicis brevis muscles (Fig. 36-2). Patients with significant muscle weakness secondary to ulnar nerve entrapment at the elbow also exhibit a positive Wartenberg's sign, with patients often complaining that the little finger gets caught outside the pants pocket when reaching for car keys (Fig. 36-3).

TESTING

Electromyography and nerve conduction velocity studies are extremely sensitive tests, and a skilled electromyographer can diagnose ulnar nerve entrapment at the elbow with a high degree of accuracy as well as distinguish other neuropathic causes of pain that may mimic it, including radiculopathy and plexopathy. Plain radiographs are indicated in all patients who present with ulnar nerve entrapment at the elbow to rule out occult bony pathology. If surgery is contemplated, magnetic resonance imaging (MRI) of the affected elbow may

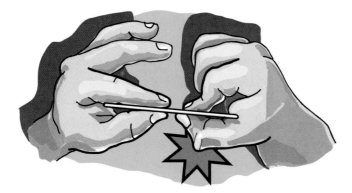

Figure 36–2. Froment's sign is elicited by asking the patient to lightly grasp a piece of paper between the thumb and index finger of each hand and monitoring flexion of the thumb interphalangeal joint on the affected side. (From Waldman SD: Physical Diagnosis of Pain: An Atlas of Signs and Symptoms. Philadelphia, Saunders, 2006, p 126.)

further delineate the pathologic process responsible for the nerve entrapment (e.g., bone spur, aponeurotic band thickening) (Fig. 36-4). If Pancoast's tumor or some other tumor of the brachial plexus is suspected, chest radiographs with apical lordotic views may be helpful. If the

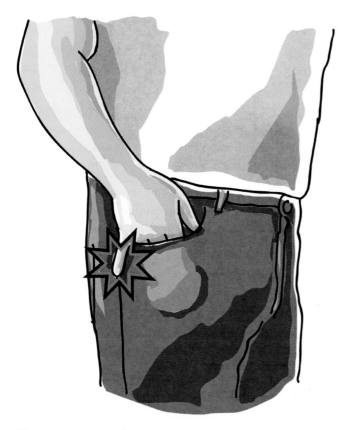

Figure 36–3. Wartenberg's sign for ulnar nerve entrapment at the elbow. (From Waldman SD: Physical Diagnosis of Pain: An Atlas of Signs and Symptoms. Philadelphia, Saunders, 2006, p 128.)

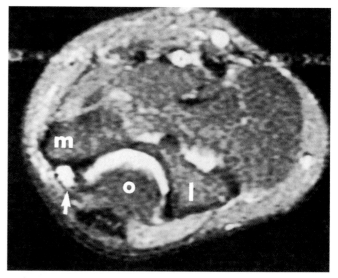

Figure 36–4. Entrapment neuropathy: cubital tunnel syndrome. A transaxial T2-weighted spin echo magnetic resonance image, obtained with fat suppression, shows increased signal intensity in the ulnar nerve *(arrow)* within the cubital tunnel. The medial (m) and lateral (l) epicondyles of the humerus and the olecranon process (o) of the ulna are indicated. A joint effusion is present. (From Resnick D: Diagnosis of Bone and Joint Disorders, 4th ed. Philadelphia, Saunders, 2002, p 3065.)

diagnosis is in question, screening laboratory tests consisting of a complete blood count, erythrocyte sedimentation rate, antinuclear antibody testing, and automated blood chemistry should be performed to rule out other causes of the patient's pain. The injection technique described later serves as both a diagnostic and a therapeutic maneuver.

DIFFERENTIAL DIAGNOSIS

Ulnar nerve entrapment at the elbow is often misdiagnosed as golfer's elbow, which explains why many patients with "golfer's elbow" fail to respond to conservative measures (see Chapter 32). With cubital tunnel syndrome, the maximal tenderness to palpation is over the ulnar nerve 1 inch below the medial epicondyle, whereas with golfer's elbow, the maximal tenderness to palpation is directly over the medial epicondyle. Cubital tunnel syndrome should also be differentiated from cervical radiculopathy involving the C7 or C8 roots. Further, cervical radiculopathy and ulnar nerve entrapment may coexist as the "double crush" syndrome. The double crush syndrome is seen most commonly with median nerve entrapment at the wrist or carpal tunnel syndrome.

TREATMENT

A short course of conservative therapy consisting of simple analgesics, nonsteroidal anti-inflammatory drugs, or cyclooxygenase-2 inhibitors, along with splinting to avoid elbow flexion, is indicated in patients who present with ulnar nerve entrapment at the elbow. If there is no marked improvement in symptoms within 1 week, careful injection of the ulnar nerve at the elbow using the following technique is a reasonable next step.

Ulnar nerve injection at the elbow is carried out by placing the patient in the supine position with the arm fully adducted at the patient's side, the elbow slightly flexed, and the dorsum of the hand resting on a folded towel. A total of 5 to 7 mL local anesthetic is drawn up in a 12-mL sterile syringe. For the first block, 80 mg methylprednisolone is added to the local anesthetic; 40 mg depot steroid is added with subsequent blocks. The clinician identifies the olecranon process and the medial epicondyle of the humerus; the ulnar nerve sulcus is located between these two bony landmarks. After preparation of the skin with antiseptic solution, a $\frac{5}{8}$-inch, 25-gauge needle is inserted just proximal to the sulcus and slowly advanced with a slightly cephalad trajectory. When the needle has advanced approximately $\frac{1}{2}$ inch, a strong paresthesia in the distribution of the ulnar nerve will be elicited. The patient should be warned to expect this and to say "There!" as soon as the paresthesia is felt. After the paresthesia is elicited and its distribution is identified, gentle aspiration is carried out to identify blood. If the aspiration test is negative and no persistent paresthesia in the distribution of the ulnar nerve remains, 5 to 7 mL of solution is slowly injected while the patient is monitored closely for signs of local anesthetic toxicity. If no paresthesia can be elicited, a similar amount of solution is slowly injected in a fanlike manner just proximal to the notch, with care being taken to avoid intravascular injection.

If the patient does not respond to these treatments or experiences progressive neurologic deficits, surgical decompression of the ulnar nerve is indicated. As mentioned earlier, MRI of the affected elbow can clarify the pathology responsible for the ulnar nerve compression.

COMPLICATIONS AND PITFALLS

Failure to promptly identify and treat ulnar nerve entrapment at the elbow can result in permanent neurologic deficit. To avoid harm to the patient, it is also important to rule out other causes of pain and numbness that may mimic the symptoms of ulnar nerve entrapment, such as Pancoast's tumor.

Ulnar nerve block at the elbow is relatively safe, with the major complications being inadvertent intravascular injection into the ulnar artery and persistent paresthesia secondary to needle-induced trauma to the nerve. Because the nerve passes through the ulnar nerve sulcus and is enclosed by a dense fibrous band, care should be taken to slowly inject just proximal to the sulcus to avoid additional compromise of the nerve.

Clinical Pearls

Ulnar nerve entrapment at the elbow is often misdiagnosed as golfer's elbow. It must also be differentiated from cervical radiculopathy involving the C8 spinal root; however, cervical radiculopathy and ulnar nerve entrapment may coexist in the double crush syndrome. Pancoast's tumor invading the medial cord of the brachial plexus may also mimic ulnar nerve entrapment and must be ruled out by apical lordotic chest radiography.

If cubital tunnel syndrome is suspected, injection of the ulnar nerve at the elbow with local anesthetic and steroid provides almost instantaneous relief. This is a simple and safe technique for the evaluation and treatment of ulnar nerve entrapment. Before performing ulnar nerve block, a careful neurologic examination should be done to identify preexisting neurologic deficits that might later be attributed to the nerve block. There seems to be a propensity for the development of persistent paresthesia when the nerve is blocked at this level. The incidence of this complication can be decreased by blocking the nerve proximal to the ulnar nerve sulcus and injecting slowly.

Chapter 37

Lateral Antebrachial Cutaneous Nerve Entrapment at the Elbow

ICD-9 CODE 354.8

THE CLINICAL SYNDROME

The lateral antebrachial cutaneous nerve may be entrapped by the biceps tendon or the brachialis muscle (Fig. 37-1). Clinically, patients complain of pain and paresthesias radiating from the elbow to the base of the thumb. Dull aching of the radial aspect of the forearm is also common. The pain of lateral antebrachial cutaneous nerve entrapment at the elbow may develop after an acute twisting injury to the elbow or direct trauma to the soft tissues overlying the lateral antebrachial cutaneous nerve; in other cases, the onset of pain is more insidious, without an obvious inciting factor. The pain is constant and becomes worse with use of the elbow. Patients with lateral antebrachial cutaneous nerve entrapment often note an increase in pain when using a computer keyboard or playing the piano (Fig. 37-2). Sleep disturbance is common.

SIGNS AND SYMPTOMS

On physical examination, there is tenderness to palpation of the lateral antebrachial cutaneous nerve at a point just lateral to the biceps tendon (Fig. 37-3). Elbow range of motion is normal. Patients with lateral antebrachial cutaneous nerve entrapment experience pain with active resisted flexion or rotation of the forearm.

TESTING

Electromyography and nerve conduction velocity studies are extremely sensitive tests, and a skilled electromyographer can diagnose lateral antebrachial cutaneous nerve entrapment with a high degree of accuracy as well as distinguish other neuropathic causes of pain that may mimic it, including radiculopathy and plexopathy. Plain radiographs are indicated in all patients who present

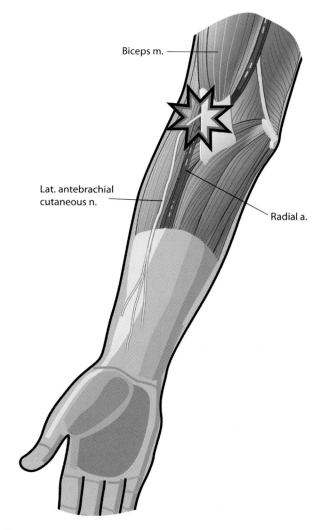

Figure 37–1. Lateral antebrachial cutaneous nerve entrapment: relevant soft tissue anatomy. (From Waldman SD: Physical Diagnosis of Pain: An Atlas of Signs and Symptoms. Philadelphia, Saunders, 2006, p 130.)

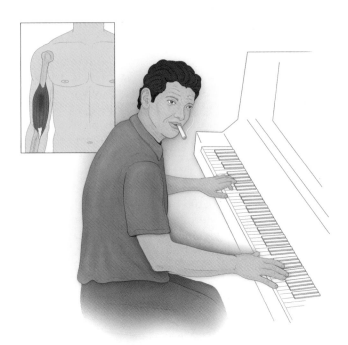

Figure 37–2. Patients with lateral antebrachial cutaneous nerve entrapment at the elbow often note increased pain when using a computer keyboard or playing the piano.

with lateral antebrachial cutaneous nerve entrapment to rule out occult bony pathology. If surgery is contemplated, magnetic resonance imaging (MRI) of the affected elbow may further delineate the pathologic process responsible for the nerve entrapment (e.g., bone spur, aponeurotic band thickening). If Pancoast's tumor or some other tumor of the brachial plexus is suspected, chest radiographs with apical lordotic views may be helpful. If the diagnosis is in question, screening laboratory tests consisting of a complete blood count, erythrocyte sedimentation rate, antinuclear antibody testing, and automated blood chemistry should be performed to rule out other causes of the patient's pain. Injection of the nerve serves as both a diagnostic and a therapeutic maneuver.

DIFFERENTIAL DIAGNOSIS

Cervical radiculopathy and tennis elbow can mimic nerve entrapment. With lateral antebrachial cutaneous nerve entrapment, the maximal tenderness to palpation is at the level of the biceps tendon, whereas with tennis elbow, the maximal tenderness to palpation is over the lateral epicondyle (see Chapter 31). Electromyography can distinguish cervical radiculopathy and lateral antebrachial cutaneous nerve entrapment from tennis elbow. Further, it should be remembered that cervical radiculopathy and lateral antebrachial cutaneous nerve entrap-

ment may coexist as the "double crush" syndrome. The double crush syndrome is seen most commonly with median nerve entrapment at the wrist or carpal tunnel syndrome.

TREATMENT

A short course of conservative therapy consisting of simple analgesics, nonsteroidal anti-inflammatory drugs, or cyclooxygenase-2 inhibitors, along with splinting to avoid elbow flexion, is indicated in patients who present with lateral antebrachial cutaneous nerve entrapment at the elbow. If there is no marked improvement in symptoms within 1 week, careful injection of the lateral antebrachial cutaneous nerve at the elbow is a reasonable next step.

If the patient does not respond to these treatments or experiences progressive neurologic deficits, surgical decompression of the lateral antebrachial cutaneous nerve is indicated. As mentioned, MRI of the affected elbow can clarify the pathology responsible for nerve compression.

COMPLICATIONS AND PITFALLS

Failure to promptly identify and treat lateral antebrachial cutaneous nerve entrapment at the elbow can result in

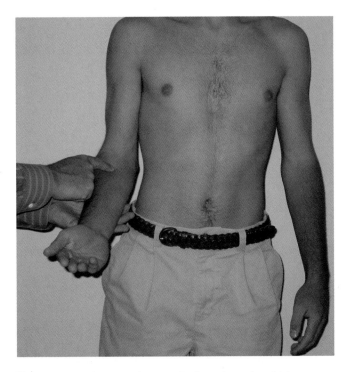

Figure 37–3. Compression test for lateral antebrachial cutaneous nerve entrapment. (From Waldman SD: Physical Diagnosis of Pain: An Atlas of Signs and Symptoms. Philadelphia, Saunders, 2006, p 131.)

permanent neurologic deficit. To avoid harm to the patient, it is also important to rule out other causes of pain and numbness that may mimic the symptoms of lateral antebrachial cutaneous nerve entrapment, such as Pancoast's tumor.

Lateral antebrachial cutaneous nerve block at the elbow is relatively safe, with the major complications being inadvertent intravascular injection into the lateral antebrachial cutaneous artery and persistent paresthesia secondary to needle-induced trauma to the nerve. Because the nerve passes through the lateral antebrachial cutaneous nerve sulcus and is enclosed by a dense fibrous band, care should be taken to slowly inject just proximal to the sulcus to avoid additional compromise of the nerve.

Clinical Pearls

Lateral antebrachial cutaneous nerve entrapment at the elbow is often misdiagnosed as tennis elbow, which explains why many patients with "tennis elbow" fail to respond to conservative measures. Lateral antebrachial cutaneous nerve block at the elbow is a simple and safe technique for the evaluation and treatment of this condition. Before performing the nerve block, a careful neurologic examination should be done to identify preexisting neurologic deficits that might later be attributed to the nerve block. The incidence of persistent paresthesia can be decreased by blocking the nerve proximal to the lateral antebrachial cutaneous nerve sulcus and injecting slowly.

Chapter 38

Olecranon Bursitis

ICD-9 CODE 726.33

THE CLINICAL SYNDROME

Olecranon bursitis may develop gradually due to repetitive irritation of the olecranon bursa or acutely due to trauma or infection. The olecranon bursa lies in the posterior aspect of the elbow between the olecranon process of the ulna and the overlying skin. It may exist as a single bursal sac or, in some patients, as a multisegmented series of loculated sacs. With overuse or misuse, these bursae may become inflamed, enlarged, and, on rare occasions, infected. The swelling associated with olecranon bursitis may be quite impressive, and the patient may complain about being unable to wear a long-sleeved shirt.

The olecranon bursa is vulnerable to injury from both acute trauma and repeated microtrauma. Acute injuries are often caused by direct trauma to the elbow in patients who play sports such as hockey or who fall directly onto the olecranon process. Repeated pressure from leaning on the elbow, such as when working long hours at a drafting table, may result in inflammation and swelling of the olecranon bursa (Fig. 38-1). Rarely, gout or bacterial infection precipitates acute olecranon bursitis. If inflammation of the olecranon bursa becomes chronic, calcification of the bursa may occur, resulting in residual nodules called "gravel."

SIGNS AND SYMPTOMS

Patients suffering from olecranon bursitis frequently complain of swelling and pain with any movement of the elbow, but especially with extension. The pain is localized to the olecranon area, with referred pain often noted above the elbow joint. Often, the patient is more concerned about the swelling than the pain. Physical examination reveals point tenderness over the olecranon and swelling of the bursa that may be extensive (Fig. 38-2). Passive extension and resisted flexion reproduce the pain, as does any pressure over the bursa. Fever and chills usually accompany infection of the bursa.

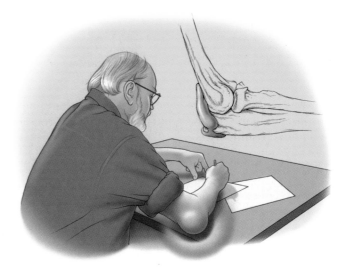

Figure 38–1. Olecranon bursitis is often caused by repeated pressure on the elbow.

TESTING

The diagnosis of olecranon bursitis is usually made on clinical grounds alone. Plain radiographs of the posterior elbow are indicated if there is a history of elbow trauma or if arthritis of the elbow is suspected. Plain radiographs may also reveal calcification of the bursa and associated structures, consistent with chronic inflammation. Magnetic resonance imaging is indicated if joint instability is suspected or if the diagnosis of olecranon bursitis is in question. A complete blood count, automated chemistry profile including uric acid level, erythrocyte sedimentation rate, and antinuclear antibody testing should be performed if collagen vascular disease is suspected. If infection is suspected, aspiration, Gram stain, and culture of the bursal fluid, followed by treatment with appropriate antibiotics, are required on an emergency basis (Fig. 38-3).

DIFFERENTIAL DIAGNOSIS

Olecranon bursitis is usually a straightforward clinical diagnosis. Occasionally, rheumatoid nodules or gouty arthritis of the elbow may confuse the clinical picture. Also, synovial cysts of the elbow may mimic olecranon

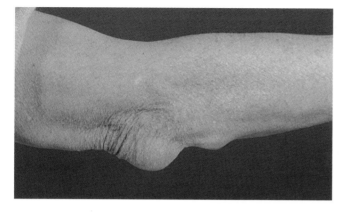

Figure 38-2. Olecranon bursitis in a patient with rheumatoid arthritis; a rheumatoid nodule is also shown. (From Klippel JH, Dieppe PA: Rheumatology, 2nd ed. London, Mosby, 1998)

bursitis. It should be remembered that coexistent tendinitis (e.g., tennis elbow, golfer's elbow) may require additional treatment.

TREATMENT

A short course of conservative therapy consisting of simple analgesics, nonsteroidal anti-inflammatory drugs, or cyclooxygenase-2 inhibitors, along with an elbow protector to prevent further trauma, is the initial treatment for patients suffering from olecranon bursitis. If rapid improvement fails to occur, the following injection technique is a reasonable next step.

The patient is placed in the supine position with the arm fully adducted at the patient's side, the elbow flexed, and the palm of the hand resting on the patient's abdomen. A total of 2 mL local anesthetic and 40 mg methylprednisolone is drawn up in a 5-mL sterile syringe. After sterile preparation of the skin overlying the posterior aspect of the joint, the olecranon process and overlying bursa are identified. Using strict aseptic technique, a 1-inch, 25-gauge needle is inserted through the skin and subcutaneous tissues directly into the bursa in the midline. If bone is encountered, the needle is withdrawn into the bursa. The contents of the syringe is gently injected; there should be little resistance to injection. The needle is removed, and a sterile pressure dressing and ice pack are applied to the injection site.

Physical modalities, including local heat and gentle range-of-motion exercises, should be introduced several days after injection for elbow pain. Vigorous exercises should be avoided, because they will exacerbate the patient's symptoms.

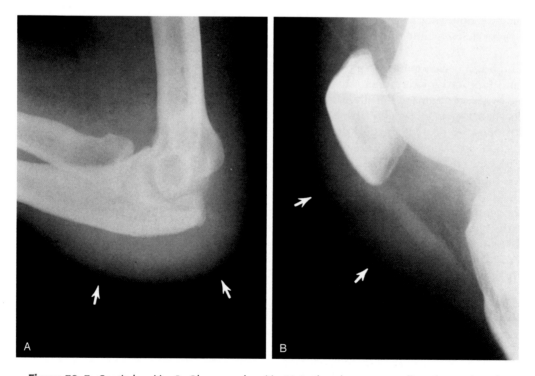

Figure 38-3. Septic bursitis. **A,** Olecranon bursitis. Note the olecranon swelling *(arrows)* and soft tissue edema due to *Staphylococcus aureus* infection. Previous surgery and trauma caused the adjacent bony abnormalities. **B,** Prepatellar bursitis. This 28-year-old carpenter who worked on his knees for prolonged periods developed tender swelling in front of the knee *(arrows)*. Inflammatory fluid that was culture positive for *Staphylococcus aureus* was recovered from the bursa. (From Resnick D: Diagnosis of Bone and Joint Disorders, 4th ed. Philadelphia, Saunders, 2002, p 2438.)

COMPLICATIONS AND PITFALLS

Failure to adequately treat olecranon bursitis may result in chronic pain and loss of elbow range of motion. The injection technique is safe if careful attention is paid to the clinically relevant anatomy. In particular, the ulnar nerve is susceptible to damage at the elbow; this can be avoided by keeping the needle trajectory in the midline. Sterile technique must be used to avoid infection, along with universal precautions to minimize any risk to the operator. The major complication of bursal injection is infection, although it should be exceedingly rare if strict aseptic technique is followed. The incidence of ecchymosis and hematoma formation can be decreased if pressure is applied to the injection site immediately after injection. Approximately 25% of patients complain of a transient increase in pain after injection of the olecranon bursa, and they should be warned of this possibility.

Clinical Pearls

The injection technique described is extremely effective in the treatment of pain and swelling secondary to olecranon bursitis. Coexistent tendinitis and epicondylitis may contribute to elbow pain, necessitating additional treatment with more localized injection of local anesthetic and methylprednisolone. Simple analgesics and nonsteroidal anti-inflammatory drugs can be used concurrently with the injection technique.

Section 6

Pain Syndromes of the Wrist

Chapter 39

Arthritis Pain of the Wrist

ICD-9 CODE **715.93**

THE CLINICAL SYNDROME

Arthritis of the wrist is a common complaint that can cause significant pain and suffering. The wrist joint is susceptible to the development of arthritis from a variety of conditions that have in common the ability to damage joint cartilage. Patients with arthritis of the wrist present with pain, swelling, and decreasing function of the wrist. Decreased grip strength is also a common finding. Osteoarthritis is the most common form of arthritis that results in wrist joint pain. However, rheumatoid arthritis, post-traumatic arthritis, and psoriatic arthritis are also common causes of arthritic wrist pain. These types of arthritis can result in significant alteration in the biomechanics of the wrist because they affect not only the joint but also the tendons and other connective tissues that make up the functional unit.

SIGNS AND SYMPTOMS

The majority of patients presenting with wrist pain secondary to osteoarthritis or post-traumatic arthritis complain of pain that is localized around the wrist and hand. Activity makes the pain worse, whereas rest and heat provide some relief. The pain is constant and is characterized as aching in nature; it may interfere with sleep. Some patients complain of a grating or popping sensation with use of the joint, and crepitus may be present on physical examination. If the pain and dysfunction are secondary to rheumatoid arthritis, the metacarpophalangeal joints are often involved, with characteristic deformity.

In addition to pain, patients suffering from arthritis of the wrist joint often experience a gradual reduction in functional ability because of decreasing wrist range of motion, making simple everyday tasks such as using a computer keyboard, holding a coffee cup, turning a doorknob, or unscrewing a bottle cap quite difficult (Fig. 39-1). With continued disuse, muscle wasting may occur, and adhesive capsulitis with subsequent ankylosis may develop.

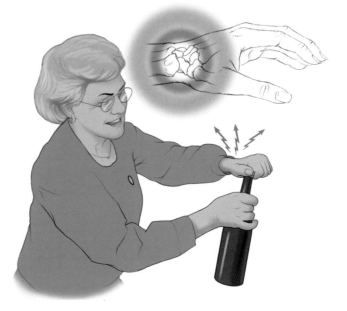

Figure 39–1. Arthritis of the wrist often makes simple everyday tasks such as opening a bottle painful.

TESTING

Plain radiographs are indicated in all patients who present with wrist pain. Based on the patient's clinical presentation, additional testing may be warranted, including a complete blood count, erythrocyte sedimentation rate, and antinuclear antibody testing. Magnetic resonance imaging of the wrist is indicated if joint instability is thought to be present (Fig. 39-2). If infection is suspected, Gram stain and culture of the synovial fluid should be performed on an emergency basis, and treatment with appropriate antibiotics should be started.

DIFFERENTIAL DIAGNOSIS

Osteoarthritis is the most common form of arthritis that results in wrist joint pain. However, rheumatoid arthritis and post-traumatic arthritis are also common causes of wrist pain. Less common causes of arthritis-induced wrist pain include collagen vascular diseases, infection,

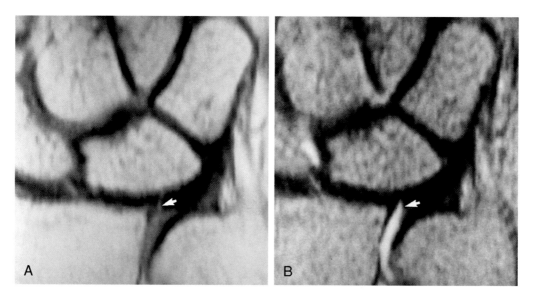

Figure 39–2. Triangular fibrocartilage complex with a communicating defect. **A,** Coronal intermediate-weighted spin echo magnetic resonance image. Note the linear region of increased signal intensity *(arrow)* in the triangular fibrocartilage. **B,** T2-weighted spin echo magnetic resonance image. Fluid of high signal intensity is present in the defect *(arrow)* in the triangular fibrocartilage and in the distal radioulnar joint. Fluid is also present in the midcarpal joint. (From Resnick D: Diagnosis of Bone and Joint Disorders, 4th ed. Philadelphia, Saunders, 2002, p 3033.)

villonodular synovitis, and Lyme disease. Acute infectious arthritis is usually accompanied by significant systemic symptoms, including fever and malaise, and should be easily recognized and treated with antibiotics. Collagen vascular diseases generally present as a polyarthropathy rather than a monoarthropathy limited to the wrist joint; however, wrist pain secondary to collagen vascular disease responds exceedingly well to the intra-articular injection technique described here.

TREATMENT

Initial treatment of the pain and functional disability associated with osteoarthritis of the wrist includes a combination of nonsteroidal anti-inflammatory drugs or cyclooxygenase-2 inhibitors and physical therapy. Local application of heat and cold may also be beneficial. Splinting the wrist in the neutral position may provide symptomatic relief and protect the joint from additional trauma. For patients who do not respond to these treatment modalities, intra-articular injection of local anesthetic and steroid is a reasonable next step.

Intra-articular injection of the wrist is performed by placing the patient in the supine position with the arm fully adducted at the patient's side, the elbow slightly flexed, and the palm of the hand resting on a folded towel. A total of 1.5 mL local anesthetic and 40 mg methylprednisolone is drawn up in a 5-mL sterile syringe. After sterile preparation of the skin overlying the dorsal

joint, the midcarpus proximal to the indentation of the capitate bone is identified. Just proximal to the capitate bone is an indentation that allows easy access to the wrist joint. Using strict aseptic technique, a 1-inch, 25-gauge needle is inserted in the center of the midcarpal indentation through the skin, subcutaneous tissues, and joint capsule and into the joint. If bone is encountered, the needle is withdrawn into the subcutaneous tissues and redirected superiorly. After entering the joint space, the contents of the syringe is gently injected. There should be little resistance to injection. If resistance is encountered, the needle is probably in a ligament or tendon and should be advanced slightly into the joint space until the injection can proceed without significant resistance. The needle is then removed, and a sterile pressure dressing and ice pack are applied to the injection site.

Physical modalities, including local heat and gentle range-of-motion exercises, should be introduced several days after the patient begins treatment for arthritis of wrist. Vigorous exercises should be avoided, because they will exacerbate the patient's symptoms.

COMPLICATIONS AND PITFALLS

Joint protection is especially important in patients suffering from inflammatory arthritis of the wrist, because repetitive trauma can result in further damage to the joint, tendons, and connective tissues. The major complication of intra-articular injection of the wrist is infection, although it should be exceedingly rare if strict aseptic technique is followed. The injection technique is safe if careful attention is paid to the clinically relevant anatomy; the ulnar nerve is especially susceptible to damage at the wrist. Approximately 25% of patients complain of a transient increase in pain after intra-articular injection of the wrist joint, and they should be warned of this possibility.

Clinical Pearls

The injection technique described is extremely effective in the treatment of pain secondary to arthritis of the wrist joint. Simple analgesics and nonsteroidal anti-inflammatory drugs can be used concurrently with the injection technique. Coexistent bursitis and tendinitis may contribute to wrist pain and necessitate additional treatment with more localized injection of local anesthetic and methylprednisolone.

Chapter 40

Carpal Tunnel Syndrome

ICD-9 CODE 354.0

THE CLINICAL SYNDROME

Carpal tunnel syndrome is the most common entrapment neuropathy encountered in clinical practice. It is caused by compression of the median nerve as it passes through the carpal canal at the wrist. The most common causes of compression of the median nerve at this location include flexor tenosynovitis, rheumatoid arthritis, pregnancy, amyloidosis, and other space-occupying lesions that compromise the median nerve as it passes through this closed space. This entrapment neuropathy presents as pain, numbness, paresthesias, and associated weakness in the hand and wrist that radiate to the thumb, index finger, middle finger, and radial half of the ring finger. These symptoms may also radiate proximal to the entrapment into the forearm. Untreated, progressive motor deficit and, ultimately, flexion contracture of the affected fingers can result. Symptoms usually begin after repetitive wrist motions or repeated pressure on the wrist, such as resting the wrists on the edge of a computer keyboard (Fig. 40-1). Direct trauma to the median nerve as it enters the carpal tunnel may result in a similar clinical presentation.

SIGNS AND SYMPTOMS

Physical findings include tenderness over the median nerve at the wrist. A positive Tinel's sign is usually present over the median nerve as it passes beneath the flexor retinaculum (Fig. 40-2). A positive Phalen's maneuver is highly suggestive of carpal tunnel syndrome. Phalen's maneuver is performed by having the patient place the wrists in complete unforced flexion for at least 30 seconds (Fig. 40-3). If the median nerve is entrapped at the wrist, this maneuver reproduces the symptoms of carpal tunnel syndrome. Weakness of thumb opposition and wasting of the thenar eminence are often seen in advanced cases of carpal tunnel syndrome; however, because of the complex motion of the thumb, subtle motor deficits can easily be missed (Fig. 40-4). Early in

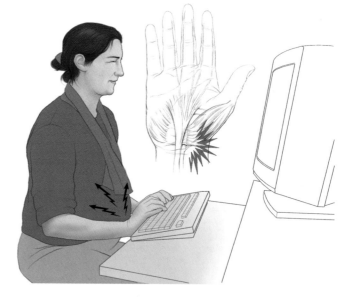

Figure 40–1. Poor positioning of the hand and wrist during keyboarding can result in carpal tunnel syndrome.

the course of carpal tunnel syndrome, the only physical finding other than tenderness over the median nerve may be the loss of sensation in the above-mentioned fingers.

TESTING

Electromyography can distinguish cervical radiculopathy and diabetic polyneuropathy from carpal tunnel syndrome. Plain radiographs are indicated in all patients who present with carpal tunnel syndrome to rule out occult bony pathology. Based on the patient's clinical presentation, additional testing may be warranted, including a complete blood count, uric acid level, erythrocyte sedimentation rate, and antinuclear antibody testing. Magnetic resonance imaging of the wrist is indicated if joint instability or a space-occupying lesion is suspected or to confirm the actual cause of median nerve compression (Fig. 40-5). The injection technique described later serves as both a diagnostic and a therapeutic maneuver.

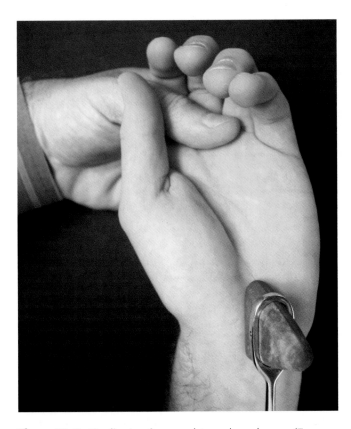

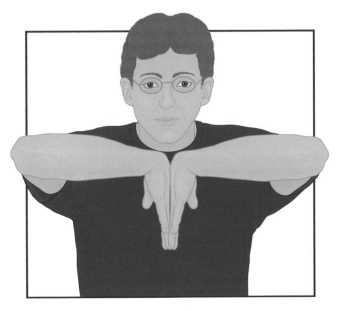

Figure 40–3. A positive Phalen's maneuver is highly indicative of carpal tunnel syndrome. (From Waldman SD: Atlas of Pain Management Injection Techniques. Philadelphia, Saunders, 2000.)

Figure 40–2. Tinel's sign for carpal tunnel syndrome. (From Waldman SD: Physical Diagnosis of Pain: An Atlas of Signs and Symptoms. Philadelphia, Saunders, 2006, p 178.)

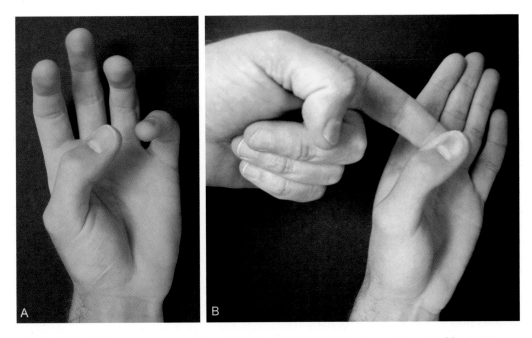

Figure 40–4. The opponens weakness test for carpal tunnel syndrome. (From Waldman SD: Physical Diagnosis of Pain: An Atlas of Signs and Symptoms. Philadelphia, Saunders, 2006, p 180.)

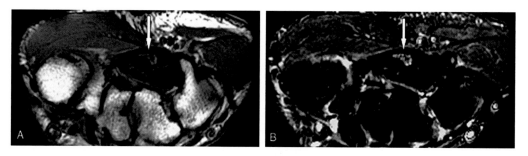

Figure 40–5. Axial T1-weighted **(A)** and short tau inversion recovery **(B)** images of a patient with carpal tunnel syndrome without marked nerve enlargement. (From Edelman RR, Hessellink JR, Zlatkin MB, Crues JV: Clinical Magnetic Resonance Imaging, 3rd ed. Philadelphia, Saunders, 2006, p 2381.)

DIFFERENTIAL DIAGNOSIS

Carpal tunnel syndrome is often misdiagnosed as arthritis of the carpometacarpal joint of the thumb, cervical radiculopathy, or diabetic polyneuropathy. Patients with arthritis of the carpometacarpal joint of the thumb have a positive Watson test and radiographic evidence of arthritis. Most patients suffering from cervical radiculopathy have reflex, motor, and sensory changes associated with neck pain; in contrast, patients with carpal tunnel syndrome have no reflex changes, and motor and sensory changes are limited to the distal median nerve. Diabetic polyneuropathy generally presents as a symmetrical sensory deficit involving the entire hand rather than being limited to the distribution of the median nerve. It should be remembered that cervical radiculopathy and median nerve entrapment may coexist as the "double crush" syndrome. Further, carpal tunnel syndrome is commonly seen in patients with diabetes, and it is not uncommon for diabetic polyneuropathy to be present as well.

TREATMENT

Mild cases of carpal tunnel syndrome usually respond to conservative therapy; surgery should be reserved for more severe cases. Initial treatment of carpal tunnel syndrome consists of simple analgesics, nonsteroidal anti-inflammatory drugs, or cyclooxygenase-2 inhibitors and splinting of the wrist. At a minimum, the splint should be worn at night, but 24 hours a day is ideal. Avoidance of the repetitive activities that are thought to be responsible for carpal tunnel syndrome (e.g., keyboarding, hammering) can also help ameliorate the patient's symptoms. If the patient fails to respond to these conservative measures, a next reasonable step is injection of the carpal tunnel with local anesthetic and steroid.

Carpal tunnel injection is performed by placing the patient in the supine position with the arm fully abducted at the patient's side, the elbow slightly flexed, and the dorsum of the hand resting on a folded towel. A total of

3 mL local anesthetic and 40 mg methylprednisolone is drawn up in a 5-mL sterile syringe. The patient is then told to make a fist and at the same time flex his or her wrist to aid in identifying the palmaris longus tendon. After preparation of the skin with antiseptic solution, a 5/8-inch, 25-gauge needle is inserted just medial to the tendon and just proximal to the crease of the wrist at a 30-degree angle (Fig. 40-6). The needle is slowly advanced until the tip is just beyond the tendon. Paresthesia in the distribution of the median nerve is often elicited, and the patient should be warned to expect this and to say

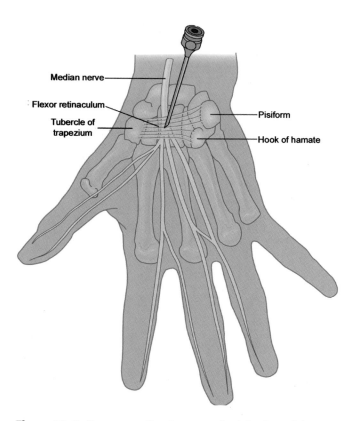

Figure 40–6. Proper needle placement for injection of the carpal tunnel. (From Waldman SD: Atlas of Pain Management Injection Techniques. Philadelphia, Saunders, 2000.)

"There!" as soon as the paresthesia is felt. If a paresthesia is elicited, the needle is withdrawn slightly away from the median nerve. Gentle aspiration is then carried out to identify blood. If the aspiration test is negative and there is no persistent paresthesia in the distribution of the median nerve, 3 mL of solution is slowly injected while the patient is monitored closely for signs of local anesthetic toxicity. If no paresthesia is elicited and the needle tip hits bone, the needle is withdrawn out of the periosteum and, after careful aspiration, 3 mL of solution is slowly injected.

When these treatment modalities fail, surgical release of the median nerve at the carpal tunnel is indicated. Endoscopic techniques are showing promise and appear to result in less postoperative pain and dysfunction.

COMPLICATIONS AND PITFALLS

Failure to adequately treat carpal tunnel syndrome can result in permanent pain, numbness, and functional disability. The problem can be exacerbated if coexistent reflex sympathetic dystrophy is not aggressively treated with sympathetic neural blockade. Injection of the carpal tunnel is a relatively safe technique, with the major complications being inadvertent intravascular injection and persistent paresthesia secondary to needle-induced trauma to the nerve. This technique can be safely performed in the presence of anticoagulation by using a 25- or 27-gauge needle, albeit with an increased risk of hematoma formation. The incidence of this complication can be decreased if manual pressure is applied to the area immediately after injection. The application of cold packs for 20 minutes after injection can also decrease the amount of postprocedure pain and bleeding.

Clinical Pearls

Carpal tunnel syndrome should always be differentiated from cervical radiculopathy involving the cervical nerve roots, which may mimic median nerve compression. Further, it should be remembered that cervical radiculopathy and median nerve entrapment may coexist in the double crush syndrome.

Carpal tunnel injection is a simple and safe technique. Before initiating median nerve block at the wrist, a careful neurologic examination should be performed to identify preexisting neurologic deficits that may later be attributed to the nerve block, especially in patients with clinical symptoms of diabetes or clinically significant carpal tunnel syndrome.

Care should be taken to place the needle just beyond the flexor retinaculum and to inject slowly to allow the solution to flow easily into the carpal tunnel without further compromising the median nerve.

Chapter 41

De Quervain's Tenosynovitis

ICD-9 CODE 727.04

THE CLINICAL SYNDROME

De Quervain's tenosynovitis is caused by inflammation and swelling of the tendons of the abductor pollicis longus and extensor pollicis brevis at the level of the radial styloid process. It is usually the result of trauma to the tendon from repetitive twisting motions. If the inflammation and swelling become chronic, the tendon sheath thickens, resulting in its constriction. A triggering phenomenon may occur, with the tendon catching within the sheath and causing the thumb to lock, or "trigger." Arthritis and gout of the first metacarpal joint may coexist with de Quervain's tenosynovitis and exacerbate the associated pain and disability.

De Quervain's tenosynovitis occurs in patients engaged in repetitive activities such as handshaking or high-torque wrist turning (e.g., when scooping ice cream). De Quervain's tenosynovitis may also develop without obvious antecedent trauma.

The pain of de Quervain's tenosynovitis is localized to the region of the radial styloid. It is constant and is made worse with active pinching activities of the thumb or ulnar deviation of the wrist (Fig. 41-1). Patients note an inability to hold a coffee cup or turn a screwdriver. Sleep disturbance is common.

SIGNS AND SYMPTOMS

On physical examination, there is tenderness and swelling over the tendons and tendon sheaths along the distal radius, with point tenderness over the radial styloid. Many patients with de Quervain's tenosynovitis note a creaking sensation with flexion and extension of the thumb. Range of motion of the thumb may be decreased due to the pain, and a trigger thumb phenomenon may be noted. Patients with de Quervain's tenosynovitis demonstrate a positive Finkelstein test (Fig. 41-2). The Finkelstein test is performed by stabilizing the patient's forearm, having the patient fully flex his or her thumb into the palm, and then actively forcing the wrist toward the ulna. Sudden severe pain is highly suggestive of de Quervain's tenosynovitis.

TESTING

The diagnosis is generally made on clinical grounds, but magnetic resonance imaging (MRI) can confirm the presence of tensoynovitis (Fig. 41-3). Electromyography can distinguish de Quervain's tenosynovitis from neuropathic processes such as cervical radiculopathy and cheiralgia paresthetica. Plain radiographs are indicated in all patients who present with de Quervain's tenosynovitis to rule out occult bony pathology. Based on the patient's clinical presentation, additional testing may be warranted, including a complete blood count, uric acid level, erythrocyte sedimentation rate, and antinuclear antibody testing. MRI of the wrist is also indicated if joint instability is suspected. The injection technique described later serves as both a diagnostic and a therapeutic maneuver.

DIFFERENTIAL DIAGNOSIS

Entrapment of the lateral antebrachial cutaneous nerve, arthritis of the first metacarpal joint, gout, cheiralgia paresthetica (caused by entrapment of the superficial branch of the radial nerve at the wrist), and occasionally C6-7 radiculopathy can mimic de Quervain's tenosynovitis. All these painful conditions can also coexist with de Quervain's tenosynovitis.

TREATMENT

Initial treatment of the pain and functional disability associated with de Quervain's tenosynovitis includes a combination of nonsteroidal anti-inflammatory drugs or cyclooxygenase-2 inhibitors and physical therapy. Local application of heat and cold may also be beneficial. Any repetitive activity that may exacerbate the patient's symptoms should be avoided. Nighttime splinting of the affected thumb may help avoid the trigger phenomenon that can occur on awakening in many patients suffering from this condition. For patients who do not respond to

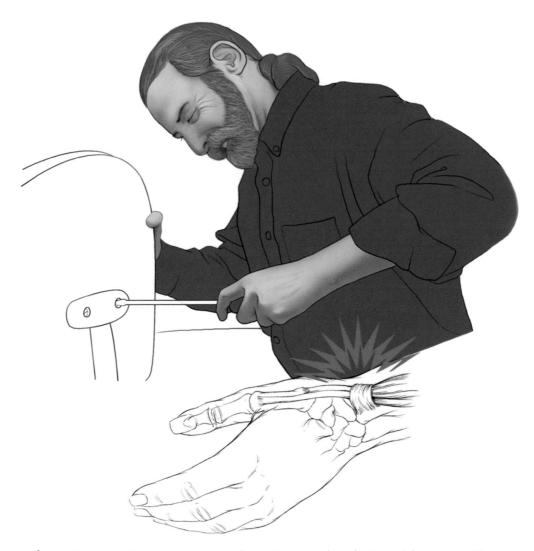

Figure 41–1. Repetitive microtrauma to the wrist can result in de Quervain's tenosynovitis.

these treatment modalities, the following injection technique is a reasonable next step.

Injection for de Quervain's tenosynovitis is carried out by placing the patient in the supine position with the arm fully adducted at the patient's side and the ulnar surface of the wrist and hand resting on a folded towel to relax the affected tendons. A total of 2 mL local anesthetic and 40 mg methylprednisolone is drawn up in a 5-mL sterile syringe. After sterile preparation of the skin overlying the affected tendons, the radial styloid is identified. Using strict aseptic technique, a 1-inch, 25-gauge needle is inserted at a 45-degree angle toward the radial styloid through the skin and into the subcutaneous tissue overlying the affected tendon. If bone is encountered, the needle is withdrawn into the subcutaneous tissue. The contents of the syringe are then gently injected. There should be little resistance to injection. If resistance is encountered, the needle is probably in the

tendon and should be withdrawn until the injection can proceed without significant resistance. The needle is then removed, and a sterile pressure dressing and ice pack are applied to the injection site.

Physical modalities, including local heat and gentle range-of-motion exercises, should be introduced several days after the patient undergoes injection. Vigorous exercises should be avoided, because they will exacerbate the patient's symptoms.

COMPLICATIONS AND PITFALLS

The injection technique is safe if careful attention is paid to the clinically relevant anatomy. The radial artery and superficial branch of the radial nerve are susceptible to damage if the needle is placed too medially, so care must be taken to avoid these structures. The major complications associated with injection are related to trauma to

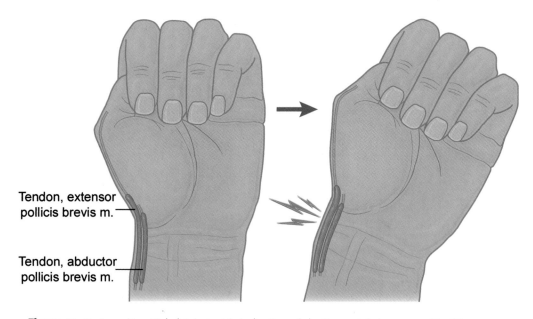

Figure 41–2. A positive Finkelstein test is indicative of de Quervain's tenosynovitis. (From Waldman SD: Atlas of Pain Management Injection Techniques. Saunders, Philadelphia, 2000.)

the inflamed and previously damaged tendons. These tendons may rupture if they are injected directly, so the needle position should be confirmed to be outside the tendon before injection. Another complication of injection is infection, although it should be exceedingly rare if strict aseptic technique is followed, as well as universal precautions to minimize any risk to the operator. The incidence of ecchymosis and hematoma formation can be decreased if pressure is applied to the injection site immediately after injection. Approximately 25% of patients complain of a transient increase in pain after injection, and they should be warned of this possibility.

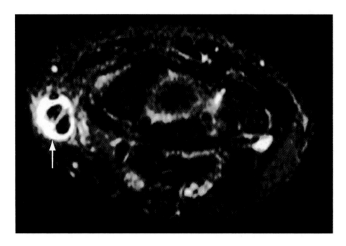

Figure 41–3. Axial short tau inversion recovery image demonstrating de Quervain's tenosynovitis. Note the thickened first extensor compartment tendons, with prominent tendon sheath fluid *(arrow)*. (From Edelman RR, Hessellink JR, Zlatkin MB, Crues JV: Clinical Magnetic Resonance Imaging, 3rd ed. Philadelphia, Saunders, 2006, p 3357.)

Clinical Pearls

The injection technique described is extremely effective in the treatment of pain secondary to de Quervain's tenosynovitis. A hand splint to immobilize the thumb may also help relieve the symptoms. Simple analgesics and nonsteroidal anti-inflammatory drugs can be used concurrently with the injection technique. Coexistent arthritis and gout may contribute to the pain, necessitating additional treatment with more localized injection of local anesthetic and methylprednisolone. Arthritis of the first metacarpal joint, gout, cheiralgia paresthetica, and cervical radiculopathy may mimic de Quervain's tenosynovitis and must be ruled out.

Chapter 42

Arthritis Pain of the Carpometacarpal Joint

ICD-9 CODE 715.94

THE CLINICAL SYNDROME

The carpometacarpal joints of the fingers are synovial plane joints that serve as the articulation between the carpals and the metacarpals and allow the bases of the metacarpal bones to articulate with one another. Movement of the joints is limited to a slight gliding motion, with the carpometacarpal joint of the little finger possessing the greatest range of motion. The primary function of these joints is to optimize the grip function of the hand. In most patients, there is a common joint space (Fig. 42-1).

Pain and dysfunction from arthritis of the carpometacarpal joints are common complaints. These joints are susceptible to the development of arthritis from a variety of conditions that have in common the ability to damage joint cartilage. Osteoarthritis is the most common form of arthritis that results in carpometacarpal joint pain. It occurs more commonly in females, and although the thumb is most commonly affected, arthritis may develop in the other carpometacarpal joints as well, especially after trauma. Rheumatoid arthritis, post-traumatic arthritis, and psoriatic arthritis are also common causes of carpometacarpal pain. Less common causes of arthritis-induced carpometacarpal pain include collagen vascular diseases, infection, and Lyme disease. Acute infectious arthritis is usually accompanied by significant systemic symptoms, including fever and malaise, and should be easily recognized; it is treated with culture and antibiotics rather than injection therapy. Collagen vascular diseases generally present as a polyarthropathy rather than a monoarthropathy limited to the carpometacarpal joint; however, carpometacarpal pain secondary to collagen vascular disease responds exceedingly well to the intra-articular injection technique described here.

SIGNS AND SYMPTOMS

The majority of patients presenting with carpometacarpal pain secondary to osteoarthritis or post-traumatic arthritis complain of pain that is localized to the dorsum of the wrist. Activity associated with flexion, extension, and ulnar deviation of the carpometacarpal joints exacerbates the pain, whereas rest and heat provide some relief. The pain is constant and is characterized as aching in nature; it may interfere with sleep. Some patients complain of a grating or popping sensation with use of the joint, and crepitus may be present on physical examination.

In addition to pain, patients suffering from arthritis of the carpometacarpal joint often experience a gradual reduction in functional ability because of decreasing pinch and grip strength, making everyday tasks such as using a pencil or opening a jar quite difficult (Fig. 42-2). With continued disuse, muscle wasting may occur, and adhesive capsulitis with subsequent ankylosis may develop.

TESTING

Plain radiographs are indicated in all patients who present with carpometacarpal pain. Based on the patient's clinical presentation, additional testing may be warranted, including a complete blood count, erythrocyte sedimentation rate, and antinuclear antibody testing. Magnetic resonance imaging (MRI) of the carpometacarpal joint is indicated if joint instability is thought to be present. If infection is suspected, Gram stain and culture of the synovial fluid should be performed on an emergency basis, and treatment with appropriate antibiotics should be started. If there is a history of trauma, MRI or radionuclide bone scanning may be useful (Fig. 42-3), because fractures of the navicular bone are often missed on plain radiographs of the wrist.

147

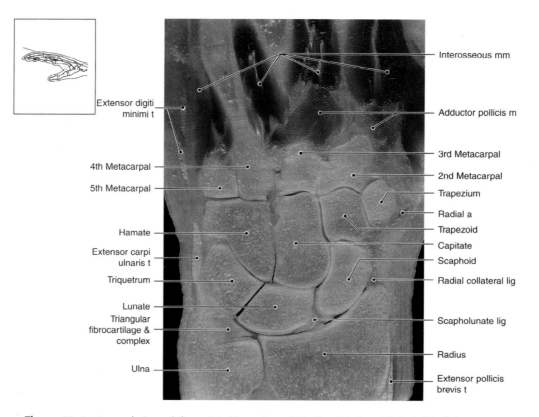

Figure 42–1. Coronal view of the wrist. (From Kang HS, Ahn JM, Resnick D: MRI of the Extremities: An Anatomic Atlas, 2nd ed. Philadelphia, Saunders, 2002, p 163.)

DIFFERENTIAL DIAGNOSIS

Arthritis pain of the carpometacarpal joints is usually diagnosed on clinical grounds, with plain radiographs confirming the clinical findings. Occasionally, arthritis pain of the carpometacarpal joints may be confused with de Quervain's tenosynovitis or other forms of tendinitis involving the wrist and fingers. These painful conditions, as well as gout, may coexist and make the diagnosis more difficult. If trauma is present, occult fractures of the metacarpals should always be considered.

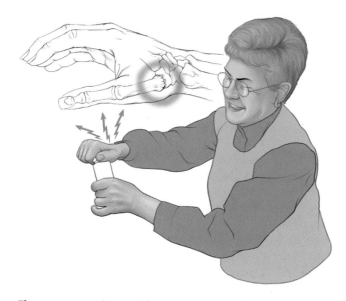

Figure 42–2. Arthritis of the carpometacarpal joints may cause pain and decreased grip strength.

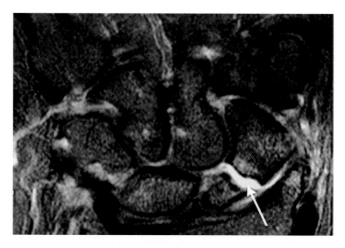

Figure 42–3. Coronal long TR/TE fast spin echo image with fat saturation shows nonunion of a proximal pole scaphoid fracture *(arrow)*, outlined by fluid signal in the fracture. (From Edelman RR, Hessellink JR, Zlatkin MB, Crues JV: Clinical Magnetic Resonance Imaging, 3rd ed. Philadelphia, Saunders, 2006, p 3344.)

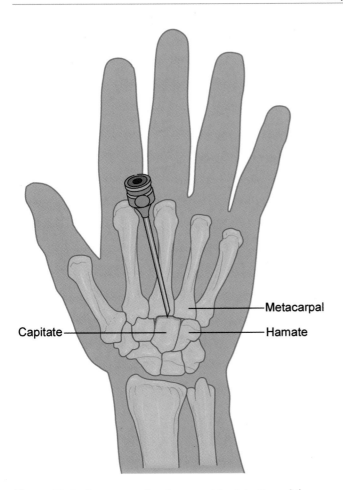

Capitate — Metacarpal — Hamate

Figure 42–4. Proper needle placement for injection of the carpometacarpal joints. (From Waldman SD: Atlas of Pain Management Injection Techniques. Philadelphia, Saunders, 2000.)

TREATMENT

Initial treatment of the pain and functional disability associated with osteoarthritis of the carpometacarpal joints includes a combination of nonsteroidal anti-inflammatory drugs or cyclooxygenase-2 inhibitors and physical therapy. Local application of heat and cold may also be beneficial. Splinting the wrist in the neutral position may provide symptomatic relief and protect the joint from additional trauma. For patients who do not respond to these treatment modalities, intra-articular injection of local anesthetic and steroid is a reasonable next step.

Intra-articular injection of the carpometacarpal joint is performed by placing the patient in the supine position with the arm fully adducted at the patient's side and the hand in a neutral position, with the palmar aspect resting on a folded towel. A total of 1.5 mL local anesthetic and 40 mg methylprednisolone is drawn up in a 5-mL sterile syringe. After sterile preparation of the skin overlying the affected carpometacarpal joint, the space between the carpal and metacarpal joints is identified. The joint can be more easily identified by gliding it back and forth. Using strict aseptic technique, a 1-inch, 25-gauge needle is inserted through the skin, subcutaneous tissues, and joint capsule and into the center of the joint (Fig. 42-4). If bone is encountered, the needle is withdrawn into the subcutaneous tissues and redirected medially. After entering the joint space, the contents of the syringe are gently injected. There should be little resistance to injection. If resistance is encountered, the needle is probably in a tendon and should be advanced slightly into the joint space until the injection can proceed without significant resistance. The needle is then removed, and a sterile pressure dressing and ice pack are applied to the injection site.

Physical modalities, including local heat and gentle range-of-motion exercises, should be introduced several days after the patient begins treatment for arthritis of the carpometacarpal joints. Vigorous exercises should be avoided, because they will exacerbate the patient's symptoms.

COMPLICATIONS AND PITFALLS

Joint protection is especially important in patients suffering from inflammatory arthritis of the carpometacarpal joints, because repetitive trauma can result in further damage to the joints, tendons, and connective tissues. The major complication associated with the intra-articular injection technique is infection, although it should be exceedingly rare if strict aseptic technique is followed. Approximately 25% of patients complain of a transient increase in pain after intra-articular injection of the carpometacarpal joints, and they should be warned of this possibility.

Clinical Pearls

The injection technique described is extremely effective in the treatment of arthritis pain of the carpometacarpal joints, and it is safe as long as careful attention is paid to the clinically relevant anatomy. Simple analgesics and nonsteroidal anti-inflammatory drugs can be used concurrently with the injection technique. Coexistent bursitis and tendinitis may contribute to the patient's pain, necessitating additional treatment with more localized injection of local anesthetic and methylprednisolone.

Section 7

Pain Syndromes of the Hand

Chapter 43

Trigger Thumb

ICD-9 CODE **727.03**

THE CLINICAL SYNDROME

Trigger thumb is caused by inflammation and swelling of the tendon of the flexor pollicis longus due to compression by the head of the first metacarpal bone. Sesamoid bones in this region may also compress and cause trauma to the tendon. Trauma is usually caused by repetitive motion or pressure on the tendon as it passes over these bony prominences. If the inflammation and swelling become chronic, the tendon sheath may thicken, resulting in constriction. Frequently, nodules develop on the tendon, and they can often be palpated when the patient flexes and extends the thumb. Such nodules may catch in the tendon sheath and produce a triggering phenomenon that causes the thumb to catch or lock. Trigger thumb occurs in patients engaged in repetitive activities, such as handshaking by politicians, or activities that require repetitive pinching movements of the thumb, such as playing video games or frequent card playing (Fig. 43-1).

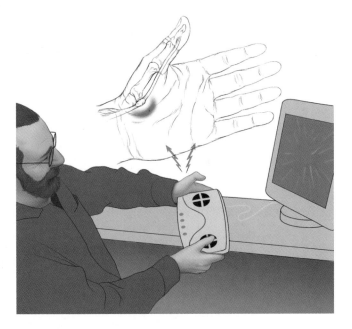

Figure 43–1. Trigger thumb is caused by microtrauma from repetitive pinching movements of the thumb.

SIGNS AND SYMPTOMS

The pain of trigger thumb is localized to the palmar aspect of the base of the thumb (unlike the pain of de Quervain's tenosynovitis, which is most pronounced more proximally, over the radial styloid). The pain of trigger thumb is constant and is made worse with active pinching of the thumb. Patients note the inability to hold a coffee cup or a pen. Sleep disturbance is common, and patients often awaken to find that the thumb has become locked in a flexed position.

On physical examination, tenderness and swelling are noted over the tendon, with maximal point tenderness over the base of the thumb. Many patients with trigger thumb experience a creaking sensation with flexion and extension of the thumb. Range of motion of the thumb may be decreased due to pain, and a triggering phenomenon may be present. As mentioned earlier, patients with trigger thumb often have nodules on the flexor pollicis longus tendon.

TESTING

Plain radiographs are indicated in all patients who present with trigger thumb to rule out occult bony pathology (Fig. 43-2). Based on the patient's clinical presentation, additional testing may be warranted, including a complete blood count, uric acid level, erythrocyte sedimentation rate, and antinuclear antibody testing. Magnetic resonance imaging of the hand is indicated if first metacarpal joint instability is suspected. The injection technique described later serves as both a diagnostic and a therapeutic maneuver.

DIFFERENTIAL DIAGNOSIS

The diagnosis of trigger thumb is usually made on clinical grounds. Arthritis or gout of the first metacarpal joint may accompany trigger thumb and exacerbate the patient's pain. The nidus of pain from trigger thumb is

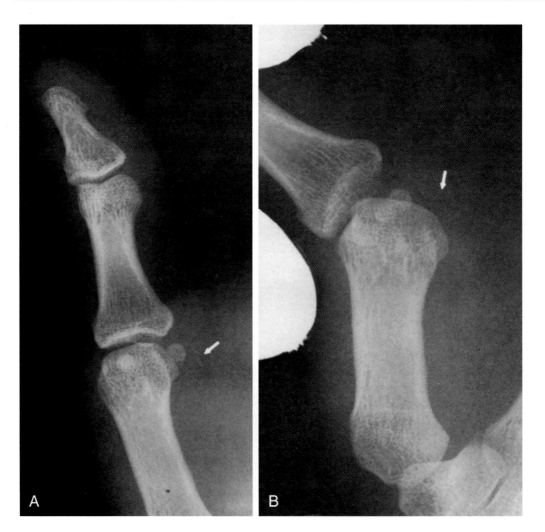

Figure 43–2. Gamekeeper's thumb. **A,** The initial radiograph outlines small osseous fragments adjacent to the first metacarpophalangeal joint *(arrow)*. **B,** A radiograph obtained during radial stress reveals subluxation of the phalanx on the metacarpal bone. The fracture fragments are shown *(arrow)*. (From Resnick D: Diagnosis of Bone and Joint Disorders, 4th ed. Philadelphia, Saunders, 2002, p 2583.)

the flexor pollicis longus tendon at the level of the base of the first metacarpal; occasionally, this may be confused with de Quervain's tenosynovitis.

TREATMENT

Initial treatment of the pain and functional disability associated with trigger thumb includes a combination of nonsteroidal anti-inflammatory drugs or cyclooxygenase-2 inhibitors and physical therapy. A quilter's glove to protect the thumb may also help relieve the patient's symptoms. If these treatments fail, the following injection technique is a reasonable next step.

Injection of trigger thumb is carried out by placing the patient in the supine position with the arm fully adducted at the patient's side and the dorsal surface of the hand resting on a folded towel. A total of 2 mL local

anesthetic and 40 mg methylprednisolone is drawn up in a 5-mL sterile syringe. After sterile preparation of the skin overlying the affected tendon, the metacarpophalangeal joint of the thumb is identified. Using strict aseptic technique, at a point just proximal to the joint, a 1-inch, 25-gauge needle is inserted at a 45-degree angle parallel to the affected tendon through the skin and into the subcutaneous tissue overlying the tendon. If bone is encountered, the needle is withdrawn into the subcutaneous tissue. The contents of the syringe is then gently injected. The tendon sheath should distend as the injection proceeds. There should be little resistance to injection; if resistance is encountered, the needle is probably in the tendon and should be withdrawn until the injection can be accomplished without significant resistance. The needle is then removed, and a sterile pressure dressing and ice pack are applied to the injection site.

Physical modalities, including local heat and gentle range-of-motion exercises, should be introduced several days after the patient undergoes injection. Vigorous exercises should be avoided, because they will exacerbate the patient's symptoms.

COMPLICATIONS AND PITFALLS

Failure to adequately treat trigger thumb early in its course can result in permanent pain and functional disability due to continued trauma to the tendon and tendon sheath. The major complications associated with injection are related to trauma to the inflamed and previously damaged tendon. The tendon may rupture if it is injected directly, so a needle position outside the tendon should be confirmed before proceeding with the injection. Further, the radial artery and superficial branch of the radial nerve are susceptible to damage if the needle is placed too far medially. Another complication of injection is infection, although it should be exceedingly rare if strict aseptic technique is followed. Approximately 25% of patients complain of a transient increase in pain after injection, and they should be warned of this possibility.

Clinical Pearls

The injection technique described is extremely effective in the treatment of pain secondary to trigger thumb. Coexistent arthritis and gout may contribute to the patient's pain, necessitating additional treatment with more localized injection of local anesthetic and methylprednisolone. The injection technique is safe if careful attention is paid to the clinically relevant anatomy, including the radial artery and the superficial branch of the radial nerve. De Quervain's tenosynovitis may be confused with trigger thumb, but it can be distinguished by the location of the pain and the motions that cause the triggering phenomenon.

Chapter 44

Trigger Finger

ICD-9 CODE 727.03

THE CLINICAL SYNDROME

Trigger finger is caused by inflammation and swelling of the tendon of the flexor digitorum superficialis due to compression by the head of the metacarpal bone. Sesamoid bones in this region may also compress and cause trauma to the tendon. Trauma is usually the result of repetitive motion or pressure on the tendon as it passes over these bony prominences. If the inflammation and swelling become chronic, the tendon sheath may thicken, resulting in constriction. Frequently, nodules develop on the tendon, and they can often be palpated when the patient flexes and extends the fingers. Such nodules may catch in the tendon sheath as they pass under a restraining tendon pulley, producing a triggering phenomenon that causes the finger to catch or lock. Trigger finger occurs in patients engaged in repetitive activities such as hammering, gripping a steering wheel, or holding a horse's reins too tightly (Fig. 44-1).

SIGNS AND SYMPTOMS

The pain of trigger finger is localized to the distal palm, and tender nodules can often be palpated. The pain is constant and is made worse with active gripping motions of the hand. Patients note significant stiffness when flexing the fingers. Sleep disturbance is common, and patients often awaken to find that the finger has become locked in a flexed position.

On physical examination, tenderness and swelling are noted over the tendon, with maximal point tenderness over the head of the metacarpal. Many patients with trigger finger experience a creaking sensation with flexion and extension of the fingers. Range of motion of the fingers may be decreased due to pain, and a triggering phenomenon may be noted. A catching tendon sign may also be elicited by having the patient clench the affected hand for 30 seconds and then relax but not open the hand. The examiner then passively extends the affected finger, and if he or she appreciates a locking,

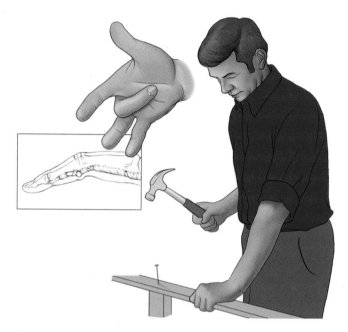

Figure 44–1. Trigger finger is caused by repetitive microtrauma from repeated clenching of the hand.

popping, or catching of the tendon as the finger is straightened, the sign is positive (Fig. 44-2).

TESTING

Plain radiographs are indicated in all patients who present with trigger finger to rule out occult bony pathology (Fig. 44-3). Based on the patient's clinical presentation, additional testing may be warranted, including a complete blood count, uric acid level, erythrocyte sedimentation rate, and antinuclear antibody testing. Magnetic resonance imaging of the hand is indicated if joint instability or some other abnormality is suspected. The injection technique described later serves as both a diagnostic and a therapeutic maneuver.

DIFFERENTIAL DIAGNOSIS

The diagnosis of trigger finger is usually made on clinical grounds. Arthritis or gout of the metacarpal or interphalangeal joints may accompany trigger finger and exacer-

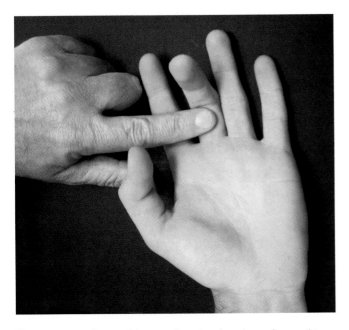

Figure 44–2. The catching tendon sign for trigger finger. (From Waldman SD: Physical Diagnosis of Pain: An Atlas of Signs and Symptoms. Philadelphia, Saunders, 2006, p 195.)

bate the patient's pain. Occult fractures occasionally confuse the clinical presentation.

TREATMENT

Initial treatment of the pain and functional disability associated with trigger finger includes a combination of nonsteroidal anti-inflammatory drugs or cyclooxygenase-2 inhibitors and physical therapy. A nighttime splint to protect the fingers may also help relieve the symptoms. If these treatments fail, the following injection technique is a reasonable next step.

Injection of trigger finger is carried out by placing the patient in the supine position with the arm fully adducted at the patient's side and the dorsal surface of the hand resting on a folded towel. A total of 2 mL local anesthetic and 40 mg methylprednisolone is drawn up in a 5-mL sterile syringe. After sterile preparation of the skin overlying the affected tendon, the head of the metacarpal beneath the tendon is identified. Using strict aseptic technique, at a point just proximal to the joint, a 1-inch, 25-gauge needle is inserted at a 45-degree angle parallel to the affected tendon through the skin and into the subcutaneous tissue overlying the tendon. If bone is encountered, the needle is withdrawn into the subcutaneous tissue. The contents of the syringe is then gently injected. The tendon sheath should distend as the injection proceeds. There should be little resistance to injection; if resistance is encountered, the needle is probably in the tendon and should be withdrawn until the injection can be accomplished without significant resistance. The needle is then removed, and a sterile pressure dressing and ice pack are applied to the injection site.

Physical modalities, including local heat and gentle range-of-motion exercises, should be introduced several days after the patient undergoes injection. Vigorous exercises should be avoided, because they will exacerbate the patient's symptoms.

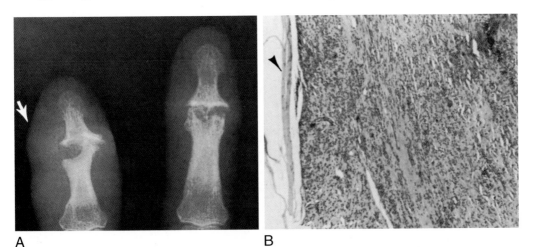

A   B

Figure 44–3. Giant cell tumor of the tendon sheath. **A,** In this 55-year-old woman with a 2-year history of pain and gradual swelling of the fingers, a soft tissue mass (arrow) can be identified at one distal interphalangeal joint. Underlying inflammatory osteoarthritis of the articulations is evident, and this combination of findings would suggest that the mass is a mucous cyst. However, biopsy of the affected joint demonstrated a giant cell tumor of the tendon sheath. **B,** Photomicrograph (×86) in a different patient reveals a tendon capsule tumor (arrowhead) associated with moderately vascularized stroma, plump spindle-shaped or ovoid cells, and multinucleated giant cells. (From Resnick D: Diagnosis of Bone and Joint Disorders, 4th ed. Philadelphia, Saunders, 2002, p 4248.)

Surgical treatment should be considered for patients who fail to respond to the aforementioned treatment modalities.

COMPLICATIONS AND PITFALLS

Failure to adequately treat trigger finger early in its course can result in permanent pain and functional disability due to continued trauma to the tendon and tendon sheath. The major complications associated with injection are related to trauma to the inflamed and previously damaged tendon. The tendon may rupture if it is injected directly, so a needle position outside the tendon should be confirmed before proceeding with the injection. Further, the radial artery and superficial branch of the radial nerve are susceptible to damage if the needle is placed too far medially. Another complication of injection is infection, although it should be exceedingly rare if strict aseptic technique is used, along with universal precautions to minimize any risk to the operator. The incidence of ecchymosis and hematoma formation can be decreased if pressure is applied to the injection site immediately after injection. Approximately 25% of patients complain of a transient increase in pain after injection, and they should be warned of this possibility.

Clinical Pearls

The injection technique described is extremely effective in the treatment of pain secondary to trigger finger. Coexistent arthritis or gout may contribute to the patient's pain, necessitating additional treatment with more localized injection of local anesthetic and methylprednisolone. A hand splint to protect the fingers may also help relieve the symptoms of trigger finger. Simple analgesics and nonsteroidal anti-inflammatory drugs can be used concurrently with the injection technique.

Chapter 45

Ganglion Cysts of the Hand and Wrist

ICD-9 CODE 727.41

THE CLINICAL SYNDROME

The dorsum of the wrist is especially susceptible to the development of ganglion cysts. These cysts usually occur in the area overlying the extensor tendons or the joint space, with a predilection for the joint space of the lunate or the tendon sheath of the extensor carpi radialis (Fig. 45-1). Ganglion cysts are thought to result from the herniation of synovium-containing tissue from the joint capsules or tendon sheaths. This tissue then becomes irritated and begins to produce increasing amounts of synovial fluid, which can pool in cystlike cavities overlying the tendons and joint space. A one-way valve phenomenon may cause these cystlike cavities to expand because the fluid cannot flow back into the synovial cavity. Although the dorsum of the wrist is the most common site, ganglion cysts can appear overlying any synovial joint.

SIGNS AND SYMPTOMS

Activity, especially extreme flexion and extension, makes the pain worse, whereas rest and heat provide some relief. The pain is constant and is characterized as aching in nature. However, it is often the unsightly nature of the ganglion cyst rather than the pain that causes the patient to seek medical attention. The ganglion is smooth to palpation and transilluminates with a penlight, in contradistinction to solid tumors, which do not transilluminate. Palpation of the ganglion may increase the pain.

TESTING

Plain radiographs of the wrist are indicated in all patients who present with ganglion cysts to rule out bony abnormalities, including tumors. Based on the patient's clinical presentation, additional testing may be warranted, including a complete blood count, erythrocyte sedimentation

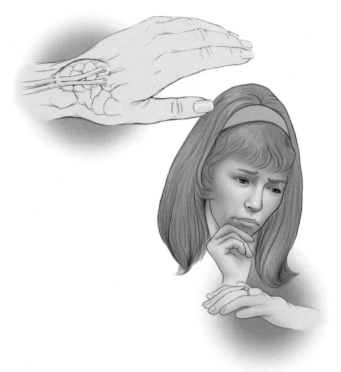

Figure 45–1. Ganglion cysts usually appear on the dorsum of the wrist, overlying the extensor tendon or joint space. Patients often seek medical attention out of a fear of cancer.

rate, and antinuclear antibody testing. Magnetic resonance imaging (MRI) of the wrist is indicated if the cause of the mass is suspect (Fig. 45-2).

DIFFERENTIAL DIAGNOSIS

Ganglion cysts of the wrist and hand generally present in a clinically distinct manner, making diagnosis easy. However, coexistent bursitis and tendinitis may confuse the clinical picture if the ganglion cyst is small. Noncystic masses should always undergo MRI to rule out primary or metastatic tumor.

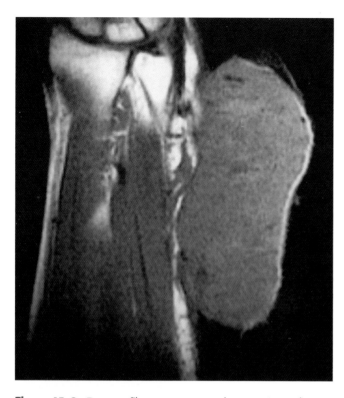

Figure 45-2. Dermatofibrosarcoma protuberans. Coronal T1-weighted spin echo magnetic resonance image in a 31-year-old man shows a large polypoid lesion in the ulnar aspect of the forearm. The signal intensity is similar to that of muscle. (From Resnick D: Diagnosis of Bone and Joint Disorders, 4th ed. Philadelphia, Saunders, 2002, p 4186.)

TREATMENT

Initial treatment of the pain and functional disability associated with ganglion cysts includes a combination of nonsteroidal anti-inflammatory drugs or cyclooxygenase-2 inhibitors and physical therapy. A nighttime splint to protect the fingers may also help relieve the symptoms. If the patient does not respond to these conservative measures, a trial of injection therapy with local anesthetic and steroid is a reasonable next step.

To inject a ganglion cyst, the patient is placed in the supine position with the arm fully adducted at the patient's side, the elbow slightly flexed, and the palm of the hand resting on a folded towel. A total of 1.5 mL local anesthetic and 40 mg methylprednisolone is drawn up in a 5-mL sterile syringe. After sterile preparation of the skin overlying the ganglion, a 1-inch, 22-gauge needle is inserted in the center of the ganglion, and the contents of the cyst are aspirated. If bone is encountered, the needle is withdrawn into the ganglion cyst, and aspiration is carried out. After aspiration, the contents of the syringe are gently injected. There should be little resistance to injection. The needle is then removed, and a sterile pressure dressing and ice pack are applied to the injection site.

Physical modalities, including local heat and gentle range-of-motion exercises, should be introduced several days after the patient undergoes injection. Vigorous exercises should be avoided, because they will exacerbate the patient's symptoms.

If the ganglion cyst reappears, surgical treatment may ultimately be required.

COMPLICATIONS AND PITFALLS

The injection technique is safe if careful attention is paid to the clinically relevant anatomy. Care must be taken to avoid injecting directly into the tendon, which may already be inflamed and irritated from the ganglion rubbing against it. Sterile technique must be used to avoid infection, as well as universal precautions to minimize any risk to the operator. The incidence of ecchymosis and hematoma formation can be decreased if pressure is applied to the injection site immediately after injection. The major complication of ganglion cyst injection is infection, although it should be exceedingly rare if strict aseptic technique is followed.

Clinical Pearls

An initial trial of conservative therapy is indicated for ganglion cysts. It this fails, the injection technique described is extremely effective in the treatment of pain secondary to ganglion cysts. Coexistent bursitis and tendinitis may contribute to wrist pain, necessitating additional treatment with more localized injection of local anesthetic and methylprednisolone. Simple analgesics and nonsteroidal anti-inflammatory drugs can be used concurrently with the injection technique. Ultimately, however, ganglion cysts of the wrist and hand often require surgical treatment.

Chapter 46

Sesamoiditis of the Hand

ICD-9 CODE 733.99

THE CLINICAL SYNDROME

Sesamoid bones are small, rounded structures embedded in the flexor tendons of the hand, usually in close proximity to the joints. These bones serve to decrease the friction and pressure of the flexor tendon as it passes in proximity to a joint. Sesamoid bones of the thumb occur in almost all patients suffering from sesamoiditis, and they are present in the flexor tendons of the index finger in a small number of patients.

Sesamoiditis is characterized by tenderness and pain over the flexor aspect of the thumb or, much less commonly, the index finger (Fig. 46-1). The patient often feels that he or she has a foreign body embedded in the affected digit when grasping something. The pain of sesamoiditis worsens with repeated flexion and extension of the affected digit. When the thumb is affected, it is usually on the radial side, where the condyle of the adjacent metacarpal is less obtrusive. Patients suffering from psoriatic arthritis may have a higher incidence of sesamoiditis of the hand.

SIGNS AND SYMPTOMS

On physical examination, pain can be reproduced by pressure on the sesamoid bone. With sesamoiditis, the tender area moves with the flexor tendon when the patient actively flexes the thumb or finger, whereas with occult bony pathology of the phalanges, the tender area remains over the pathologic area. With acute trauma to the sesamoid, ecchymosis over the flexor surface of the affected digit may be present.

TESTING

Plain radiographs (Fig. 46-2) and magnetic resonance imaging (MRI) are indicated in all patients who present with sesamoiditis to rule out fractures and identify sesa-

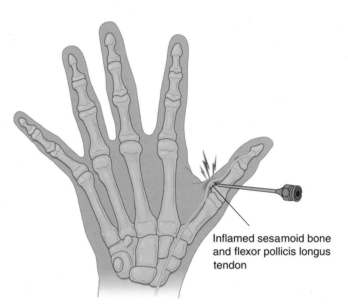

Inflamed sesamoid bone and flexor pollicis longus tendon

Figure 46–1. Sesamoiditis is characterized by tenderness and pain over the flexor aspect of the thumb. (From Waldman SD: Atlas of Pain Management Injection Techniques, 2nd ed. Philadelphia, Saunders, 2007, p 238.)

moid bones that may have become inflamed. Based on the patient's clinical presentation, additional testing may be warranted, including a complete blood count, erythrocyte sedimentation rate, and antinuclear antibody testing. MRI of the fingers and wrist is indicated if joint instability, occult mass, occult fracture, infection, or tumor is suspected. Radionuclide bone scanning may be useful to identify stress fractures of the thumb and fingers or sesamoid bones that might be missed on plain radiographs of the hand.

DIFFERENTIAL DIAGNOSIS

The tentative diagnosis of sesamoiditis is made on clinical grounds and confirmed by radiographic testing. Arthritis, tenosynovitis, or gout of the affected digit may accompany sesamoiditis and exacerbate the patient's

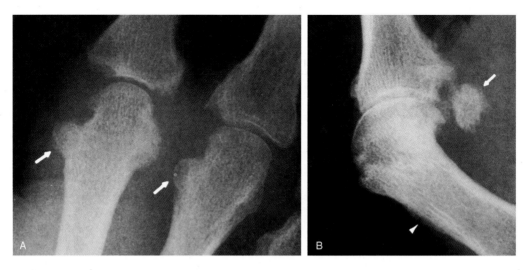

Figure 46–2. Radiographic abnormalities of the metacarpophalangeal joints. **A,** Startling osseous excrescences *(arrows)* around the metacarpal heads are associated with soft tissue swelling, joint space narrowing, and bony erosion and proliferation in the phalanges. **B,** At the first metacarpophalangeal joint, irregular bone formation in the metacarpal head, proximal phalanx, and adjacent sesamoid *(arrow)* can be seen. Periostitis of the metacarpal diaphysis is also evident *(arrowhead).* (From Resnick D: Diagnosis of Bone and Joint Disorders, 4th ed. Philadelphia, Saunders, 2002, p 1087.)

pain. Occult fractures occasionally confuse the clinical presentation.

TREATMENT

Initial treatment of the pain and functional disability associated with sesamoiditis of the hand includes a combination of nonsteroidal anti-inflammatory drugs or cyclooxygenase-2 inhibitors and physical therapy. A nighttime splint to protect the fingers may also help relieve the symptoms. If the patient does not respond to these conservative measures, a trial of injection therapy with local anesthetic and steroid is a reasonable next step.

To perform injection of the sesamoid bone, the patient is placed in the supine position with the palmar surface of the hand exposed. The skin overlying the tender sesamoid bone is prepared with antiseptic solution. A sterile syringe containing 2 mL of 0.25% preservative-free bupivacaine and 40 mg methylprednisolone is attached to a $\frac{5}{8}$-inch, 25-gauge needle using strict aseptic technique. The needle is carefully advanced through the palmar surface of the affected digit until the needle tip rests against the sesamoid bone (see Fig. 46-1). The needle is then withdrawn slightly out of the periosteum and substance of the tendon. Once the needle is in the correct position next to the affected sesamoid bone and aspiration for blood is negative, the contents of the syringe is

gently injected. There may be slight resistance to injection, given the closed nature of the space. If significant resistance is encountered, the needle is probably in a ligament or tendon and should be advanced or withdrawn slightly until the injection can proceed without significant resistance. The needle is then removed, and a sterile pressure dressing and ice pack are applied to the injection site. The ice should not be left on for longer than 10 minutes to avoid freezing injuries.

Physical modalities, including local heat and gentle range-of-motion exercises, should be introduced several days after the patient undergoes injection. Vigorous exercises should be avoided, because they will exacerbate the patient's symptoms.

COMPLICATIONS AND PITFALLS

The injection technique is safe if careful attention is paid to the clinically relevant anatomy. The major complication of injection is infection, which should be exceedingly rare if strict aseptic technique is followed; in addition, universal precautions should be used to minimize any risk to the operator. The incidence of ecchymosis and hematoma formation can be decreased if pressure is applied to the injection site immediately after injection. Approximately 25% of patients complain of a transient increase in pain after injection of sesamoid bones, and they should be warned of this possibility.

Clinical Pearls

Pain emanating from the hand is a common problem. Sesamoiditis must be distinguished from stress fractures and other occult pathology of the phalanges, as well as fractures of the sesamoid bones. Although the injection technique described provides pain relief, patients often require resting hand splints to aid in rehabilitation of the affected finger. Padded gloves may be useful to take pressure off the affected sesamoid bone and overlying soft tissue. Coexisting bursitis and tendinitis may contribute to the patient's pain, necessitating additional treatment with more localized injection of local anesthetic and steroid. Simple analgesics and nonsteroidal anti-inflammatory agents can be used concurrently with the injection technique.

Chapter 47

Plastic Bag Palsy

ICD-9 CODE 354.9

THE CLINICAL SYNDROME

Plastic bag palsy is an entrapment neuropathy of the digital nerves caused by compression of the nerves against the bony phalanges by the handles of a plastic bag. The common digital nerves arise from fibers of the median and ulnar nerves. The thumb also has contributions from superficial branches of the radial nerve. The common digital nerves pass along the metacarpal bones and divide as they reach the distal palm. The volar digital nerves supply the majority of sensory innervation to the fingers and run along the ventrolateral aspect of the finger beside the digital vein and artery. The smaller dorsal digital nerves contain fibers from the ulnar and radial nerves and supply the dorsum of the fingers as far as the proximal joints.

Plastic bag palsy has increased in frequency as stores have switched from paper bags to plastic ones. Compression by the handles of a heavy plastic bag is the inciting cause, and the most common clinical feature is the presence of painful digital nerves at the point of compression (Fig. 47-1). Plastic bag palsy may present in either an acute or a chronic form. Pain may develop from an acute injury to the nerves after carrying a heavy bag on too few fingers, or it may occur from direct trauma to the soft tissues overlying the digital nerves if the fingers get caught in a bag handle twisted around them. Plastic bag palsy is occasionally seen in homeless people who carry their possessions around in bags, using the same hand day after day. The affected nerves may be thickened, and inflammation of the nerve and overlying soft tissues may be seen. In addition to pain, patients may complain of paresthesias and numbness just below the point of nerve compromise.

SIGNS AND SYMPTOMS

The pain of plastic bag palsy is constant and is made worse with compression of the affected digital nerves. Patients often note the inability to hold objects with the affected fingers. Sleep disturbance is common.

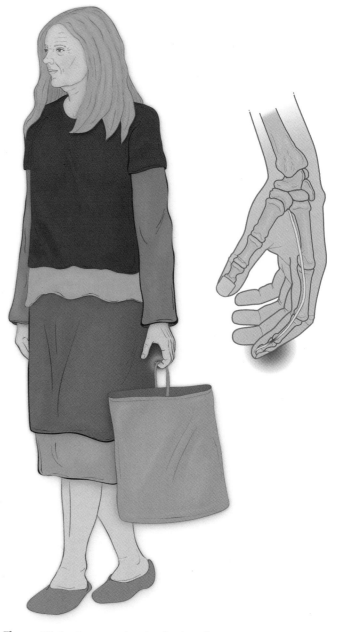

Figure 47–1. Compression by the handles of a heavy plastic bag can cause plastic bag palsy.

On physical examination, there is tenderness to palpation of the affected digital nerves. Palpation can also cause paresthesias, and continued pressure on the nerves may induce numbness distal to the point of compression. Range of motion of the thumb is normal. With acute trauma to the sesamoid, ecchymosis of the skin overlying the affected digital nerves may be present.

TESTING

Plain radiographs are indicated in all patients who present with plastic bag palsy to rule out occult bony pathology such as bone spurs or cysts that may be compressing the digital nerves. Electromyography can distinguish other causes of hand numbness. Based on the patient's clinical presentation, additional testing may be indicated, including a complete blood count, uric acid level, erythrocyte sedimentation rate, and antinuclear antibody testing. Magnetic resonance imaging of the hand can rule out soft tissue tumors that may be compressing the digital nerves (Fig. 47-2). Injection of the nerve serves as both a diagnostic and a therapeutic maneuver.

DIFFERENTIAL DIAGNOSIS

The tentative diagnosis of plastic bag palsy is made on clinical grounds and confirmed by electromyography. Arthritis, tenosynovitis, or gout of the affected digits may accompany plastic bag palsy and exacerbate the patient's pain. Occult fractures occasionally confuse the clinical presentation.

TREATMENT

The first step in the treatment of the pain and functional disability associated with plastic bag palsy is to remove the offending compression of the digital nerves. Nonsteroidal anti-inflammatory drugs, simple analgesics, or cyclooxygenase-2 inhibitors may be prescribed as well. If the patient complains of significant dysesthesias or paresthesias, the addition of gabapentin should be considered. Gabapentin is started at a bedtime dose of 300 mg; it is then titrated upward to 3600 mg in divided doses, as side effects allow. Physical modalities, including local heat and gentle range-of-motion exercises, should be introduced to avoid loss of function. Vigorous exercises should be avoided, because they will exacerbate the patient's symptoms. A nighttime splint to protect the fingers may be helpful, and wearing padded gloves can take pressure off the affected digital nerves and overlying soft tissue. If sleep disturbance is present, low-dose tricyclic antidepressants are indicated. If the patient does not respond to these conservative modalities, a trial of injection therapy with local anesthetic and steroid is a reasonable next step. Rarely, surgical exploration and neuroplasty of the affected nerves are required for symptomatic relief.

COMPLICATIONS AND PITFALLS

Injection of the affected digital nerves is safe if careful attention is paid to the clinically relevant anatomy. Sterile technique must be used to avoid infection, as well as universal precautions to minimize any risk to the operator. The incidence of ecchymosis and hematoma formation can be decreased if pressure is applied to the injection site immediately after injection. The major complication of injection is infection, which should be exceedingly rare if strict aseptic technique is followed. Approximately 25% of patients complain of a transient increase in pain after injection of the affected digital nerves, and they should be warned of this possibility.

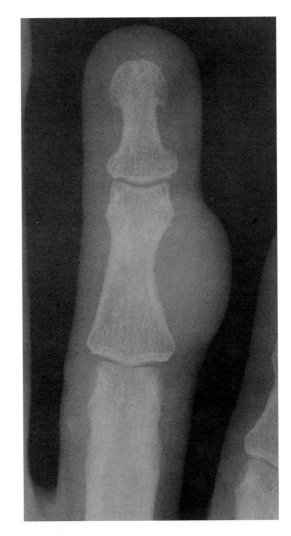

Figure 47-2. Fibrous xanthoma. A soft tissue mass adjacent to the middle phalanx has produced erosion of the adjacent bone. This pattern of bony resorption is indicative of pressure atrophy and is not a sign of malignancy. (From Resnick D: Diagnosis of Bone and Joint Disorders, 4th ed. Philadelphia, Saunders, 2002, p 4190.)

Clinical Pearls

Pain emanating from the hand is a common problem. Plastic bag palsy must be distinguished from stress fractures and other occult pathology of the phalanges, as well as sesamoiditis and occult fractures of the sesamoid bones. Coexistent bursitis and tendinitis may contribute to the patient's pain, necessitating additional treatment with more localized injection of local anesthetic and steroid.

Chapter 48

Carpal Boss Syndrome

ICD-9 CODE 726.4

THE CLINICAL SYNDROME

Carpal boss syndrome, or os styloideum, is characterized by localized tenderness and sharp pain over the junction of the second and third carpometacarpal joints (Fig. 48-1). The pain of carpal boss is due to exostosis of the second and third carpometacarpal joints or, more uncommonly, a loose body involving the intra-articular space (Fig. 48-2). Patients often report that the pain is worse *after* rigorous physical activity involving the hand rather than during the activity itself. The pain of carpal boss may also radiate locally, confusing the clinical presentation.

SIGNS AND SYMPTOMS

On physical examination, pain can be reproduced by applying pressure to the soft tissue overlying the carpal boss. Patients with carpal boss demonstrate a positive hunchback sign; that is, the examiner can appreciate a bony prominence when he or she palpates the carpal boss (Fig. 48-3). With acute trauma to the dorsum of the hand, ecchymosis over the carpal boss of the affected joint or joints may be present.

TESTING

Plain radiographs are indicated in all patients who present with carpal boss to rule out fractures and identify exostoses responsible for the symptoms (see Fig. 48-2). Based on the patient's clinical presentation, additional testing may be warranted to rule out inflammatory arthritis, including a complete blood count, erythrocyte sedimentation rate, uric acid level, and antinuclear antibody testing. Magnetic resonance imaging of the fingers and wrist is indicated if joint instability, occult mass, occult fracture, infection, or tumor is suspected. Radionuclide bone scanning may be useful to identify stress fractures.

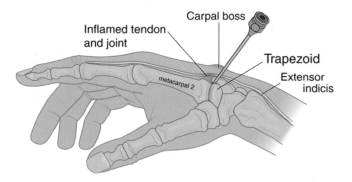

Figure 48–1. Carpal boss, or os styloideum, is characterized by localized tenderness and sharp pain over the junction of the second and third carpometacarpal joints. (From Waldman SD: Atlas of Pain Management Injection Techniques, 2nd ed. Philadelphia, Saunders, 2007, p 268.)

DIFFERENTIAL DIAGNOSIS

The tentative diagnosis of carpal boss is made on clinical grounds and confirmed by radiographic testing. Arthritis, tenosynovitis, or gout of the affected digits may accompany carpal boss and exacerbate the patient's pain. Occult fractures occasionally confuse the clinical presentation.

TREATMENT

Initial treatment of the pain and functional disability associated with carpal boss consists of nonsteroidal anti-inflammatory drugs, simple analgesics, or cyclooxygenase-2 inhibitors. Physical modalities, including local heat and gentle range-of-motion exercises, should be introduced to avoid loss of function. Vigorous exercises should be avoided, because they will exacerbate the patient's symptoms. A nighttime splint to protect the fingers may be helpful. If sleep disturbance is present, low-dose tricyclic antidepressants are indicated. If the patient does not respond to these conservative modalities, a trial of injection therapy with local anesthetic and steroid is a reasonable next step. Rarely, surgical

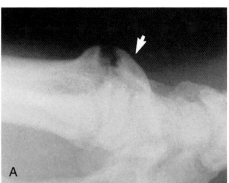

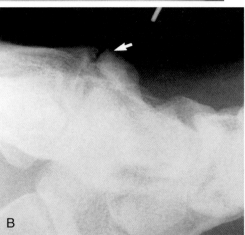

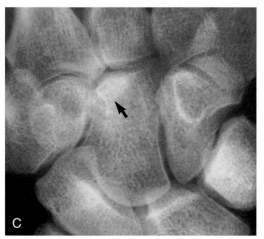

Figure 48–2. Radiographic manifestations of os styloideum. A lateral radiograph of the hand **(A)** demonstrates the "osteophytic" appearance of the extra ossification center *(arrow)*. Clinically, a painless soft tissue lump is often evident. In another patient, a similar outgrowth *(arrows)* is evident on lateral **(B)** and frontal **(C)** radiographs. (From Resnick D: Diagnosis of Bone and Joint Disorders, 4th ed. Philadelphia, Saunders, 2002, p 1312.)

exploration and removal of the carpal boss are required for symptomatic relief.

COMPLICATIONS AND PITFALLS

The major complication of injection with local anesthetic and steroid is infection, which should be exceedingly rare if strict aseptic technique is followed. Approximately 25% of patients complain of a transient increase in pain after injection, and they should be warned of this possibility. The clinician should always keep in mind that occult fracture or tumor may mimic the clinical symptoms of carpal boss.

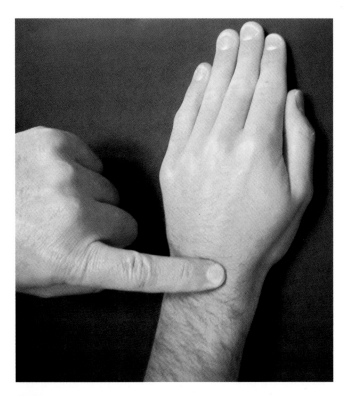

Figure 48–3. The hunchback sign for carpal boss. (From Waldman SD: Physical Diagnosis of Pain: An Atlas of Signs and Symptoms. Philadelphia, Saunders, 2006, p 189.)

Clinical Pearls

Pain emanating from the hand is a common problem. Carpal boss must be distinguished from stress fracture, arthritis, and other occult pathology of the wrist and hand. Although injection with local anesthetic and steroid palliates the pain of carpal boss, patients may ultimately require surgical removal of the exostosis to obtain long-lasting relief. Coexistent bursitis and tendinitis may contribute to the patient's pain, necessitating additional treatment with more localized injection of local anesthetic and steroid.

Chapter 49

Dupuytren's Contracture

ICD-9 CODE 728.6

THE CLINICAL SYNDROME

Dupuytren's contracture is a common complaint. Although it is initially painful, the pain seems to decrease as the condition progresses. As a result, patients suffering from Dupuytren's contracture generally seek medical attention owing to functional disability rather than pain.

Dupuytren's contracture is caused by progressive fibrosis of the palmar fascia. Initially, the patient may notice fibrotic nodules along the course of the flexor tendons of the hand that are tender to palpation. As the disease advances, these nodules coalesce and form fibrous bands that gradually thicken and contract around the flexor tendons; this has the effect of drawing the affected fingers into flexion. Although any finger can develop Dupuytren's contracture, the ring and little fingers are most commonly affected (Fig. 49-1). If untreated, the fingers can develop permanent flexion contractures. The plantar fascia may be affected concurrently.

Dupuytren's contracture is thought to have a genetic basis and occurs most frequently in males of northern Scandinavian descent. The disease may also be associated with trauma to the palm, diabetes, alcoholism, and chronic barbiturate use. The disease rarely occurs before the fourth decade.

SIGNS AND SYMPTOMS

In the early stages of the disease, hard fibrotic nodules along the path of the flexor tendons can be palpated. These nodules are often misdiagnosed as calluses or warts. At this early stage, pain is invariably present. As the disease progresses, taut fibrous bands form; they may cross the metacarpophalangeal joint and ultimately the proximal interphalangeal joint (Fig. 49-2). These bands are not painful to palpation, and although they limit finger extension, finger flexion remains relatively normal. It is at this point that patients often seek medical advice

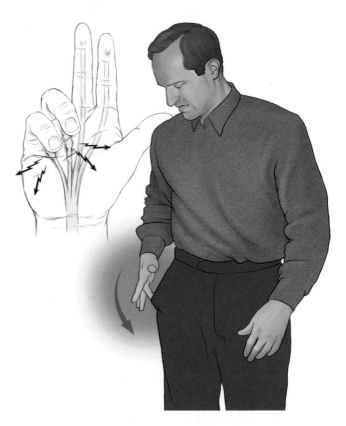

Figure 49–1. Dupuytren's contracture usually affects the fourth and fifth digits in men older than 40 years.

because of difficulty putting on gloves and reaching into their pockets. In the final stages of the disease, flexion contracture develops, with its negative impact on function. Arthritis, gout of the metacarpal and interphalangeal joints, and trigger finger may coexist with Dupuytren's contracture and exacerbate the patient's pain and disability.

TESTING

Plain radiographs are indicated for all patients who present with Dupuytren's contracture to rule out occult bony pathology (Fig. 49-3). Based on the patient's clinical presentation, additional testing may be warranted,

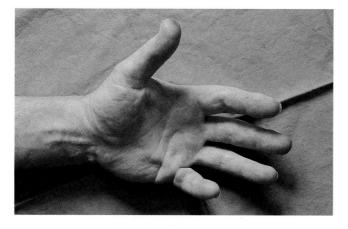

Figure 49–2. Dupuytren's contracture of the palmar fascia. (From Klippel JH, Dieppe PA: Rheumatology, 2nd ed. London, Mosby, 1998, p 4-9.7.)

including a complete blood count, uric acid level, erythrocyte sedimentation rate, and antinuclear antibody testing. Magnetic resonance imaging of the hand is indicated if joint instability or tumor is suspected. Electromyography is indicated if coexistent ulnar or carpal tunnel syndrome is suspected.

DIFFERENTIAL DIAGNOSIS

Dupuytren's contracture is a clinically distinct entity that is rarely misdiagnosed once the syndrome is well established. Coexisting flexor tendinitis or trigger finger may be confused with Dupuytren's contracture early in the course of the disease.

TREATMENT

Initial treatment of the pain and functional disability associated with Dupuytren's contracture includes a combination of nonsteroidal anti-inflammatory drugs or cyclooxygenase-2 inhibitors and physical therapy. A nighttime splint to protect the fingers may be helpful. If greater symptomatic relief is required, the following injection technique is a reasonable next step.

Injection of Dupuytren's contracture is carried out by placing the patient in the supine position with the arm fully adducted at the patient's side and the dorsal surface of the hand resting on a folded towel. A total of 2 mL local anesthetic and 40 mg methylprednisolone is drawn up in a 5-mL sterile syringe. The skin overlying the fibrous band or nodule is prepared with antiseptic solution. At a point just lateral to the fibrosis, a 1-inch, 25-gauge needle is inserted at a 45-degree angle parallel to the fibrosis, through the skin, and into the subcutaneous tissue overlying the fibrotic area. If bone is encountered, the needle is withdrawn into the subcutaneous tissue and advanced again in proximity to the fibrosis. The contents of the syringe is then gently injected. There may be some resistance to injection due to fibrosis of the surrounding tissue. If significant resistance is encountered, the needle is probably in the tendon or

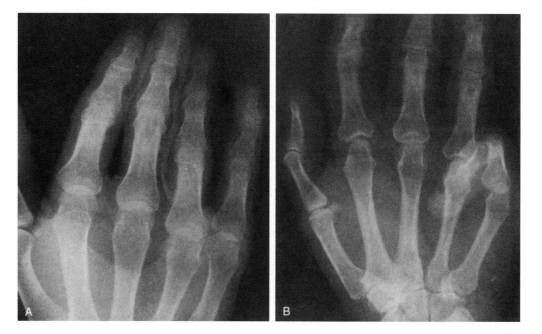

Figure 49–3. Radiographic manifestations of Dupuytren's contracture. **A,** Flexion deformities of the metacarpophalangeal joints of the four ulnar digits are demonstrated. **B,** Severe flexion contracture is evident in the fifth finger, with minor changes in the other digits. (From Resnick D: Diagnosis of Bone and Joint Disorders, 4th ed. Philadelphia, Saunders, 2002, p 4667.)

nodule and should be withdrawn until the injection can proceed without significant resistance. The needle is then removed, and a sterile pressure dressing and ice pack are applied to the injection site.

Physical modalities, including local heat and gentle range-of-motion exercises, should be introduced several days after the patient undergoes injection. Vigorous exercises should be avoided, because they will exacerbate the patient's symptoms.

Although these treatment modalities provide symptomatic relief, Dupuytren's contracture usually requires surgical treatment.

COMPLICATIONS AND PITFALLS

The injection technique is safe if careful attention is paid to the clinically relevant anatomy. Sterile technique must be used to avoid infection, as well as universal precautions to minimize any risk to the operator. The incidence of ecchymosis and hematoma formation can be decreased if pressure is applied to the injection site immediately after injection. The major complications associated with injection are related to trauma to an inflamed or previ-

ously damaged tendon. Such tendons may rupture if they are injected directly, so a needle position outside the tendon should be confirmed before proceeding with the injection. Another complication of injection is infection, although it should be exceedingly rare if strict aseptic technique is followed. Approximately 25% of patients complain of a transient increase in pain after injection, and they should be warned of this possibility.

Clinical Pearls

The aforementioned treatment modalities are useful in providing symptomatic relief of the pain and disability of Dupuytren's contracture. However, most patients ultimately require surgical treatment. Co-existent arthritis or gout may contribute to the patient's pain, necessitating additional treatment with more localized injection of local anesthetic and methylprednisolone. Simple analgesics and nonsteroidal anti-inflammatory drugs can be used concurrently with this injection technique.

Pain Syndromes of the Chest Wall

Chapter 50

Costosternal Syndrome

ICD-9 CODE **733.6**

THE CLINICAL SYNDROME

A significant number of patients with noncardiogenic chest pain are suffering from costosternal joint pain. Most commonly, the costosternal joints become painful due to inflammation as a result of overuse or misuse or due to trauma secondary to acceleration-deceleration injuries or blunt trauma to the chest wall (Fig. 50-1). With severe trauma, the joints may subluxate or dislocate. The costosternal joints are susceptible to the development of osteoarthritis, rheumatoid arthritis, ankylosing spondylitis, Reiter's syndrome, and psoriatic arthritis. The joints are also subject to invasion by tumor from primary malignancies, including thymoma, or from metastatic disease.

SIGNS AND SYMPTOMS

Physical examination reveals that the patient vigorously attempts to splint the joints by keeping the shoulders stiffly in a neutral position. Pain is reproduced with active protraction or retraction of the shoulder, deep inspiration, and full elevation of the arm. Shrugging of the shoulder may also reproduce the pain. Coughing may be difficult, leading to inadequate pulmonary toilet in patients who have sustained trauma to the anterior chest wall. The costosternal joints and adjacent intercostal muscles may be tender to palpation. The patient may also complain of a clicking sensation with movement of the joint.

TESTING

Plain radiographs are indicated for all patients who present with pain that is thought to be emanating from the costosternal joints to rule out occult bony pathology, including tumor (Fig. 50-2). If trauma is present, radionuclide bone scanning may be useful to rule out occult

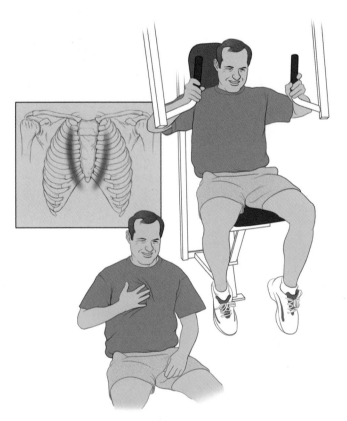

Figure 50–1. Irritation of the costosternal joints from overuse of exercise equipment can cause costosternal syndrome.

fractures of the ribs or sternum. Based on the patient's clinical presentation, additional testing may be indicated, including a complete blood count, prostate-specific antigen level, erythrocyte sedimentation rate, and antinuclear antibody testing. Laboratory evaluation for collagen vascular disease is indicated in patients suffering from costosternal joint pain if other joints are involved. Magnetic resonance imaging of the joints is indicated if joint instability or occult mass is suspected or to further elucidate the cause of the pain. The injection technique

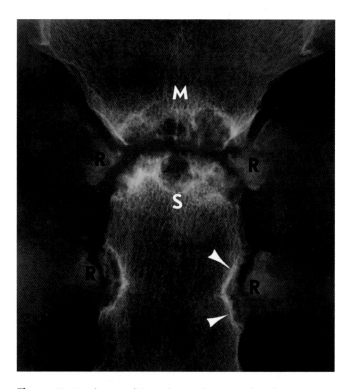

Figure 50-2. Abnormalities of manubriosternal and sternocostal joints in rheumatoid arthritis. Radiograph of a sternum from a cadaver with rheumatoid arthritis shows large erosions of the articular surface of both the manubrium (M) and the body of the sternum (S). Subtle irregularities of the second and third sternocostal joints are evident, most prominently in the sternal facet of the left third sternocostal joint *(arrowheads)*. R, ossified costal cartilage. (From Resnick D: Diagnosis of Bone and Joint Disorders, 4th ed. Philadelphia, Saunders, 2002, p 854.)

described later serves as both a diagnostic and a therapeutic maneuver.

DIFFERENTIAL DIAGNOSIS

As mentioned, the pain of costosternal syndrome is often mistaken for pain of cardiac origin, leading to visits to the emergency department and unnecessary cardiac workups. If trauma has occurred, costosternal syndrome may coexist with fractured ribs or fractures of the sternum itself, which can be missed on plain radiographs and may require radionuclide bone scanning for proper identification. Tietze's syndrome, which is painful enlargement of the upper costochondral cartilage associated with viral infection, may be confused with costosternal syndrome.

Neuropathic pain involving the chest wall may also be confused or coexist with costosternal syndrome. Examples of such neuropathic pain include diabetic polyneuropathies and acute herpes zoster involving the

thoracic nerves. Diseases of the structures of the mediastinum are possible and may be difficult to diagnose. Pathologic processes that inflame the pleura, such as pulmonary embolus, infection, and Bornholm disease, may also confuse the diagnosis and complicate treatment.

TREATMENT

Initial treatment of the pain and functional disability associated with costosternal syndrome includes a combination of nonsteroidal anti-inflammatory drugs or cyclooxygenase-2 inhibitors. The local application of heat and cold may also be beneficial. Use of an elastic rib belt may provide symptomatic relief and protect the costosternal joints from additional trauma. For patients who do not respond to these treatment modalities, injection with local anesthetic and steroid is a reasonable next step.

Intra-articular injection of the costosternal joint is performed by placing the patient in the supine position. The skin overlying the affected costosternal joints is prepared with antiseptic solution. A sterile syringe containing 1 mL of 0.25% preservative-free bupivacaine for each joint to be injected and 40 mg methylprednisolone is attached to a 1½-inch, 25-gauge needle using strict aseptic technique. The costosternal joints are identified; they should be easily palpable as a slight bulging at the point where the rib attaches to the sternum. The needle is then carefully advanced through the skin and subcutaneous tissues medially, with a slight cephalad trajectory, into proximity with the joint (Fig. 50-3). If bone is encountered, the needle is withdrawn from the periosteum. After the needle is in proximity to the joint, 1 mL of solution is gently injected. There should be limited resistance to injection. If significant resistance is encountered, the needle should be withdrawn slightly until the injection can proceed with only limited resistance. This procedure is repeated for each affected joint. The needle is then removed, and a sterile pressure dressing and ice pack are applied to the injection site.

Physical modalities, including local heat and gentle range-of-motion exercises, should be introduced several days after the patient undergoes injection for costosternal joint pain. Vigorous exercises should be avoided, because they will exacerbate the patient's symptoms. Simple analgesics and nonsteroidal anti-inflammatory drugs may be used concurrently with this injection technique.

COMPLICATIONS AND PITFALLS

Because many pathologic processes can mimic the pain of costosternal syndrome, the clinician must carefully rule out underlying cardiac disease and diseases of the

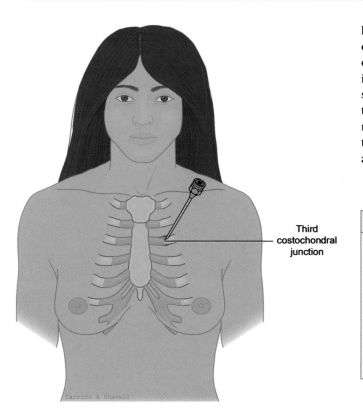

Figure 50-3. Correct needle placement for injection of the costosternal joints. (From Waldman SD: Atlas of Pain Management Injection Techniques. Philadelphia, Saunders, 2000.)

Third costochondral junction

lung and structures of the mediastinum. Failure to do so could lead to disastrous results. The major complication of the injection technique is pneumothorax if the needle is placed too laterally or deeply and invades the pleural space. Infection, though rare, can occur if strict aseptic technique is not followed. Trauma to the contents of the mediastinum is also a possibility. Risk of this complication can be greatly decreased with strict attention to accurate needle placement.

Clinical Pearls

Patients suffering from pain emanating from the costosternal joints often believe that they are having a heart attack. Reassurance is required, although it should be remembered that musculoskeletal pain syndromes and coronary artery disease can coexist. Tietze's syndrome may be confused with costosternal syndrome, although both respond to the aforementioned injection technique.

Chapter 51

Manubriosternal Syndrome

ICD-9 CODE 786.52

THE CLINICAL SYNDROME

The manubrium articulates with the body of the sternum via the manubriosternal joint at the angle of Louis. The manubriosternal joint is a fibrocartilaginous joint or synchondrosis, which lacks a true joint cavity. The joint allows protraction and retraction of the thorax.

Pain originating from the manubriosternal joint can mimic pain of cardiac origin. The manubriosternal joint is susceptible to the development of osteoarthritis, rheumatoid arthritis, ankylosing spondylitis, Reiter's syndrome, and psoriatic arthritis. The joint can also be traumatized during acceleration-deceleration injuries and blunt trauma to the chest (Fig. 51-1). With severe trauma, the joint may subluxate or dislocate. Overuse or misuse can result in acute inflammation of the manubriosternal joint, which can be quite debilitating. The joint is also subject to invasion by tumor from primary malignancies, including thymoma, or from metastatic disease.

SIGNS AND SYMPTOMS

Physical examination reveals that the patient vigorously attempts to splint the joint by keeping the shoulders stiffly in a neutral position. Pain is reproduced with active protraction or retraction of the shoulder, deep inspiration, and full elevation of the arm. Shrugging of the shoulder may also reproduce the pain. Coughing may be difficult, leading to inadequate pulmonary toilet in patients who have sustained trauma to the anterior chest wall. The manubriosternal joint may be tender to palpation. The patient may also complain of a clicking sensation with movement of the joint.

TESTING

Plain radiographs are indicated for all patients who present with pain thought to be emanating from the manubriosternal joint to rule out occult bony pathology,

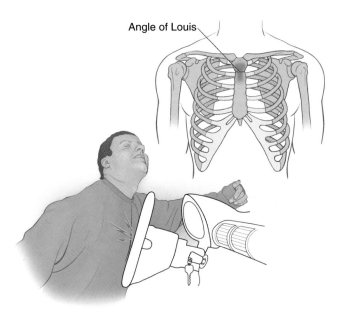

Figure 51–1. The manubriosternal joint is susceptible to the development of arthritis. It is often traumatized during acceleration-deceleration injuries and blunt trauma to the chest.

including tumor. If trauma is present, radionuclide bone scanning may be useful to rule out occult fractures of the ribs or sternum. Based on the patient's clinical presentation, additional testing may be indicated, including a complete blood count, prostate-specific antigen level, erythrocyte sedimentation rate, and antinuclear antibody testing. Laboratory evaluation for collagen vascular disease is indicated in patients suffering from manubriosternal joint pain if other joints are involved. Magnetic resonance imaging or computed tomography of the joint is indicated if joint instability or occult mass is suspected or to further elucidate the cause of the pain (Fig. 51-2). The injection technique described later serves as both a diagnostic and a therapeutic maneuver.

DIFFERENTIAL DIAGNOSIS

As mentioned, the pain of manubriosternal syndrome is often mistaken for pain of cardiac origin, leading to visits to the emergency department and unnecessary cardiac

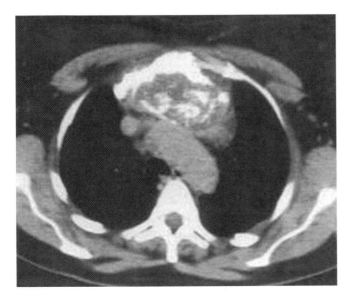

Figure 51–2. Chondrosarcoma of the sternum. Computed tomography clearly demonstrates manubrial irregularity and a preaortic soft tissue mass with chondral calcification. Nearly all sternal tumors are malignant. (From Grainger RG, Allison DJ, Adam A, Dixon AK: Grainger & Allison's Diagnostic Radiology: A Textbook of Medical Imaging, 4th ed. Philadelphia, Churchill Livingstone, 2002, p 253.)

workups. If trauma has occurred, manubriosternal syndrome may coexist with fractured ribs or fractures of the sternum itself, which can be missed on plain radiographs and may require radionuclide bone scanning for proper identification. Tietze's syndrome, which is painful enlargement of the upper costochondral cartilage associated with viral infection, may be confused with manubriosternal syndrome.

Neuropathic pain involving the chest wall may also be confused or coexist with manubriosternal syndrome. Examples of such neuropathic pain include diabetic polyneuropathies and acute herpes zoster involving the thoracic nerves. Diseases of the structures of the mediastinum are possible and can be difficult to diagnose. Pathologic processes that inflame the pleura, such as pulmonary embolus, infection, and Bornholm disease, may also confuse the diagnosis and complicate treatment.

TREATMENT

Initial treatment of the pain and functional disability associated with manubriosternal syndrome includes a combination of nonsteroidal anti-inflammatory drugs or cyclooxygenase-2 inhibitors. The local application of heat and cold may also be beneficial. Use of an elastic rib belt may also provide symptomatic relief and protect the manubriosternal joint from additional trauma. For patients who do not respond to these treatment modali-

ties, injection with local anesthetic and steroid is a reasonable next step.

The patient is placed in the supine position, and the skin overlying the angle of the sternum is prepared with antiseptic solution. A sterile syringe containing 1 mL of 0.25% preservative-free bupivacaine and 40 mg methylprednisolone is attached to a 1½-inch, 25-gauge needle using strict aseptic technique. The angle of the sternum is identified; the manubriosternal joint should be easily palpable as a slight indentation at this point. The needle is then carefully advanced through the skin and subcutaneous tissues medially, with a slight cephalad trajectory, into the joint (Fig. 51-3). If bone is encountered, the needle is withdrawn into the subcutaneous tissues and redirected slightly more cephalad. After entering the joint, the contents of the syringe are gently injected. There should be some resistance to injection owing to the fibrocartilaginous nature of the joint. If significant resistance is encountered, the needle should be advanced or withdrawn slightly into the joint until the injection can proceed with only limited resistance. The needle is then removed, and a sterile pressure dressing and ice pack are applied to the injection site.

Physical modalities, including local heat and gentle range-of-motion exercises, should be introduced several days after the patient undergoes injection for manubriosternal joint pain. Vigorous exercises should be avoided, because they will exacerbate the patient's symptoms. Simple analgesics and nonsteroidal anti-inflammatory drugs may be used concurrently with this injection technique.

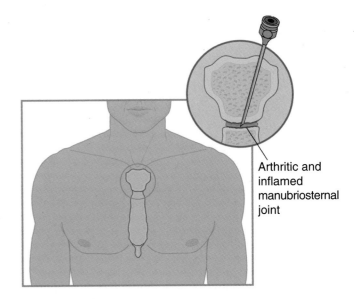

Arthritic and inflamed manubriosternal joint

Figure 51–3. Correct needle placement for injection of the manubriosternal joint. (From Waldman SD: Atlas of Pain Management Injection Techniques, 2nd ed. Philadelphia, Saunders, 2000.)

COMPLICATIONS AND PITFALLS

Because many pathologic processes can mimic the pain of manubriosternal syndrome, the clinician must carefully rule out underlying cardiac disease and diseases of the lung and structures of the mediastinum. Failure to do so could lead to disastrous results. The major complication of the injection technique is pneumothorax if the needle is placed too laterally or deeply and invades the pleural space. Infection, though rare, can occur if strict aseptic technique is not followed. Trauma to the contents of the mediastinum is also a possibility. This complication can be greatly decreased with strict attention to accurate needle placement.

Clinical Pearls

Patients suffering from pain emanating from the manubriosternal joint often believe that they are having a heart attack. Reassurance is required, although it should be remembered that musculoskeletal pain syndromes and coronary artery disease can coexist. Tietze's syndrome may be confused with manubriosternal syndrome, although both respond to the aforementioned injection technique.

Chapter 52

Intercostal Neuralgia

ICD-9 CODE 353.8

THE CLINICAL SYNDROME

Whereas most other causes of chest wall pain are musculoskeletal in nature, the pain of intercostal neuralgia is neuropathic. As with costosternal joint pain, Tietze's syndrome, and rib fractures, a significant number of patients who suffer from intercostal neuralgia seek medical attention because they believe they are having a heart attack. If the subcostal nerve is involved, gallbladder disease may be suspected. The pain of intercostal neuralgia is due to damage to or inflammation of the intercostal nerves. The pain is constant and burning in nature and may involve any of the intercostal nerves, as well as the subcostal nerve of the 12th rib. The pain usually begins at the posterior axillary line and radiates anteriorly into the distribution of the affected intercostal or subcostal nerves, or both (Fig. 52-1). Deep inspiration or movement of the chest wall may slightly increase the pain of intercostal neuralgia, but to a much lesser extent than with musculoskeletal causes of chest wall pain.

SIGNS AND SYMPTOMS

Physical examination generally reveals minimal findings unless there is a history of previous thoracic or subcostal surgery or cutaneous evidence of herpes zoster involving the thoracic dermatomes. Unlike patients with musculoskeletal causes of chest wall and subcostal pain, those with intercostal neuralgia do not attempt to splint or protect the affected area. Careful sensory examination of the affected dermatomes may reveal decreased sensation or allodynia. With significant motor involvement of the subcostal nerve, the patient may complain that his or her abdomen bulges out.

TESTING

Plain radiographs are indicated for all patients who present with pain thought to be emanating from the

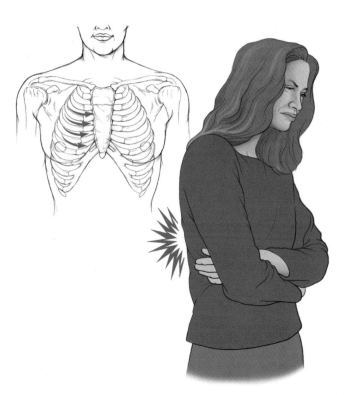

Figure 52–1. The pain of intercostal neuralgia is neuropathic rather than musculoskeletal in origin.

intercostal nerve to rule out occult bony pathology, including tumor (Fig. 52-2). If trauma is present, radionuclide bone scanning may be useful to rule out occult fractures of the ribs or sternum. Based on the patient's clinical presentation, additional testing may be indicated, including a complete blood count, prostate-specific antigen level, erythrocyte sedimentation rate, and antinuclear antibody testing. Computed tomography of the thoracic contents is indicated if occult mass is suspected. The injection technique described later serves as both a diagnostic and a therapeutic maneuver.

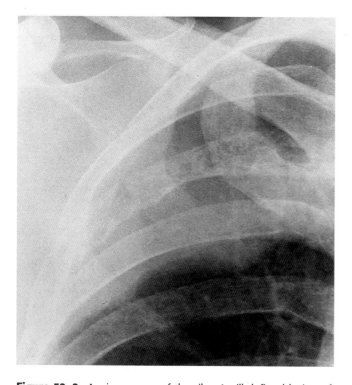

Figure 52–2. Angiosarcoma of the ribs. An ill-defined lesion of the posterior aspect of the fourth rib is associated with a coarsened trabecular pattern and a large soft tissue mass. The osseous changes are consistent with a vascular lesion. The extent of the soft tissue involvement suggests an aggressive process. (From Resnick D: Diagnosis of Bone and Joint Disorders, 4th ed. Philadelphia, Saunders, 2002, p 4006.)

DIFFERENTIAL DIAGNOSIS

As mentioned, the pain of intercostal neuralgia is often mistaken for pain of cardiac or gallbladder origin, leading to visits to the emergency department and unnecessary cardiac and gastrointestinal workups. If trauma has occurred, intercostal neuralgia may coexist with fractured ribs or fractures of the sternum itself, which can be missed on plain radiographs and may require radionuclide bone scanning for proper identification. Tietze's syndrome, which is painful enlargement of the upper costochondral cartilage associated with viral infection, may be confused with intercostal neuralgia.

Other types of neuropathic pain involving the chest wall may be confused or coexist with intercostal neuralgia. Examples of such neuropathic pain include diabetic polyneuropathies and acute herpes zoster involving the thoracic nerves. Diseases of the structures of the mediastinum are possible and can be difficult to diagnose. Pathologic processes that inflame the pleura, such as pulmonary embolus, infection, and Bornholm disease, may also confuse the diagnosis and complicate treatment.

TREATMENT

Initial treatment of intercostal neuralgia includes a combination of simple analgesics and nonsteroidal anti-inflammatory drugs or cyclooxygenase-2 inhibitors. If these medications do not adequately control the patient's symptoms, a tricyclic antidepressant or gabapentin should be added.

Traditionally, tricyclic antidepressants have been a mainstay in the palliation of pain caused by intercostal neuralgia. Controlled studies have demonstrated the efficacy of amitriptyline, and nortriptyline and desipramine have also proved to be clinically useful. Unfortunately, this class of drugs is associated with significant anticholinergic side effects, including dry mouth, constipation, sedation, and urinary retention. They should be used with caution in patients suffering from glaucoma, cardiac arrhythmia, and prostatism. To minimize side effects and encourage compliance, the physician should start amitriptyline or nortriptyline at a 10-mg dose at bedtime; the dose can then be titrated upward to 25 mg at bedtime, as side effects allow. Subsequently, upward titration in 25-mg increments can be carried out each week, as side effects allow. Even at lower doses, patients generally report a rapid improvement in sleep disturbance and begin to experience some pain relief in 10 to 14 days. If the patient does not show any improvement in pain as the dose is being titrated upward, the addition of gabapentin alone or in combination with nerve blocks is recommended (see later). The selective serotonin reuptake inhibitors such as fluoxetine have also been used to treat the pain of intercostal neuralgia, and although these drugs are better tolerated than the tricyclic antidepressants, they appear to be less efficacious.

If the antidepressant compounds are ineffective or contraindicated, gabapentin is a reasonable alternative. Gabapentin is started at a 300-mg dose at bedtime for 2 nights. The patient should be cautioned about potential side effects, including dizziness, sedation, confusion, and rash. The drug is then increased in 300-mg increments given in equally divided doses over 2 days, as side effects allow, until pain relief is obtained or a total dosage of 2400 mg/day is reached. At this point, if the patient has experienced partial pain relief, blood values are measured, and the drug is carefully titrated upward using 100-mg tablets. Rarely is a dose greater than 3600 mg/day required.

The local application of heat and cold or the use of an elastic rib belt may also provide symptomatic relief. For patients who do not respond to these treatment modalities, injection using local anesthetic and steroid is a reasonable next step.

The patient is placed in the prone position with the arms hanging loosely off the sides of the table. Alternatively, this block can be done with the patient in the sitting or lateral position. The rib to be blocked is identified by palpating its path at the posterior axillary line. The operator's index and middle fingers are then placed on the rib, bracketing the site of needle insertion, and the skin is prepared with antiseptic solution. A 1½-inch, 22-gauge needle is attached to a 12-mL syringe and advanced perpendicular to the skin, aiming for the middle of the rib between the operator's index and middle fingers. The needle should impinge on bone after being advanced approximately ¾ inch. Once bony contact is made, the needle is withdrawn into the subcutaneous tissues, and the skin and subcutaneous tissues are retracted with the palpating fingers inferiorly. This allows the needle to be walked off the inferior margin of the rib. As soon as bony contact is lost, the needle is slowly advanced approximately 2 mm deeper. This places the needle in proximity to the costal groove, which contains the intercostal nerve as well as the intercostal artery and vein. After careful aspiration reveals no blood or air, 3 to 5 mL of 1% preservative-free lidocaine is injected. If there is an inflammatory component to the pain, the local anesthetic is combined with 80 mg methylprednisolone and injected in incremental doses. Subsequent daily nerve blocks are carried out in a similar manner, substituting 40 mg methylprednisolone for the initial 80-mg dose. Because of the overlapping innervation of the chest and upper abdominal wall, the intercostal nerves above and below the nerve suspected of causing the pain must be blocked as well.

COMPLICATIONS AND PITFALLS

The major problem in the treatment of patients thought to be suffering from intercostal neuralgia is failure to identify potentially serious pathology of the thorax or upper abdomen. Given the proximity of the pleural space, pneumothorax after intercostal nerve block is a distinct possibility. The incidence of this complication is less than 1%, but it occurs with greater frequency in patients with chronic obstructive pulmonary disease. Owing to the proximity to the intercostal nerve and artery, the clinician must carefully calculate the total dosage of local anesthetic administered, because vascular uptake via these vessels is high. Although uncommon, infection is always a possibility, especially in immunocompromised patients with cancer. Early detection of infection is crucial to avoid potentially life-threatening sequelae.

Clinical Pearls

Intercostal neuralgia is a commonly encountered cause of chest wall and thoracic pain. Correct diagnosis is necessary to properly treat this painful condition and to avoid overlooking serious intrathoracic or intra-abdominal pathology. Pharmacologic agents generally provide adequate pain control. If necessary, intercostal nerve block is a simple technique that can produce dramatic pain relief, but the proximity of the intercostal nerve to the pleural space makes careful attention to technique mandatory.

Chapter 53

Diabetic Truncal Neuropathy

ICD-9 CODE 354.5

THE CLINICAL SYNDROME

Diabetic neuropathy is a term used by clinicians to describe a heterogeneous group of diseases that affect the autonomic and peripheral nervous systems of patients suffering from diabetes mellitus. Diabetic neuropathy is now thought to be the most common form of peripheral neuropathy that afflicts humankind, with an estimated 220 million people worldwide suffering from this malady.

One of the most commonly encountered forms of diabetic neuropathy is diabetic truncal neuropathy. In this condition, pain and motor dysfunction are often incorrectly attributed to intrathoracic or intra-abdominal pathology, leading to extensive workups for appendicitis, cholecystitis, renal calculi, and so on. The onset of symptoms frequently coincides with periods of extreme hypoglycemia or hyperglycemia or with weight loss or gain. Patients who present with diabetic truncal neuropathy complain of severe dysesthetic pain with patchy sensory deficits in the distribution of the lower thoracic or upper thoracic dermatomes. The pain is often worse at night, causing significant sleep disturbance. The symptoms of diabetic truncal neuropathy often resolve spontaneously over 6 to 12 months. However, because of the severity of symptoms, aggressive treatment with pharmacotherapy and neural blockade is indicated.

SIGNS AND SYMPTOMS

Physical examination generally reveals minimal findings unless there is a history of previous thoracic or subcostal surgery or cutaneous evidence of herpes zoster involving the thoracic dermatomes. Unlike patients with musculoskeletal causes of chest wall and subcostal pain, those with diabetic truncal neuropathy do not attempt to splint or protect the affected area. Careful sensory examination of the affected dermatomes may reveal decreased sensation or allodynia. With significant motor involvement of

the subcostal nerve, the patient may complain that his or her abdomen bulges out (Fig. 53-1).

TESTING

The presence of diabetes should lead to a high index of suspicion for diabetic truncal neuropathy. If the diagnosis of diabetic truncal neuropathy is suspected based on the targeted history and physical examination, screening laboratory tests, including a complete blood count, chemistry profile, erythrocyte sedimentation rate, thyroid function studies, antinuclear antibody testing, and urinalysis, should rule out most other peripheral neuropathies that are easily treatable. Electromyography and nerve conduction velocity testing are indicated in all patients suffering from peripheral neuropathy to identify treatable entrapment neuropathies and further delineate the type of peripheral neuropathy present; these tests

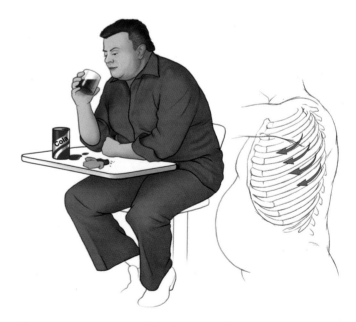

Figure 53–1. The pain of diabetic truncal neuropathy is neuropathic in nature and is often made worse by poorly controlled blood sugar levels.

may also be able to quantify the severity of peripheral or entrapment neuropathy. Additional laboratory testing is indicated as the clinical situation dictates (e.g., Lyme disease titers, heavy metal screens). Magnetic resonance imaging of the spinal canal and cord should be performed if myelopathy is suspected. Nerve or skin biopsy is occasionally indicated if no cause for the peripheral neuropathy can be ascertained. Lack of response to the therapies discussed later should lead to a reconsideration of the diagnosis and the repetition of testing, as clinically indicated.

DIFFERENTIAL DIAGNOSIS

Diseases other than diabetic neuropathy may cause peripheral neuropathies in diabetic patients. These diseases may exist alone or may coexist with diabetic truncal neuropathy, making their identification and treatment difficult.

Although uncommon in the United States, Hansen's disease is a common cause of peripheral neuropathy worldwide that may mimic or coexist with diabetic truncal neuropathy. Other infectious causes of peripheral neuropathies include Lyme disease and human immunodeficiency virus infection. Substances that are toxic to nerves, including alcohol, heavy metals, chemotherapeutic agents, and hydrocarbons, may also cause peripheral neuropathies that are indistinguishable from diabetic neuropathy on clinical grounds. Heritable disorders such as Charcot-Marie-Tooth disease and other familial diseases of the peripheral nervous system must also be considered, although treatment options are somewhat limited. Metabolic and endocrine causes of peripheral neuropathy that must be ruled out include vitamin deficiencies, pernicious anemia, hypothyroidism, uremia, and acute intermittent porphyria. Other causes of peripheral neuropathy that may confuse the clinical picture include Guillain-Barré syndrome, amyloidosis, entrapment neuropathies, carcinoid syndrome, paraneoplastic syndromes, and sarcoidosis. Because many of these diseases are treatable, it is imperative that the clinician rule them out before attributing a patient's symptoms solely to diabetes.

Intercostal neuralgia and musculoskeletal causes of chest wall and subcostal pain may also be confused with diabetic truncal neuropathy. In all these conditions, the patient's pain may be erroneously attributed to cardiac or upper abdominal pathology, leading to unnecessary testing and treatment.

TREATMENT

Control of Blood Sugar

Current thinking is that the better the patient's glycemic control, the less severe the symptoms of diabetic truncal

neuropathy. Significant swings in blood sugar levels seem to predispose diabetic patients to the development of clinically significant diabetic truncal neuropathy. Some investigators believe that although oral hypoglycemic agents control blood sugar levels, they do not protect patients from diabetic truncal neuropathy as well as insulin does. In fact, some patients taking hypoglycemic agents experience an improvement in the symptoms of diabetic truncal neuropathy when they are switched to insulin.

Pharmacologic Treatment

Antidepressants

Traditionally, tricyclic antidepressants have been a mainstay in the palliation of pain caused by diabetic truncal neuropathy. Controlled studies have demonstrated the efficacy of amitriptyline, and nortriptyline and desipramine have also proved to be clinically useful. Unfortunately, this class of drugs is associated with significant anticholinergic side effects, including dry mouth, constipation, sedation, and urinary retention. They should be used with caution in patients suffering from glaucoma, cardiac arrhythmia, and prostatism. To minimize side effects and encourage compliance, the physician should start amitriptyline or nortriptyline at a 10-mg dose at bedtime; the dose can then be titrated upward to 25 mg at bedtime, as side effects allow. Subsequently, upward titration in 25-mg increments can be carried out each week, as side effects allow. Even at lower doses, patients generally report a rapid improvement in sleep disturbance and begin to experience some pain relief in 10 to 14 days. If the patient does not show any improvement in pain as the dose is being titrated upward, the addition of gabapentin alone or in combination with nerve blocks is recommended (see later). The selective serotonin reuptake inhibitors such as fluoxetine have also been used to treat the pain of diabetic truncal neuropathy, and although these drugs are better tolerated than the tricyclic antidepressants, they appear to be less efficacious.

Anticonvulsants

Anticonvulsants have long been used to treat neuropathic pain, including that of diabetic truncal neuropathy. Both phenytoin and carbamazepine have been used with varying degrees of success, either alone or in combination with antidepressants. Unfortunately, the side effects of these drugs have limited their clinical usefulness. The anticonvulsant gabapentin is highly efficacious in the treatment of a variety of painful neuropathic conditions, including postherpetic neuralgia and diabetic truncal neuropathy. Used properly, gabapentin is extremely well tolerated, and in most pain centers, it has become the adjuvant analgesic of choice in the treatment of diabetic truncal neuropathy. Gabapentin has a large therapeutic window, but the physician is cautioned to start at the low end of the dosage spectrum and titrate upward slowly to avoid central nervous system side effects, including sedation and fatigue. The following recommended dosage schedule can minimize side effects and encourage compliance: A single bedtime dose of 300 mg for 2 nights is followed by 300 mg twice a day for an additional 2 days. If the patient is tolerating this twice-daily dosing, the dosage may be increased to 300 mg three times a day. Most patients begin to experience pain relief at this dosage. Additional titration upward can be carried out in 300-mg increments, as side effects allow. A total greater than 3600 mg/day in divided doses is not currently recommended. The use of 600- or 800-mg tablets can simplify maintenance dosing after titration has been completed. Clinical trials are under way with a gabapentin analogue that may provide additional therapeutic options for patients suffering from diabetic truncal neuropathy.

Antiarrhythmics

Mexiletine is an antiarrhythmic drug that may be effective in the management of diabetic truncal neuropathy. Some pain specialists believe that mexiletine is especially useful in patients with primarily sharp, lancinating pain or burning pain. Unfortunately, this drug is poorly tolerated by most patients and should be reserved for those who do not respond to first-line pharmacologic treatments such as gabapentin or nortriptyline alone or in combination with neural blockade.

Topical Agents

Some clinicians have reported the successful treatment of diabetic truncal neuropathy with topical application of capsaicin. An extract of chili peppers, capsaicin is thought to relieve neuropathic pain by depleting substance P. The side effects of capsaicin include significant burning and erythema, however, limiting its use.

Topical lidocaine administered via transdermal patch or in a gel can also provide short-term relief of the pain of diabetic truncal neuropathy. This drug should be used with caution in patients taking mexiletine, because there is the potential for cumulative local anesthetic toxicity. Whether topical lidocaine has a role in the long-term treatment of diabetic truncal neuropathy remains to be seen.

Analgesics

In general, neuropathic pain responds poorly to analgesic compounds. The simple analgesics, including acet-

aminophen and aspirin, can be used in combination with antidepressants and anticonvulsants, but care must be taken not to exceed the recommended daily dose, because renal or hepatic side effects may occur. The nonsteroidal anti-inflammatory drugs may also provide a modicum of pain relief when used with antidepressants and anticonvulsants; however, because of the nephrotoxicity of this class of drugs, they should be used with extreme caution in diabetic patients, given the high incidence of diabetic nephropathy even early in the course of the disease. The role of cyclooxygenase-2 inhibitors in the palliation of the pain of diabetic truncal neuropathy has not been adequately studied.

The pain of diabetic truncal neuropathy responds poorly to treatment with opioid analgesics. Given the significant central nervous system and gastrointestinal side effects, coupled with the problems of tolerance, dependence, and addiction, narcotic analgesics should rarely if ever be used as a primary treatment for the pain of diabetic truncal neuropathy. If a narcotic analgesic is being considered, however, tramadol may be a reasonable choice; it binds weakly to the opioid receptors and may provide some symptomatic relief. Tramadol should be used with care in combination with antidepressants to avoid the increased risk of seizures.

Neural Blockade

Neural blockade with local anesthetic alone or in combination with steroid can be useful in the management of both acute and chronic pain associated with diabetic truncal neuropathy. Thoracic epidural or intercostal nerve block with local anesthetic, steroid, or both may be beneficial. Occasionally, neuroaugmentation via spinal cord stimulation may provide significant pain relief in patients who have not been helped by more conservative measures. Neurodestructive procedures are rarely if ever indicated to treat the pain of diabetic truncal neuropathy; they often worsen the patient's pain and cause functional disability.

COMPLICATIONS AND PITFALLS

The major problem in the care of patients thought to be suffering from diabetic truncal neuropathy is failure to identify potentially serious pathology of the thorax or upper abdomen. Given the proximity of the pleural space, pneumothorax after intercostal nerve block is a distinct possibility. The incidence of the complication is less than 1%, but it occurs with greater frequency in patients with chronic obstructive pulmonary disease. Owing to the proximity to the intercostal nerve and artery, the clinician must carefully calculate the total dosage of local anesthetic administered, because vascular uptake via these vessels is high. Although uncommon, infection is always a possibility, especially in immuno-compromised patients with cancer. Early detection of infection is crucial to avoid potentially life-threatening sequelae.

Clinical Pearls

Diabetic truncal neuropathy is a commonly encountered cause of thoracic and subcostal pain. Correct diagnosis is necessary to properly treat this painful condition and to avoid overlooking serious intrathoracic or intra-abdominal pathology. Pharmacologic agents generally provide adequate pain control. If necessary, intercostal or epidural nerve block is a simple technique that can produce dramatic pain relief, but the proximity of the intercostal nerve to the pleural space makes careful attention to technique mandatory.

Chapter 54

Tietze's Syndrome

ICD-9 CODE 733.6

THE CLINICAL SYNDROME

Tietze's syndrome is a frequent cause of chest wall pain. Distinct from the more common costosternal syndrome, Tietze's syndrome was first described in 1921 and is characterized by acute, painful swelling of the costal cartilage. In fact, painful swelling of the second and third costochondral joints is the sine qua non of Tietze's syndrome (Fig. 54-1); such swelling is absent in costosternal syndrome. Also distinguishing the two syndromes is the age of onset: whereas costosternal syndrome usually occurs no earlier than the fourth decade of life, Tietze's syndrome is a disease of the second and third decades. The onset is acute and is often associated with a concurrent viral infection of the respiratory tract. It has been postulated that microtrauma to the costosternal joints from serve coughing or heavy labor may be the cause of Tietze's syndrome.

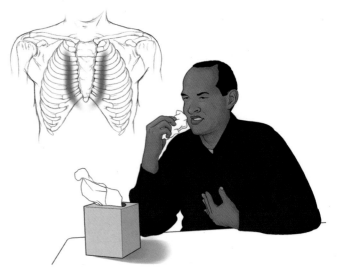

Figure 54–1. Swelling of the second and third costochondral joints is pathognomonic of Tietze's syndrome.

SIGNS AND SYMPTOMS

Physical examination reveals that patients suffering from Tietze's syndrome vigorously attempt to splint the joints by keeping the shoulders stiffly in a neutral position. Pain is reproduced with active protraction or retraction of the shoulder, deep inspiration, and full elevation of the arm. Shrugging of the shoulder may also reproduce the pain. Coughing may be difficult, leading to inadequate pulmonary toilet in some patients. The costosternal joints, especially the second and third, are swollen and exquisitely tender to palpation. This swollen costochondral joint sign is pathognomonic for Tietze's syndrome (Fig. 54-2). The adjacent intercostal muscles may also be tender to palpation. The patient may complain of a clicking sensation with movement of the joint.

TESTING

Plain radiographs are indicated for all patients who present with pain thought to be emanating from the costosternal joints to rule out occult bony pathology, including tumor. If trauma is present, radionuclide bone scanning should be considered to rule out occult fractures of the ribs or sternum. Based on the patient's clinical presentation, additional testing may be indicated, including a complete blood count, prostate-specific antigen level, erythrocyte sedimentation rate, and antinuclear antibody testing. Laboratory evaluation for collagen vascular disease is indicated in patients suffering from costosternal joint pain if other joints are involved. Magnetic resonance imaging of the joints is indicated if joint instability or occult mass is suspected or to confirm the diagnosis (Fig. 54-3). The injection technique

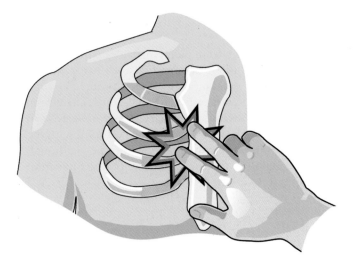

Figure 54–2. Inspection of the costosternal joint for swelling indicative of Tietze's syndrome. (From Waldman SD: Physical Diagnosis of Pain: An Atlas of Signs and Symptoms. Philadelphia, Saunders, 2006, p 209.)

described later serves as both a diagnostic and a therapeutic maneuver.

DIFFERENTIAL DIAGNOSIS

Many other painful conditions that affect the costosternal joints are much more common than Tietze's syndrome. For instance, the costosternal joints are susceptible to osteoarthritis, rheumatoid arthritis, ankylosing spon-

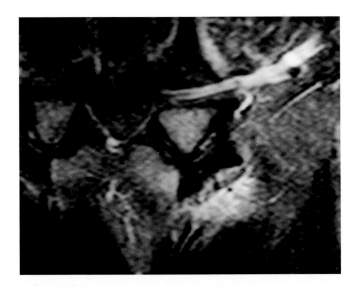

Figure 54–3. Tietze's syndrome. Coronal, short tau inversion recovery, magnetic resonance image of the thorax shows high signal intensity below the sternoclavicular joint at the costosternal junction in a 45-year-old man with pain and tenderness in this region. (From Resnick D: Diagnosis of Bone and Joint Disorders, 4th ed. Philadelphia, Saunders, 2002, p 2605.)

dylitis, Reiter's syndrome, and psoriatic arthritis. The joints are often traumatized during acceleration-deceleration injuries and blunt trauma to the chest; with severe trauma, the joints may subluxate or dislocate. Overuse or misuse can result in acute inflammation of the costosternal joint, which can be quite debilitating. The joints are also subject to invasion by tumor from primary malignancies, including thymoma, or from metastatic disease.

TREATMENT

Initial treatment of the pain and functional disability associated with Tietze's syndrome includes nonsteroidal anti-inflammatory drugs or cyclooxygenase-2 inhibitors. The local application of heat and cold may also be beneficial. Use of an elastic rib belt may provide symptomatic relief and protect the costosternal joints from additional trauma. For patients who do not respond to these treatment modalities, injection using local anesthetic and steroid is a reasonable next step.

Injection for Tietze's syndrome is performed by placing the patient in the supine position. The skin overlying the affected costosternal joints is prepared with antiseptic solution. A sterile syringe containing 1 mL of 0.25% preservative-free bupivacaine for each joint to be injected and 40 mg methylprednisolone is attached to a 1½-inch, 25-gauge needle using strict aseptic technique. The costosternal joints are identified; they should be easily palpable as a slight bulging at the point where the rib attaches to the sternum. The needle is carefully advanced through the skin and subcutaneous tissues medially, with a slight cephalad trajectory, in proximity to the joint. If bone is encountered, the needle is withdrawn out of the periosteum. After the needle is in proximity to the joint, 1 mL of solution is gently injected. There should be limited resistance to injection. If significant resistance is encountered, the needle should be withdrawn slightly until the injection can proceed with only limited resistance. This procedure is repeated for each affected joint. The needle is then removed, and a sterile pressure dressing and ice pack are applied to the injection site.

Physical modalities, including local heat and gentle range-of-motion exercises, should be introduced several days after the patient undergoes injection for Tietze's syndrome. Vigorous exercises should be avoided, because they will exacerbate the patient's symptoms. Simple analgesics and nonsteroidal anti-inflammatory drugs may be used concurrently with this injection technique.

COMPLICATIONS AND PITFALLS

Because many pathologic processes can mimic the pain of Tietze's syndrome, the clinician must carefully rule out underlying cardiac disease and diseases of the lung and structures of the mediastinum. Failure to do so could lead to disastrous results. The major complication of the injection technique is pneumothorax if the needle is placed too laterally or deeply and invades the pleural space. Trauma to the contents of the mediastinum is also a possibility. This complication can be greatly decreased with strict attention to accurate needle placement. Infection, though rare, can occur if strict aseptic technique is not followed, and universal precautions should be used to minimize risk to the operator. The incidence of ecchymosis and hematoma formation can be decreased if pressure is applied to the injection site immediately after injection.

Clinical Pearls

Patients suffering from pain emanating from the costosternal joint often believe that they are having a heart attack. Reassurance is required, although it should be remembered that musculoskeletal pain syndromes and coronary artery disease can coexist. Tietze's syndrome may be confused with the more common costosternal syndrome, although both respond to the aforementioned injection technique.

Chapter 55

Precordial Catch Syndrome

ICD-9 CODE 786.51

THE CLINICAL SYNDROME

Precordial catch syndrome, also known as Texidor's twinge, is a common cause of chest wall pain. Occurring most frequently in adolescents and young adults, precordial catch syndrome is the cause of anxiety among patients and clinicians alike, given the intensity of the pain and its frequent attribution to the heart. Precordial catch syndrome almost always occurs at rest, often while the patient is sitting in a slumped position on an old couch (Fig. 55-1).

Distinct from other causes of chest wall pain, precordial catch syndrome is characterized by sharp, stabbing, needle-like pain that is well localized in the precordial region. Symptoms begin without warning, only adding to the patient's anxiety, and they go away as suddenly as they came. The pain lasts from 30 seconds to 3 minutes, and it is often made worse by deep inspiration. Patients suffering from precordial catch syndrome usually outgrow the syndrome by the third decade of life.

SIGNS AND SYMPTOMS

There are no physical findings (e.g., flushing, pallor, diaphoresis) associated with the onset of pain, although some patients suffering from precordial catch syndrome may demonstrate tenderness to palpation in the anterior intercostal muscles overlying the painful area. Because the pain is made worse with deep inspiration, the patient may get lightheaded from prolonged shallow breathing.

TESTING

Plain radiographs are indicated for all patients who present with pain thought to be emanating from the chest wall to rule out occult bony pathology, including tumor. If trauma is present, radionuclide bone scanning should be considered to rule out occult fractures of the ribs or sternum. Given the location of the pain, an electrocardiogram is indicated, but in those with precordial

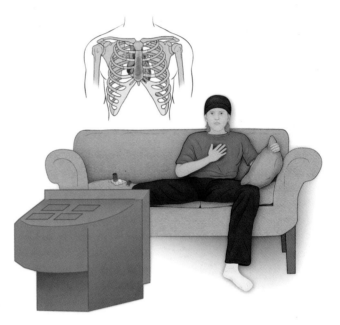

Figure 55–1. Precordial catch syndrome can be caused by prolonged sitting in a slumped position.

catch syndrome, the results are expected to be normal. Based on the patient's clinical presentation, additional testing may be indicated, including a complete blood count, prostate-specific antigen level, erythrocyte sedimentation rate, and antinuclear antibody testing. Magnetic resonance imaging of the joints is indicated if joint instability or an occult mass is suspected or to confirm the diagnosis.

DIFFERENTIAL DIAGNOSIS

Many other painful conditions that affect the chest wall occur with much greater frequency than precordial catch syndrome. The costosternal joints are susceptible to osteoarthritis, rheumatoid arthritis, ankylosing spondylitis, Reiter's syndrome, and psoriatic arthritis. The joints are often traumatized during acceleration-deceleration injuries and blunt trauma to the chest; with severe trauma, the joints may subluxate or dislocate. Overuse or misuse can result in acute inflammation of the costosternal joint, which can be quite debilitating. The joints are also subject to invasion by tumor from primary malignancies, including thymoma, or from metastatic disease. Sharp pleuritic chest pain may be associated with devil's grip, pleurisy, pneumonia, or pulmonary embolus.

TREATMENT

Treatment of precordial catch syndrome is a combination of reassurance and instructing the patient to take a deep breath as soon as the pain begins, even though this produces a sharp, stabbing pain. Improving one's posture and changing position frequently while resting or watching television should also help decrease the frequency of attacks. Pharmacologic treatment is not indicated, given the rapid onset and offset of the pain.

COMPLICATIONS AND PITFALLS

Because many pathologic processes may mimic the pain of precordial catch syndrome, the clinician must carefully rule out underlying cardiac disease and diseases of the lung and structures of the mediastinum. Failure to do so could lead to disastrous results. The biggest risk in patients suffering from precordial catch syndrome is related to unnecessary testing (e.g., cardiac catheterization) to rule out cardiac disease.

Clinical Pearls

Patients suffering from precordial catch syndrome often believe that they are having a heart attack. Reassurance is required, although it should be remembered that musculoskeletal pain syndromes and coronary artery disease can coexist.

Chapter 56

Fractured Ribs

ICD-9 CODE 807.0

THE CLINICAL SYNDROME

Fractured ribs are one of the most common causes of chest wall pain, and they are usually associated with trauma to the chest wall (Fig. 56-1). In osteoporotic patients or in those with primary tumors or metastatic disease involving the ribs, fractures may occur with coughing (tussive fractures) or spontaneously.

The pain and functional disability associated with fractured ribs are largely determined by the severity of the injury (e.g., number of ribs involved), nature of the injury (e.g., partial or complete fracture, free-floating fragments), and amount of damage to surrounding structures, including the intercostal nerves and pleura. The pain associated with fractured ribs ranges from a dull, deep ache with partial osteoporotic fractures to severe, sharp, stabbing pain that may lead to inadequate pulmonary toilet.

SIGNS AND SYMPTOMS

Rib fractures are aggravated by deep inspiration, coughing, and any movement of the chest wall. Palpation of the affected ribs may elicit pain and reflex spasm of the musculature of the chest wall. Ecchymosis overlying the fractures may be present. The clinician should be aware of the possibility of pneumothorax or hemopneumothorax. Damage to the intercostal nerves may produce severe pain and result in reflex splinting of the chest wall, further compromising the patient's pulmonary status. Failure to aggressively treat this pain and splinting may result in a negative cycle of hypoventilation, atelectasis, and ultimately pneumonia.

TESTING

Plain radiographs or computed tomography scans of the ribs and chest are indicated for all patients who present with pain from fractured ribs to rule out occult fractures and other bony pathology, including tumor, as well as pneumothorax and hemopneumothorax (Fig. 56-2). If

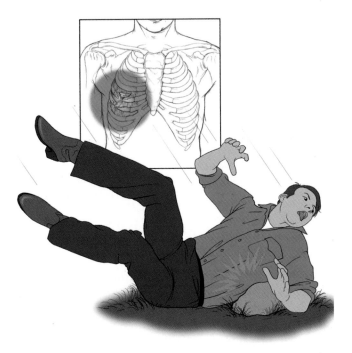

Figure 56–1. The pain of fractured ribs is amenable to intercostal nerve block with local anesthetic and steroid.

trauma is present, radionuclide bone scanning may be useful to rule out occult fractures of the ribs or sternum. If no trauma is present, bone density testing to rule out osteoporosis is appropriate, as are serum protein electrophoresis and testing for hyperparathyroidism. Based on the patient's clinical presentation, additional testing may be warranted, including a complete blood count, prostate-specific antigen level, erythrocyte sedimentation rate, and antinuclear antibody testing. Computed tomography scanning of the thoracic contents is indicated if occult mass or significant trauma to the thoracic contents is suspected (Fig. 56-3). Electrocardiography to rule out cardiac contusion is recommended for all patients with traumatic sternal fractures or significant anterior chest wall trauma. The injection technique described later should be used early to avoid pulmonary complications.

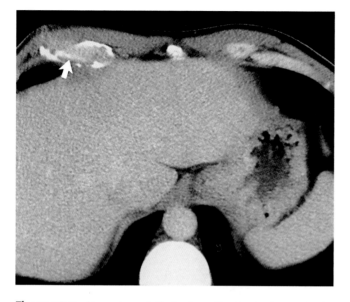

Figure 56–2. Nonunion of rib fracture. Contrast-enhanced axial computed tomography scan shows expansile right rib lesion with questionable chondroid matrix *(arrow)*. (From Haaga JR, Lanzieri CF, Gilkeson RC [eds]: CT and MR Imaging of the Whole Body, 4th ed. Philadelphia, Mosby, 2003, p 1009.)

DIFFERENTIAL DIAGNOSIS

In the setting of trauma, the diagnosis of fractured ribs is usually straightforward. In the setting of spontaneous rib fracture secondary to osteoporosis or metastatic disease, the diagnosis may be less clear-cut. In this case, the pain of occult rib fracture is often mistaken for pain of cardiac or gallbladder origin, leading to visits to the emergency department and unnecessary cardiac and

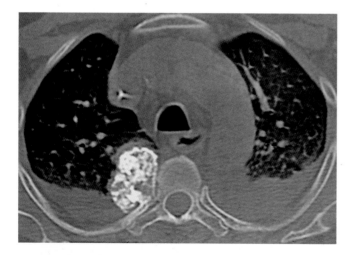

Figure 56–3. Noncontrast computed tomography scan reveals a heterogeneous, lobulated, calcified mass with a cartilaginous cap arising from the right third rib, consistent with osteochondroma. (From Haaga JR, Lanzieri CF, Gilkeson RC [eds]: CT and MR Imaging of the Whole Body, 4th ed. Philadelphia, Mosby, 2003, p 1008.)

gastrointestinal workups. Tietze's syndrome, which is painful enlargement of the upper costochondral cartilage associated with viral infection, may be confused with fractured ribs, especially if the patient has been coughing.

TREATMENT

Initial treatment of rib fracture pain includes a combination of simple analgesics and nonsteroidal anti-inflammatory drugs or cyclooxygenase-2 inhibitors. If these medications do not adequately control the patient's symptoms, short-acting opioid analgesics such as hydrocodone are a reasonable next step. Because opioid analgesics have the potential to suppress the cough reflex and respiration, the patient must be closely monitored and instructed in adequate pulmonary toilet techniques.

The local application of heat and cold or the use of an elastic rib belt may also provide symptomatic relief. For patients who do not respond to these treatment modalities, injection using local anesthetic and steroid should be implemented to avoid pulmonary complications.

The patient is placed in the prone position with the arms hanging loosely off the sides of the table. Alternatively, this injection technique can be performed with the patient in the sitting or lateral position. The rib to be blocked is identified by palpating its path at the posterior axillary line. The operator's index and middle fingers are placed on the rib, bracketing the site of needle insertion. The skin is prepared with antiseptic solution. A 1½-inch, 22-gauge needle is attached to a 12-mL syringe and advanced perpendicular to the skin, aiming for the middle of the rib, between the operator's index and middle fingers. The needle should impinge on bone after being advanced approximately ¾ inch. Once bony contact is made, the needle is withdrawn into the subcutaneous tissues, and the skin and subcutaneous tissues are retracted with the palpating fingers inferiorly. This allows the needle to be walked off the inferior margin of the rib. As soon as bony contact is lost, the needle is slowly advanced approximately 2 mm deeper. This places the needle in proximity to the costal groove, which contains the intercostal nerve as well as the intercostal artery and vein. After careful aspiration reveals no blood or air, 3 to 5 mL of 1% preservative-free lidocaine is injected. If there is an inflammatory component to the pain, the local anesthetic is combined with 80 mg methylprednisolone and is injected in incremental doses. Subsequent daily nerve blocks are carried out in a similar manner, substituting 56 mg methylprednisolone for the initial 80-mg dose. Because of the overlapping innervation of the chest and upper abdominal wall, the intercostal nerves above and below the nerve suspected of causing the pain must be blocked as well.

COMPLICATIONS AND PITFALLS

The major problem in the care of patients thought to be suffering from rib fracture is failure to identify potentially serious pathology of the thorax or upper abdomen, such as tumor, pneumothorax, or hemopneumothorax. Given the proximity of the pleural space, pneumothorax after intercostal nerve block is a distinct possibility. The incidence of this complication is less than 1%, but it occurs with greater frequency in patients with chronic obstructive pulmonary disease. Owing to the proximity to the intercostal nerve and artery, the clinician must carefully calculate the total dosage of local anesthetic administered, because vascular uptake via these vessels is high. Though uncommon, infection is always a possibility, especially in immunocompromised patients with cancer.

Early detection of infection is crucial to avoid potentially life-threatening sequelae.

Clinical Pearls

Rib fracture is a common cause of chest wall and thoracic pain. Correct diagnosis is necessary to properly treat this painful condition and to avoid overlooking serious intrathoracic or intra-abdominal pathology. Pharmacologic agents, including opioid analgesics, are usually adequate to control the pain of rib fracture. If necessary, intercostal nerve block is a simple technique that can produce dramatic pain relief. However, because of the proximity of the intercostal nerve to the pleural space, strict attention to technique is mandatory.

Chapter 57

Post-Thoracotomy Pain Syndrome

ICD-9 CODE 786.52

THE CLINICAL SYNDROME

Essentially all patients who undergo thoracotomy suffer from acute postoperative pain. This acute pain syndrome invariably responds to the rational use of systemic and spinal opioids, as well as intercostal nerve block. Unfortunately, in a small percentage of patients who undergo thoracotomy, the pain persists beyond the postoperative period and can be difficult to treat. The causes of post-thoracotomy pain syndrome are listed in Table 57-1 and include direct surgical trauma, fractured ribs, compressive neuropathy, neuroma, and stretch injuries. When the syndrome is caused by fractured ribs, it produces local pain that is worse with deep inspiration, coughing, or movement of the affected ribs. The other causes of the syndrome result in moderate to severe pain that is constant in nature and follows the distribution of the affected intercostal nerves. The pain may be characterized as neuritic and may occasionally have a dysesthetic quality.

SIGNS AND SYMPTOMS

Physical examination generally reveals tenderness along the healed thoracotomy incision (Fig. 57-1). Occasionally, palpation of the scar elicits paresthesias, suggestive of neuroma formation. Patients suffering from post-thoracotomy syndrome may attempt to splint or protect the affected area. Careful sensory examination of the affected dermatomes may reveal decreased sensation or allodynia. With significant motor involvement of the subcostal nerve, patients may complain that the abdomen bulges out. Occasionally, patients suffering from post-thoracotomy syndrome develop a reflex sympathetic dystrophy of the ipsilateral upper extremity that, if left untreated, may result in a frozen shoulder.

Table 57–1. Causes of Post-Thoracotomy Pain Syndrome

Direct surgical trauma to the intercostal nerves
Fractured ribs due to use of the rib spreader
Compressive neuropathy of the intercostal nerves due to direct compression by retractors
Cutaneous neuroma formation
Stretch injuries to the intercostal nerves at the costovertebral junction

TESTING

Plain radiographs are indicated for all patients who present with pain that is thought to be emanating from the intercostal nerve to rule out occult bony pathology, including unsuspected fracture or tumor. Radionuclide bone scanning may be useful to rule out occult fractures

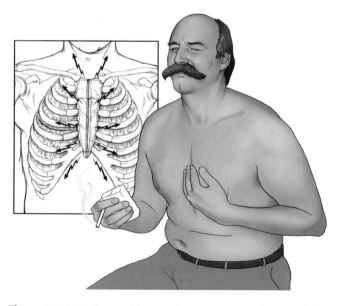

Figure 57–1. Patients with post-thoracotomy syndrome exhibit tenderness to palpation of the scar.

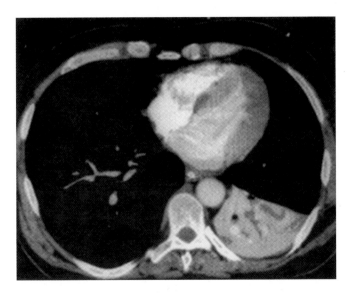

Figure 57–2. Computed tomography scan showing left lower lobe atelectasis. Some of the bronchi are open (air filled), and others are plugged (mucus filled). (From Grainger RG, Allison DJ, Adam A, Dixon AK: Grainger & Allison's Diagnostic Radiology: A Textbook of Medical Imaging, 4th ed. Philadelphia, Churchill Livingstone, 2002.)

of the ribs or sternum. Based on the patient's clinical presentation, additional testing may be warranted, including a complete blood count, prostate-specific antigen level, erythrocyte sedimentation rate, and antinuclear antibody testing. Computed tomography scanning of the thoracic contents is indicated if occult mass or pleural disease is suspected (Fig. 57-2). The injection technique described later serves as both a diagnostic and a therapeutic maneuver. Electromyography is useful in distinguishing injury of the distal intercostal nerve from stretch injuries of the intercostal nerve at the costovertebral junction.

DIFFERENTIAL DIAGNOSIS

The pain of post-thoracotomy syndrome may be mistaken for pain of cardiac or gallbladder origin, leading to visits to the emergency department and unnecessary cardiac and gastrointestinal workups. In the presence of trauma, post-thoracotomy syndrome may coexist with fractured ribs or fractures of the sternum itself, which can be missed on plain radiographs and may require radionuclide bone scanning for proper identification. Tietze's syndrome, which is painful enlargement of the upper costochondral cartilage associated with viral infection, may be confused with post-thoracotomy syndrome.

Neuropathic pain involving the chest wall may also be confused or coexist with post-thoracotomy syndrome. Examples of such neuropathic pain include diabetic polyneuropathies and acute herpes zoster involving the

thoracic nerves. Diseases of the structures of the mediastinum are possible and may be difficult to diagnose. Pathologic processes that inflame the pleura, such as pulmonary embolus, infection, and Bornholm disease, may also confuse the diagnosis and complicate treatment (Fig. 57-3).

TREATMENT

Initial treatment of post-thoracotomy syndrome includes a combination of simple analgesics and nonsteroidal anti-inflammatory drugs or cyclooxygenase-2 inhibitors. If these medications do not adequately control the patient's symptoms, a tricyclic antidepressant or gabapentin should be added.

Traditionally, tricyclic antidepressants have been a mainstay in the palliation of pain caused by post-thoracotomy syndrome. Controlled studies have demonstrated the efficacy of amitriptyline, and nortriptyline and desipramine have also proved to be clinically useful. Unfortunately, this class of drugs is associated with significant anticholinergic side effects, including dry mouth, constipation, sedation, and urinary retention. They should be used with caution in patients suffering from glaucoma, cardiac arrhythmia, and prostatism. To minimize side effects and encourage compliance, the physician should start amitriptyline or nortriptyline at a 10-mg dose at bedtime; the dose can then be titrated upward

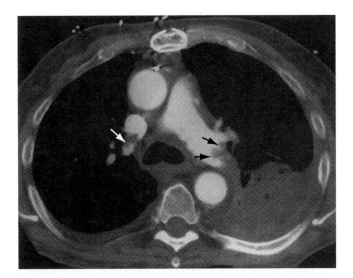

Figure 57–3. Computed tomography demonstrates bilateral pulmonary emboli in the presence of left lower lobe consolidation and bilateral pleural effusions. There is a large embolus in the left main pulmonary artery (black arrows) and a small embolus in the proximal right upper lobe pulmonary artery (white arrow). (From Grainger RG, Allison DJ, Adam A, Dixon AK: Grainger & Allison's Diagnostic Radiology: A Textbook of Medical Imaging, 4th ed. Philadelphia, Churchill Livingstone, 2002.)

to 25 mg at bedtime, as side effects allow. Subsequently, upward titration in 25-mg increments can be carried out each week, as side effects allow. Even at lower doses, patients generally report a rapid improvement in sleep disturbance and begin to experience some pain relief in 10 to 14 days. If the patient does not show any improvement in pain as the dose is being titrated upward, the addition of gabapentin alone or in combination with nerve blocks is recommended (see later). The selective serotonin reuptake inhibitors such as fluoxetine have also been used to treat the pain of post-thoracotomy syndrome, and although these drugs are better tolerated than the tricyclic antidepressants, they appear to be less efficacious.

If the antidepressant compounds are ineffective or contraindicated, gabapentin is a reasonable alternative. Gabapentin is started at a 300-mg dose at bedtime for 2 nights. The patient should be cautioned about potential side effects, including dizziness, sedation, confusion, and rash. The drug is then increased in 300-mg increments given in equally divided doses over 2 days, as side effects allow, until pain relief is obtained or a total dosage of 2400 mg/day is reached. At this point, if the patient has experienced partial pain relief, blood values are measured, and the drug is carefully titrated upward using 100-mg tablets. Rarely is a dose greater than 3600 mg/day required.

The local application of heat and cold or the use of an elastic rib belt may also provide symptomatic relief. For patients who do not respond to these treatment modalities, injection using local anesthetic and steroid is a reasonable next step.

The patient is placed in the prone position with the arms hanging loosely off the sides of the table. Alternatively, this block can be done with the patient in the sitting or lateral position. The rib to be blocked is identified by palpating its path at the posterior axillary line. The operator's index and middle fingers are placed on the rib, bracketing the site of needle insertion. The skin is prepared with antiseptic solution. A 1½-inch, 22-gauge needle is attached to a 12-mL syringe and advanced perpendicular to the skin, aiming for the middle of the rib between the operator's index and middle fingers. The needle should impinge on bone after being advanced approximately ¾ inch. Once bony contact is made, the needle is withdrawn into the subcutaneous tissues, and the skin and subcutaneous tissues are retracted with the palpating fingers inferiorly. This allows the needle to be walked off the inferior margin of the rib. As soon as bony contact is lost, the needle is slowly advanced approximately 2 mm deeper. This places the needle in proximity to the costal groove, which contains the intercostal

nerve as well as the intercostal artery and vein. After careful aspiration reveals no blood or air, 3 to 5 mL of 1% preservative-free lidocaine is injected. If there is an inflammatory component to the pain, the local anesthetic is combined with 80 mg methylprednisolone and is injected in incremental doses. Subsequent daily nerve blocks are carried out in a similar manner, substituting 40 mg methylprednisolone for the initial 80-mg dose. Because of the overlapping innervation of the chest and upper abdominal wall, the intercostal nerves above and below the nerve suspected of causing the pain must be blocked as well.

If post-thoracotomy pain syndrome is caused by stretch injury of the intercostal nerve (identified by electromyography), it may respond to thoracic epidural nerve block with steroid.

COMPLICATIONS AND PITFALLS

The major problem in the care of patients thought to be suffering from post-thoracotomy syndrome is failure to identify potentially serious pathology of the thorax or upper abdomen. Given the proximity of the pleural space, pneumothorax after intercostal nerve block is a distinct possibility. The incidence of this complication is less than 1%, but it occurs with greater frequency in patients with chronic obstructive pulmonary disease. Owing to the proximity to the intercostal nerve and artery, the clinician must carefully calculate the total dosage of local anesthetic administered, because vascular uptake via these vessels is high. Though uncommon, infection is always a possibility, especially in immunocompromised patients with cancer. Early detection of infection is crucial to avoid potentially life-threatening sequelae.

Clinical Pearls

Post-thoracotomy syndrome is a common cause of chest wall and thoracic pain. Correct diagnosis is necessary to properly treat this painful condition and to avoid overlooking serious intrathoracic or intra-abdominal pathology. Pharmacologic agents are usually adequate to control the pain of post-thoracotomy syndrome. If necessary, intercostal nerve block is a simple technique that can produce dramatic pain relief. However, because of the proximity of the intercostal nerve to the pleural space, strict attention to technique is mandatory.

Section 9

Pain Syndromes of the Thoracic Spine

Chapter 58

Acute Herpes Zoster of the Thoracic Dermatomes

ICD-9 CODE 053.9

THE CLINICAL SYNDROME

Herpes zoster is an infectious disease caused by the varicella-zoster virus (VZV). Primary infection with VZV in a nonimmune host manifests clinically as the childhood disease chickenpox. It is postulated that during the course of the primary infection, the virus migrates to the dorsal root of the thoracic nerves, where it remains dormant in the ganglia, producing no clinically evident disease. In some individuals, the virus reactivates and travels along the sensory pathways of the thoracic nerves, producing the pain and skin lesions characteristic of herpes zoster, or shingles. Although the thoracic nerve roots are the most common site for the development of acute herpes zoster, the first division of the trigeminal nerve may also be affected.

Why reactivation occurs in some individuals but not in others is not fully understood, but it is theorized that a decrease in cell-mediated immunity may play an important role in the evolution of this disease by allowing the virus to multiply in the ganglia and spread to the corresponding sensory nerves, producing clinical disease. Patients who are suffering from malignancy (particularly lymphoma) or chronic disease and those receiving immunosuppressive therapy (chemotherapy, steroids, radiation) are generally debilitated and thus much more likely than the healthy population to develop acute herpes zoster. These patients all have in common a decreased cell-mediated immune response, which may also explain why the incidence of shingles increases dramatically in patients older than 60 years and is relatively uncommon in those younger than 20.

SIGNS AND SYMPTOMS

As viral reactivation occurs, ganglionitis and peripheral neuritis cause pain that may be accompanied by flulike symptoms. The pain generally progresses from a dull, aching sensation to dysesthetic or neuritic pain in the distribution of the thoracic nerve roots (Fig. 58-1). In most patients, the pain of acute herpes zoster precedes the eruption of rash by 3 to 7 days, often leading to an erroneous diagnosis (see Differential Diagnosis). However, in most patients, the clinical diagnosis of shingles is readily made when the characteristic rash appears. Like chickenpox, the rash of herpes zoster appears in crops of macular lesions, which rapidly progress to papules and then to vesicles. Eventually, the vesicles coalesce, and crusting occurs. The affected area can be extremely painful, and the pain tends to be exacerbated by any movement or contact (e.g., with clothing or sheets). As the lesions heal, the crust falls away,

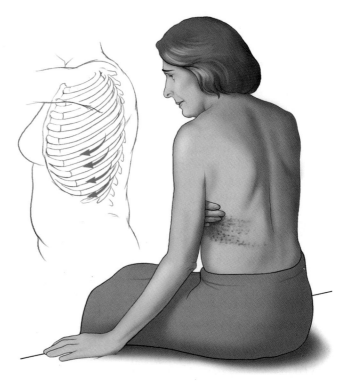

Figure 58–1. Acute herpes zoster occurs most commonly in the thoracic dermatomes.

leaving pink scars that gradually become hypopigmented and atrophic.

In most patients, the hyperesthesia and pain resolve as the skin lesions heal. In some, however, pain persists beyond lesion healing. This common and feared complication of acute herpes zoster is called postherpetic neuralgia, and the elderly are affected at a higher rate than is the general population suffering from acute herpes zoster. The symptoms of postherpetic neuralgia can vary from a mild, self-limited condition to a debilitating, constantly burning pain that is exacerbated by light touch, movement, anxiety, or temperature change. This unremitting pain may be so severe that it completely devastates the patient's life; ultimately, it can lead to suicide. To avoid this disastrous sequela to a usually benign, self-limited disease, the clinician must use all possible therapeutic efforts in patients with acute herpes zoster of the thoracic nerve roots.

TESTING

Although in most instances the diagnosis of acute herpes zoster involving the thoracic nerve roots is easily made on clinical grounds, confirmatory testing is occasionally required. Such testing may be desirable in patients with other skin lesions that confuse the clinical picture, such as those with human immunodeficieincy virus infection who are suffering from Kaposi's sarcoma. In such patients, the diagnosis of acute herpes zoster may be confirmed by obtaining a Tzanck smear from the base of a fresh vesicle, which reveals multinucleated giant cells and eosinophilic inclusions. To differentiate acute herpes zoster from localized herpes simplex infection, the clinician can obtain fluid from a fresh vesicle and submit it for immunofluorescent testing.

DIFFERENTIAL DIAGNOSIS

A careful initial evaluation, including a thorough history and physical examination, is indicated in all patients suffering from acute herpes zoster involving the thoracic nerve roots. The goal is to rule out occult malignancy or systemic disease that may be responsible for the patient's immunocompromised state. A prompt diagnosis allows early recognition of changes in clinical status that may presage the development of complications, including myelitis or dissemination of the disease. Other causes of pain in the distribution of the thoracic nerve roots include thoracic radiculopathy and peripheral neuropathy. Intrathoracic and intra-abdominal pathology may also mimic the pain of acute herpes zoster involving the thoracic dermatomes.

TREATMENT

The therapeutic challenge in patients presenting with acute herpes zoster involving the thoracic nerve roots is twofold: (1) the immediate relief of acute pain and other symptoms, and (2) the prevention of complications, including postherpetic neuralgia. It is the consensus of most pain specialists that the earlier treatment is initiated, the less likely it is that postherpetic neuralgia will develop. Further, because older individuals are at highest risk for developing postherpetic neuralgia, early and aggressive treatment of this group of patients is mandatory.

Nerve Block

Thoracic epidural nerve block with local anesthetic and steroid is the treatment of choice to relieve the symptoms of acute herpes zoster involving the thoracic nerve roots, as well as to prevent the occurrence of postherpetic neuralgia. As vesicular crusting occurs, the steroid may also reduce neural scarring. Neural blockade is thought to achieve these goals by blocking the profound sympathetic stimulation that results from viral inflammation of the nerve and dorsal root ganglion. If untreated, this sympathetic hyperactivity can cause ischemia secondary to decreased blood flow to the intraneural capillary bed. If this ischemia is allowed to persist, endoneural edema forms, increasing endoneural pressure and further reducing endoneural blood flow, resulting in irreversible nerve damage.

These sympathetic blocks should be continued aggressively until the patient is pain free and should be reimplemented if the pain returns. Failure to use sympathetic neural blockade immediately and aggressively, especially in the elderly, may sentence the patient to a lifetime of suffering from postherpetic neuralgia. Occasionally, some patients with acute herpes zoster of the thoracic nerve roots do not experience pain relief from thoracic epidural nerve block but may respond to blockade of the thoracic sympathetic nerves.

Opioid Analgesics

Opioid analgesics can be useful to relieve the aching pain that is common during the acute stages of herpes zoster, while sympathetic nerve blocks are being implemented. Opioids are less effective in relieving neuritic pain, which is also common. Careful administration of potent, long-acting narcotic analgesics (e.g., oral morphine elixir, methadone) on a time-contingent rather than an as-needed basis may be a beneficial adjunct to the pain relief provided by sympathetic neural blockade. Because many patients suffering from acute herpes zoster are elderly or have severe multisystem disease, close monitoring for the potential side effects of potent narcotic analgesics (e.g., confusion or dizziness, which may cause a patient to fall) is warranted. Daily dietary fiber supplementation and milk of magnesia should be started along with opioid analgesics to prevent constipation.

Adjuvant Analgesics

The anticonvulsant gabapentin represents a first-line treatment for the neuritic pain of acute herpes zoster of the thoracic nerve roots. Studies suggest that gabapentin may also help prevent postherpetic neuralgia. Treatment with gabapentin should begin early in the course of the disease; this drug may be used concurrently with neural blockade, opioid analgesics, and other adjuvant analgesics, including antidepressants, if care is taken to avoid central nervous system side effects. Gabapentin is started at a bedtime dose of 300 mg and is titrated upward in 300-mg increments to a maximum of 3600 mg/day given in divided doses, as side effects allow.

Carbamazepine should be considered in patients suffering from severe neuritic pain who fail to respond to nerve blocks and gabapentin. If this drug is used, strict monitoring of hematologic parameters is indicated, especially in patients receiving chemotherapy or radiation therapy. Phenytoin may also be beneficial to treat neuritic pain, but it should not be used in patients with lymphoma; the drug may induce a pseudolymphoma-like state that is difficult to distinguish from the actual lymphoma.

Antidepressants

Antidepressants may also be useful adjuncts in the initial treatment of patients suffering from acute herpes zoster. On an acute basis, these drugs help alleviate the significant sleep disturbance that is commonly seen. In addition, antidepressants may be valuable in ameliorating the neuritic component of the pain, which is treated less effectively with narcotic analgesics. After several weeks of treatment, antidepressants may exert a mood-elevating effect, which may be desirable in some patients. Care must be taken to observe closely for central nervous system side effects in this patient population. In addition, these drugs may cause urinary retention and constipation, which may mistakenly be attributed to herpes zoster myelitis.

Antiviral Agents

A limited number of antiviral agents, including famciclovir and acyclovir, can shorten the course of acute herpes zoster and may even help prevent its development. They are probably useful in attenuating the disease in immunosuppressed patients. These antiviral agents can be used in conjunction with the aforementioned treatment modalities. Careful monitoring for side effects is mandatory.

Adjunctive Treatments

The application of ice packs to the lesions of acute herpes zoster may provide relief in some patients. Application of heat increases pain in most patients, presumably because of the increased conduction of small fibers; however, it is beneficial in an occasional patient and may be worth trying if the application of cold is ineffective. Transcutaneous electrical nerve stimulation and vibration may also be effective in a limited number of patients. The favorable risk-benefit ratio of these modalities makes them reasonable alternatives for patients who cannot or will not undergo sympathetic neural blockade or cannot tolerate pharmacologic interventions.

Topical application of aluminum sulfate as a tepid soak provides excellent drying of the crusting and weeping lesions of acute herpes zoster, and most patients find these soaks soothing. Zinc oxide ointment may also be used as a protective agent, especially during the healing phase, when temperature sensitivity is a problem. Disposable diapers can be used as absorbent padding to protect healing lesions from contact with clothing and sheets.

COMPLICATIONS AND PITFALLS

In most patients, acute herpes zoster involving the thoracic nerve roots is a self-limited disease. In the elderly and the immunosuppressed, however, complications may occur. Cutaneous and visceral dissemination may range from a mild rash resembling chickenpox to an overwhelming, life-threatening infection in those already suffering from severe multisystem disease. Myelitis may cause bowel, bladder, and lower extremity paresis.

Clinical Pearls

Because the pain of herpes zoster usually precedes the eruption of skin lesions by 3 to 7 days, some other painful condition (e.g., thoracic radiculopathy, cholecystitis) may erroneously be diagnosed. In this setting, an astute clinician should advise the patient to call immediately if a rash appears, because acute herpes zoster is a possibility. Some pain specialists believe that in a small number of immunocompetent patients, when reactivation of VZV occurs, a rapid immune response attenuates the natural course of the disease, and the characteristic rash of acute herpes zoster may not appear. In this case, pain in the distribution of the thoracic nerve roots without an associated rash is called zoster sine herpete and is, by necessity, a diagnosis of exclusion. Therefore, other causes of thoracic and subcostal pain must be ruled out before invoking this diagnosis.

Chapter 59

Costovertebral Joint Syndrome

ICD-9 CODE 719.48

THE CLINICAL SYNDROME

The costovertebral joint is a true joint and is susceptible to osteoarthritis, rheumatoid arthritis, psoriatic arthritis, Reiter's syndrome, and, in particular, ankylosing spondylitis (Figs. 59-1 and 59-2). The joint is often traumatized during acceleration-deceleration injuries and blunt trauma to the chest; with severe trauma, the joint may subluxate or dislocate. Overuse or misuse can result in acute inflammation of the costovertebral joint, which can be quite debilitating. The joint is also subject to invasion by tumor from primary malignancies, including lung cancer, or from metastatic disease. Pain emanating from the costovertebral joint can mimic pain of pulmonary or cardiac origin.

SIGNS AND SYMPTOMS

On physical examination, patients attempt to splint the affected joint or joints by avoiding flexion, extension,

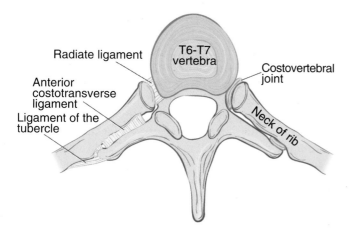

and lateral bending of the spine; they may also retract the scapulae in an effort to relieve the pain. The costovertebral joint may be tender to palpation and feel hot and swollen if it is acutely inflamed. Patients may also complain of a "clicking" sensation with movement of the joint. Because ankylosing spondylitis commonly affects both the costovertebral joint and the sacroiliac joint, many patients assume a stooped posture, which should alert the clinician to the possibility of this disease as the cause of costovertebral joint pain.

TESTING

Plain radiographs or computed tomography scans are indicated for all patients who present with pain that is thought to be emanating from the costovertebral joint to rule out occult bony pathology, including tumor (Fig. 59-3). If trauma is present, radionuclide bone scanning may be useful to rule out occult fractures of the ribs or sternum. Laboratory evaluation for collagen vascular disease and other joint diseases, including ankylosing spondylitis, is indicated for patients with costovertebral joint pain, especially if other joints are involved. Because of the high incidence of costovertebral joint abnormalities in patients with anklyosing spondylitis, HLA B-27 testing should also be considered. Based on the patient's clinical presentation, additional testing may be warranted, including a complete blood count, prostate-specific antigen level, erythrocyte sedimentation rate, and antinuclear antibody testing. Magnetic resonance imaging of the joints is indicated if joint instability or occult mass is suspected or to further elucidate the cause of the pain.

DIFFERENTIAL DIAGNOSIS

As mentioned earlier, the pain of costovertebral joint syndrome is often mistaken for pain of pulmonary or cardiac origin, leading to visits to the emergency department and unnecessary pulmonary or cardiac workups. If trauma has occurred, costovertebral joint syndrome may

Figure 59–1. Costovertebral joint. (From Waldman SD: Atlas of Pain Management Injection Techniques, 2nd ed. Philadelphia, Saunders, 2007.)

Figure 59–2. Costovertebral joint ankylosis. **A,** Photograph of the lateral aspect of the macerated thoracic spine of a spondylitic cadaver demonstrates extensive bony ankylosis *(arrows)* of the head of the ribs (R) and vertebral bodies. Disk ossification is also seen. **B,** Transaxial computed tomography scan of a thoracic vertebra in a patient with ankylosing spondylitis reveals bone erosions and partial ankylosis *(arrowhead)* of the costovertebral joints on one side. Note the involvement of the ipsilateral rib with cortical thickening *(arrows)*. (From Resnick D: Diagnosis of Bone and Joint Disorders, 4th ed. Philadelphia, Saunders, 2002, p 1045.)

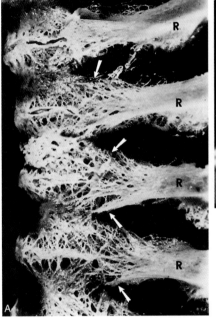
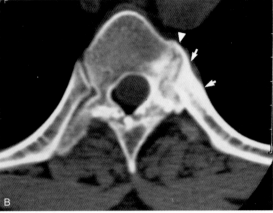

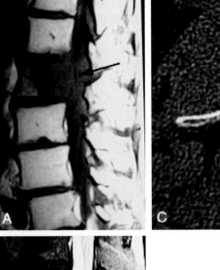
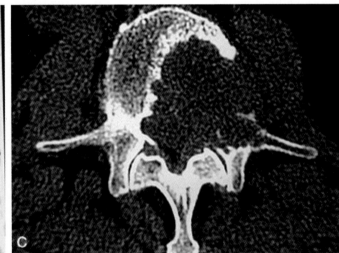
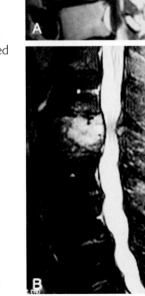

Figure 59–3. Metastatic renal carcinoma. Sagittal T1-weighted **(A)** and short tau inversion recovery **(B)** images show an expansile, destructive mass replacing a lumbar vertebra, with remodeling of the posterior margin and an epidural component *(arrow)*. Axial computed tomography scan **(C)** shows the lesion involving the pedicle and transverse process, with a significant intraspinal component. (From Edelman RR, Hessellink JR, Zlatkin MB, Crues JV: Clinical Magnetic Resonance Imaging, 3rd ed. Philadelphia, Saunders, 2006, p 2324.)

coexist with fractured ribs or fractures of the spine or sternum itself, which can be missed on plain radiographs and may require radionuclide bone scanning for proper identification.

Neuropathic pain involving the chest wall may also be confused or coexist with costovertebral joint syndrome. Examples of such neuropathic pain include diabetic polyneuropathies and acute herpes zoster involving the thoracic nerves. Diseases of the structures of the mediastinum are possible and can be difficult to diagnose. Pathologic processes that inflame the pleura, such as pulmonary embolus, infection, and Bornholm disease, may also confuse the diagnosis and complicate treatment.

TREATMENT

Initial treatment of the pain and functional disability associated with costovertebral joint syndrome is nonsteroidal anti-inflammatory drugs or cyclooxygenase-2 inhibitors. The local application of heat and cold may also be beneficial. Use of an elastic rib belt may provide symptomatic relief and protect the costovertebral joints from additional trauma. For patients who do not respond to these treatment modalities, injection of the costovertebral joint with local anesthetic and steroid is a reasonable next step (Fig. 59-4). Physical modalities, including local heat and gentle range-of-motion exercises, should be introduced several days after injection for costovertebral joint pain. Vigorous exercises should be avoided, because they will exacerbate the patient's symptoms. Simple analgesics and nonsteroidal anti-inflammatory drugs can be used concurrently with the injection technique.

COMPLICATIONS AND PITFALLS

Because many pathologic processes can mimic the pain of costovertebral joint syndrome, the clinician must carefully rule out underlying diseases of the lung, heart, and

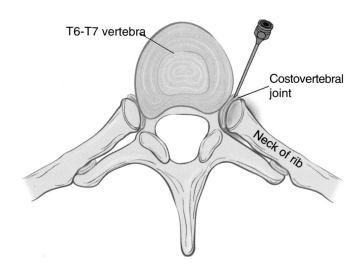

Figure 59–4. Needle placement for costovertebral joint injection. (From Waldman SD: Atlas of Pain Management Injection Techniques, 2nd ed. Philadelphia, Saunders, 2007.)

structures of the spine and mediastinum. Failure to do so could lead to disastrous results.

The major complication of the injection technique is pneumothorax if the needle is placed too laterally or deeply and invades the pleural space. Infection, though rare, can occur if strict aseptic technique is not followed. Trauma to the contents of the mediastinum is also a possibility. This complication can be greatly reduced with strict attention to accurate needle placement.

Clinical Pearls

Patients with pain emanating from the costovertebral joint may believe that they are suffering from pneumonia or having a heart attack. Reassurance is required.

Chapter 60

Postherpetic Neuralgia

ICD-9 CODE 053.13

THE CLINICAL SYNDROME

Postherpetic neuralgic is one of the most difficult pain syndromes to treat. It affects 10% of patients with acute herpes zoster. It is unknown why this painful condition occurs in some patients but not others; however, it is more common in older individuals and appears to occur more frequently after acute herpes zoster involving the trigeminal nerve as opposed to the thoracic dermatomes. Conditions that cause vulnerable nerve syndrome, such as diabetes, may also predispose patients to develop postherpetic neuralgia. It is the consensus among pain specialists that aggressive treatment of acute herpes zoster can help prevent postherpetic neuralgia.

SIGNS AND SYMPTOMS

As the lesions of acute herpes zoster heal, the crust falls away, leaving pink scars that gradually become hypopigmented and atrophic. The affected cutaneous areas are often allodynic, although hypesthesia and, rarely, anesthesia may occur. In most patients, the sensory abnormalities and pain resolve as the skin lesions heal. In some, however, pain persists beyond lesion healing.

The pain of postherpetic neuralgia is characterized as a constant dysesthetic pain that may be exacerbated by movement or stimulation of the affected cutaneous regions (Fig. 60-1). There may be sharp, shooting neuritic pain superimposed on the constant dysesthetic pain. Some patients suffering from postherpetic neuralgia also note a burning component, reminiscent of reflex sympathetic dystrophy.

TESTING

In most cases, the diagnosis of postherpetic neuralgia is made on clinical grounds. Testing is generally used to evaluate other treatable coexisting conditions, such as vertebral compression fractures, or to identify any underlying disease responsible for the patient's immunocom-

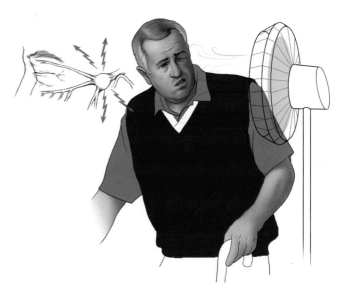

Figure 60–1. Allodynia and dysesthesia are characteristic of postherpetic neuralgia.

promised state. Such testing includes basic laboratory screening, rectal examination, mammography, and testing for collagen vascular diseases and human immunodeficiency virus infection. Skin biopsy may confirm the presence of previous infection with herpes zoster if the history is in question.

DIFFERENTIAL DIAGNOSIS

A careful initial evaluation, including a thorough history and physical examination, is indicated for all patients suffering from postherpetic neuralgia to rule out an occult malignancy or systemic disease that may be responsible for the patient's immunocompromised state. This also allows early recognition of changes in clinical status that may presage the development of complications, including myelitis or dissemination of the disease. Other causes of pain in the distribution of the thoracic nerve roots include thoracic radiculopathy and peripheral neuropathy. Intrathoracic and intra-abdominal pathology may also mimic the pain of acute herpes zoster involving the thoracic dermatomes. For pain in the distribution of the first division of the trigeminal nerve, the clinician must rule out diseases of the eye, ear, nose, and throat, as well as intracranial pathology.

TREATMENT

Ideally, rapid and aggressive treatment of acute herpes zoster is instituted in every patient, because it is the consensus of most pain specialists that the earlier treatment is initiated, the less likely it is that postherpetic neuralgia will develop. This is especially important in older individuals, who are at greatest risk for developing postherpetic neuralgia. If, despite everyone's best efforts, postherpetic neuralgia occurs, the following treatment regimens are appropriate.

Analgesics

The anticonvulsant gabapentin is first-line treatment for the pain of postherpetic neuralgia. Treatment with gabapentin should begin early in the course of the disease, and this drug may be used concurrently with neural blockade, opioid analgesics, and other analgesics, including antidepressants, if care is taken to avoid central nervous system side effects. Gabapentin is started at a dose of 300 mg at bedtime and is titrated upward in 300-mg increments to a maximum of 3600 mg/day in divided doses, as side effects allow.

Carbamazepine should be considered in patients suffering from severe neuritic pain in whom nerve blocks and gabapentin fail to provide relief. If this drug is used, rigid monitoring of hematologic parameters is indicated, especially in patients receiving chemotherapy or radiation therapy. Phenytoin may also be beneficial to treat neuritic pain, but it should not be used in patients with lymphoma; the drug may induce a pseudolymphoma-like state that is difficult to distinguish from actual lymphoma.

Antidepressants

Antidepressants may be useful adjuncts in the initial treatment of postherpetic neuralgia. On an acute basis, these drugs help alleviate the significant sleep disturbance that is common in this setting. In addition, antidepressants may be valuable in ameliorating the neuritic component of the pain, which is treated less effectively with narcotic analgesics. After several weeks of treatment, antidepressants may exert a mood-elevating effect that is desirable in some patients. Care must be taken to observe closely for central nervous system side effects in this patient population. These drugs may cause urinary retention and constipation that may mistakenly be attributed to herpes zoster myelitis.

Nerve Block

Neural blockade with local anesthetic and steroid via either epidural nerve block or blockade of the sympathetic nerves subserving the painful area is a reasonable next step if the aforementioned pharmacologic modalities fail to control the pain of postherpetic neuralgia. Although the exact mechanism of pain relief is unknown, it may be related to modulation of pain transmission at the spinal cord level. In general, neurodestructive procedures have a very low success rate and should be used only after all other treatments have failed, if at all.

Opioid Analgesics

Opioid analgesics have a limited role in the management of postherpetic neuralgia and may do more harm than good. Careful administration of potent, long-acting narcotic analgesics (e.g., oral morphine elixir, methadone) on a time-contingent rather than an as-needed basis may be a beneficial adjunct to the pain relief provided by sympathetic neural blockade. Because many patients suffering from postherpetic neuralgia are elderly or have severe multisystem disease, close monitoring for the potential side effects of narcotic analgesics (e.g., confusion or dizziness, which may cause a patient to fall) is warranted. Daily dietary fiber supplementation and milk of magnesia should be started along with opioid analgesics to prevent constipation.

Adjunctive Treatments

The application of ice packs to the affected area may provide relief in some patients. The application of heat increases pain in most patients, presumably because of increased conduction of small fibers; however, it is beneficial in an occasional patient and may be worth trying if the application of cold is ineffective. Transcutaneous electrical nerve stimulation and vibration may also be effective in a limited number of patients. The favorable risk-benefit ratio of all these modalities makes them reasonable alternatives for patients who cannot or will not undergo sympathetic neural blockade or cannot tolerate pharmacologic interventions. The topical application of capsaicin may be beneficial in some patients suffering from postherpetic neuralgia; however, it tends to burn when applied, limiting its usefulness.

COMPLICATIONS AND PITFALLS

Although there are no specific complications associated with postherpetic neuralgia itself, the consequences of the unremitting pain can be devastating. Failure to aggressively treat the pain of postherpetic neuralgia and the associated symptoms of sleep disturbance and depression can result in suicide.

Clinical Pearls

Because the pain of postherpetic neuralgia is so severe, the clinician must make every effort to avoid its occurrence by rapidly and aggressively treating acute herpes zoster. If postherpetic neuralgia develops, the aggressive treatment outlined here, with special attention to the insidious onset of severe depression, should be undertaken. If serious depression occurs, hospitalization with suicide precautions is mandatory.

Chapter **61**

Thoracic Vertebral Compression Fracture

ICD-9 CODE | **805.2 Traumatic Fractures**
733.13 Pathologic Fractures

THE CLINICAL SYNDROME

Thoracic vertebral compression fracture is one of the most common causes of dorsal spine pain. Vertebral compression fractures are most often the result of osteoporosis (Fig. 61-1), but they may also occur with trauma to the dorsal spine due to acceleration-deceleration injuries. In osteoporotic patients or in those with primary tumors or metastatic disease involving the thoracic vertebrae, fracture may occur with coughing (tussive fractures) or spontaneously.

The pain and functional disability associated with fractured vertebrae are determined largely by the severity of the injury (e.g., number of vertebrae involved) and the nature of the injury (e.g., whether the fracture causes impingement on the spinal nerves or spinal cord). The pain associated with thoracic vertebral compression fracture may range from a dull, deep ache (with minimal compression of the vertebrae and no nerve impingement) to severe, sharp, stabbing pain that limits the patient's ability to ambulate and cough.

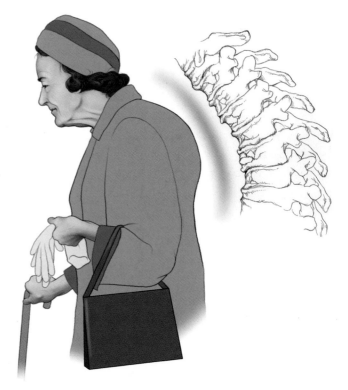

Figure 61-1. Osteoporosis is a common cause of thoracic vertebral fractures.

SIGNS AND SYMPTOMS

Compression fractures of the thoracic vertebrae are aggravated by deep inspiration, coughing, and any movement of the dorsal spine. Palpation of the affected vertebra may elicit pain and reflex spasm of the paraspinous musculature of the dorsal spine. If trauma has occurred, hematoma and ecchymosis may be present overlying the fracture site, and the clinician should be aware of the possibility of damage to the bony thorax and the intra-abdominal and intrathoracic contents. Damage to the spinal nerves may produce abdominal ileus and severe pain, resulting in splinting of the paraspinous muscles and further compromise to the patient's pulmonary

status and ability to ambulate. Failure to aggressively treat this pain and splinting may result in a negative cycle of hypoventilation, atelectasis, and, ultimately, pneumonia.

TESTING

Plain radiographs of the vertebrae are indicated to rule out other occult fractures and other bony pathology, including tumor. Magnetic resonance imaging may help characterize the nature of the fracture and distinguish benign from malignant causes of pain (Fig. 61-2). If

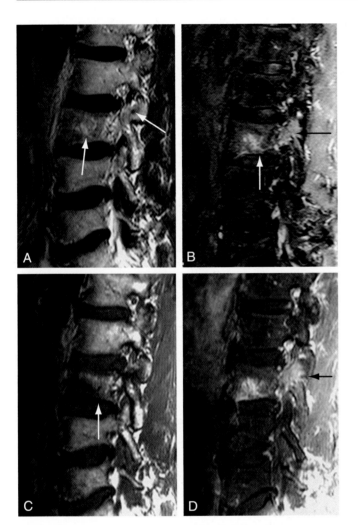

Figure 61–2. Metastasis. **A,** Parasagittal fast spin echo T2-weighted image shows an ill-defined, heterogeneous signal abnormality involving the L3 vertebral body and the pedicle *(arrows).* **B,** The lesion is more conspicuous on the sagittal short tau inversion recovery image *(arrows).* **C,** It is predominantly hypointense on the sagittal T1-weighted image. **D,** The lesion enhances on the postgadolinium T1-weighted image with fat saturation. (From Edelman RR, Hessellink JR, Zlatkin MB, Crues JV: Clinical Magnetic Resonance Imaging, 3rd ed. Philadelphia, Saunders, 2006, p 2315.)

trauma is present, radionuclide bone scanning may be useful to rule out occult fractures of the vertebrae or sternum. If no trauma is present, bone density testing to evaluate for osteoporosis is appropriate, as are serum protein electrophoresis and testing for hyperparathyroidism. Based on the patient's clinical presentation, additional testing may be warranted, including a complete blood count, prostate-specific antigen level, erythrocyte sedimentation rate, and antinuclear antibody testing. Computed tomography of the thoracic contents is indicated if occult mass or significant trauma is suspected. Electrocardiography to rule out cardiac contusion is indicated in all patients with traumatic sternal fractures or significant anterior dorsal spine trauma. The injection technique described later should be used early to avoid pulmonary complications.

DIFFERENTIAL DIAGNOSIS

In the setting of trauma, the diagnosis of thoracic vertebral compression fracture is usually straightforward. In the setting of spontaneous vertebral fracture secondary to osteoporosis or metastatic disease, the diagnosis may be less clear-cut. In this case, the pain of occult vertebral compression fracture is often mistaken for pain of cardiac or gallbladder origin, leading to visits to the emergency department and unnecessary cardiac and gastrointestinal workups. Acute sprain of the thoracic paraspinous muscles may be confused with thoracic vertebral compression fracture, especially if the patient has been coughing. Because the pain of acute herpes zoster may precede the rash by 3 to 7 days, it may erroneously be attributed to vertebral compression fracture.

TREATMENT

The initial treatment of pain secondary to compression fracture of the thoracic spine includes a combination of simple analgesics and nonsteroidal anti-inflammatory drugs or cyclooxygenase-2 inhibitors. If these medications do not adequately control the patient's symptoms, a short-acting opioid analgesic such as hydrocodone is a reasonable next step. Because the opioid analgesics have the potential to suppress the cough reflex and respiration, the patient must be closely monitored and instructed in adequate pulmonary toilet techniques.

The local application of heat and cold or the use of an orthotic device (e.g., the Cash brace) may provide symptomatic relief. For patients who do not respond to these treatment modalities, thoracic epidural block with local anesthetic and steroid is a reasonable next step. Kyphoplasty with cement fixation of the fracture is also a good option if pain and decreased mobility become a problem (Figs. 61-3 and 61-4).

COMPLICATIONS AND PITFALLS

The major problem in the care of patients thought to be suffering from compression fractures of the thoracic vertebrae is failure to identify compression of the spinal cord or to recognize that the fracture is due to metastatic disease. In patients with thoracic vertebral compression fractures due to osteoporosis, rapid pain control and early ambulation are mandatory to avoid complications such as pneumonia and thrombophlebitis.

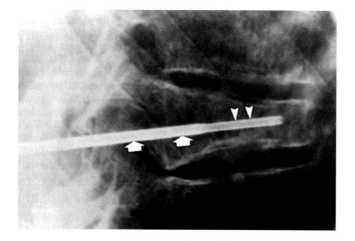

Figure 61–3. Trocar in the proper position to inject polymethyl methacrylate. (From Connors JJ, Wojak JC [eds]: Interventional Neuroradiology: Strategies and Practical Techniques. Philadelphia, Saunders, 1999, p 355.)

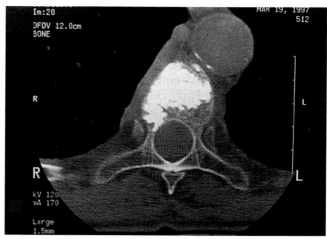

Figure 61–4. Computed tomography scan showing satisfactory injection of polymethyl methacrylate into the vertebral body. (From Connors JJ, Wojak JC [eds]: Interventional Neuroradiology: Strategies and Practical Techniques. Philadelphia, Saunders, 1999, p 350.)

Clinical Pearls

Compression fractures of the thoracic vertebrae are a common cause of dorsal spine pain. Correct diagnosis is necessary to properly treat this painful condition and to avoid overlooking serious intrathoracic or upper intra-abdominal pathology. Pharmacologic agents usually provide adequate pain control. If necessary, thoracic epidural block is a simple technique that can produce dramatic pain relief.

Pain Syndromes of the Groin and Abdomen

Chapter 62

Acute Pancreatitis

ICD-9 CODE 577.0

THE CLINICAL SYNDROME

Acute pancreatitis is one of the most common causes of abdominal pain, with an incidence of approximately 0.5% among the general population; the mortality rate is 1% to 1.5%. In the United States, acute pancreatitis is most commonly caused by excessive alcohol consumption (Fig. 62-1); gallstones are the most common cause in most European countries. There are many other causes of acute pancreatitis, including viral infection, tumor, and medications Table 62-1.

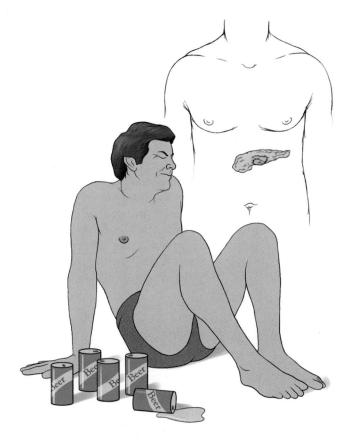

Figure 62–1. Excessive consumption of alcohol is one of the causes of acute pancreatitis.

Table 62–1. Common Causes of Acute Pancreatitis

Alcohol
Gallstones
Viral infections
Medications
Metabolic causes
Connective tissue diseases
Tumor obstructing the ampulla of Vater
Hereditary causes

Abdominal pain is a common feature of acute pancreatitis. It may range from mild to severe and is characterized by steady, boring epigastric pain that radiates to the flanks and chest. The pain is worse in the supine position, and patients with acute pancreatitis often prefer to sit with the dorsal spine flexed and the knees drawn up to the abdomen. Nausea, vomiting, and anorexia are other common features.

SIGNS AND SYMPTOMS

Patients with acute pancreatitis appear ill and anxious. Tachycardia and hypotension due to hypovolemia are common, as is low-grade fever. Saponification of subcutaneous fat is seen in approximately 15% of patients suffering from acute pancreatitis; a similar percentage of patients experiences pulmonary complications, including pleural effusion and pleuritic pain that may compromise respiration. Diffuse abdominal tenderness with peritoneal signs is invariably present. A pancreatic mass or pseudocyst due to pancreatic edema may be palpable. If hemorrhage occurs, periumbilical ecchymosis (Cullen's sign) and flank ecchymosis (Turner's sign) may be present. Both these findings suggest severe necrotizing pancreatitis and indicate a poor prognosis. If hypocalcemia is present, Chvostek's or Trousseau's sign may be present.

TESTING

Elevation of serum amylase levels is the sine qua non of acute pancreatitis. Levels tend to peak at 48 to 72 hours and then begin to drift toward normal. Serum lipase

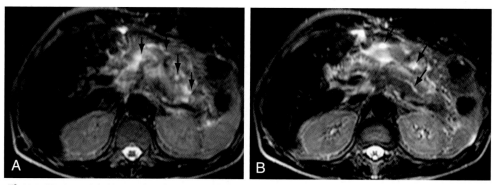

Figure 62–2. Axial T2-weighted images of acute pancreatitis. **A,** Scattered high signal *(black arrows)* surrounding the pancreas is consistent with peripancreatic edema. **B,** Normal pancreatic duct *(white arrow).* (From Edelman RR, Hessellink JR, Zlatkin MB, Crues JV: Clinical Magnetic Resonance Imaging, 3rd ed. Philadelphia, Saunders, 2006, p 2661.)

remains elevated and may correlate better with actual disease severity. Because serum amylase levels may be elevated with other diseases, such as parotitis, amylase isozymes may be necessary to confirm a pancreatic basis for this finding. Plain radiographs of the chest are indicated for all patients who present with acute pancreatitis to identify pulmonary complications, including pleural effusion. Given its extrapancreatic manifestations (e.g., acute renal or hepatic failure), serial complete blood counts, serum calcium and glucose levels, liver function tests, and electrolytes are indicated in all patients with acute pancreatitis. Computed tomography or MRI of the abdomen can identify pancreatic pseudocyst and edema and may help the clinician gauge the severity and progress of the disease (Fig. 62-2). Gallbladder evaluation with radionuclides is indicated if gallstones may be the cause of acute pancreatitis. Arterial blood gases can identify respiratory failure and metabolic acidosis.

DIFFERENTIAL DIAGNOSIS

The differential diagnosis includes perforated peptic ulcer, acute cholecystitis, bowel obstruction, renal calculi, myocardial infarction, mesenteric infarction, diabetic ketoacidosis, and pneumonia. Rarely, the collagen vascular diseases, including systemic lupus erythematosus and polyarteritis nodosa, may mimic pancreatitis. Because the pain of acute herpes zoster may precede the rash by 3 to 5 days, it may erroneously be attributed to acute pancreatitis.

TREATMENT

Most cases of acute pancreatitis are self-limited and resolve within 5 to 7 days. Initial treatment is aimed primarily at allowing the pancreas to rest, which is accomplished by giving the patient nothing by mouth to decrease serum gastrin secretion and, if ileus is present, by instituting nasogastric suction. Short-acting opioid analgesics such as hydrocodone are a reasonable next step if conservative measures do not control the patient's pain. If ileus is present, a parenteral narcotic such as meperidine is a good alternative. Because the opioid analgesics have the potential to suppress the cough reflex and respiration, the patient must be closely monitored and instructed in pulmonary toilet techniques. If symptoms persist, computed tomography–guided celiac plexus block with local anesthetic and steroid is indicated and may decrease the mortality and morbidity associated with the disease (Fig. 62-3). Alternatively, continuous thoracic epidural block with local anesthetic, opioid, or both may provide adequate pain control and allow the patient to avoid the respiratory depression associated with systemic opioid analgesics.

Hypovolemia should be treated aggressively with crystalloid and colloid infusions. For prolonged cases of acute pancreatitis, parenteral nutrition is indicated to avoid malnutrition. Surgical drainage and removal of necrotic tissue may be required if severe necrotizing pancreatitis fails to respond to these treatment modalities.

COMPLICATIONS AND PITFALLS

The major pitfall is failure to recognize the severity of the patient's condition and to identify and aggressively treat the extrapancreatic manifestations of acute pancreatitis. Hypovolemia, hypocalcemia, and renal and respiratory failure occur with sufficient frequency that the clinician must actively seek these potentially fatal complications and treat them aggressively.

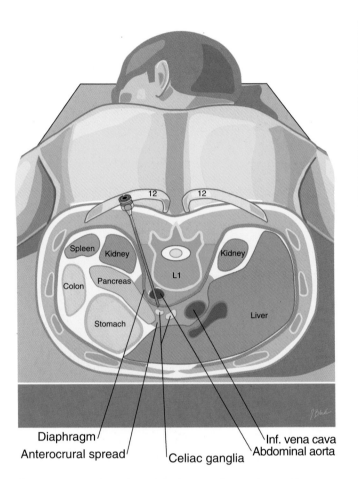

Diaphragm
Anterocrural spread
Celiac ganglia
Inf. vena cava
Abdominal aorta

Figure 62–3. Celiac plexus block using the single-needle transaortic approach. (From Waldman SD: Atlas of Interventional Pain Management, 2nd ed. Philadelphia, Saunders, 2004, p 286.)

Clinical Pearls

Acute pancreatitis is a common cause of abdominal pain. Correct diagnosis is necessary to properly treat this painful condition and to avoid overlooking serious extrapancreatic complications associated with this disease. Opioid analgesics generally provide adequate pain control. If necessary, celiac plexus block and thoracic epidural block are straightforward techniques that can produce dramatic pain relief.

Chapter 63

Chronic Pancreatitis

ICD-9 CODE **577.1**

THE CLINICAL SYNDROME

Chronic pancreatitis may present as recurrent episodes of acute inflammation of the pancreas superimposed on chronic pancreatic dysfunction, or it may be a more constant problem. As the exocrine function of the pancreas deteriorates, malabsorption with steatorrhea and azotorrhea develops. In the United States, chronic pancreatitis is most commonly caused by alcohol consumption, followed by cystic fibrosis and pancreatic malignancies. Hereditary causes such as alpha$_1$-antitrypsin deficiency are also common. In developing countries, the most common cause of chronic pancreatitis is severe protein calorie malnutrition. Chronic pancreatitis can also result from acute pancreatitis.

Abdominal pain is a common feature of chronic pancreatitis, and it mimics the pain of acute pancreatitis; it ranges from mild to severe and is characterized by steady, boring epigastric pain that radiates to the flanks and chest. The pain is worse with the consumption of alcohol and fatty meals. Nausea, vomiting, and anorexia are also common features. With chronic pancreatitis, the clinical symptoms are often subject to periods of exacerbation and remission.

SIGNS AND SYMPTOMS

Patients with chronic pancreatitis present similarly to those with acute pancreatitis but may appear more chronically ill than acutely ill (Fig. 63-1). Tachycardia and hypotension due to hypovolemia are much less common in chronic pancreatitis and are ominous prognostic indicators, or they may suggest that another pathologic process, such as perforated peptic ulcer, is present. Diffuse abdominal tenderness with peritoneal signs may be present if there is acute inflammation. A pancreatic mass or pseudocyst due to pancreatic edema may be palpable.

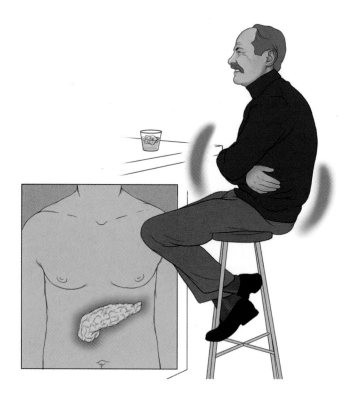

Figure 63–1. Chronic pancreatitis may present similarly to acute pancreatitis, but it can be more challenging to treat.

TESTING

Although serum amylase levels are always elevated in acute pancreatitis, they may be only mildly elevated or even within normal limits in chronic pancreatitis. Serum lipase levels are also attenuated in chronic, compared with acute, pancreatitis, although lipase may remain elevated longer than amylase in this setting and be more indicative of actual disease severity. Because serum amylase may be elevated with other diseases, such as parotitis, amylase isozymes may be necessary to confirm a pancreatic basis for this finding. Plain radiographs of the chest are indicated in all patients with chronic pancreatitis to identify pulmonary complications, including

218

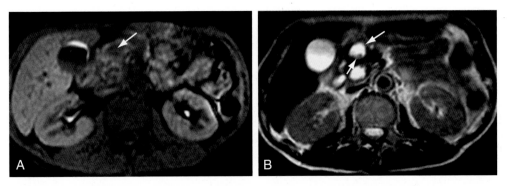

Figure 63–2. Chronic pancreatic pseudocyst. **A,** Axial T1-weighted postgadolinium magnetic resonance image shows a low-signal collection anterior to the pancreas *(arrow).* **B,** Axial T2-weighted magnetic resonance image shows a high-signal collection *(white arrow).* In a patient with a prior history of pancreatitis, this is consistent with a pseudocyst. Debris is noted within the pseudocyst *(small arrow).* (From Edelman RR, Hessellink JR, Zlatkin MB, Crues JV: Clinical Magnetic Resonance Imaging, 3rd ed. Philadelphia, Saunders, 2006, p 2666.)

pleural effusion. Given its extrapancreatic manifestations (e.g., acute renal or hepatic failure), serial complete blood counts, serum calcium and glucose levels, liver function tests, and electrolytes are indicated in all patients with chronic pancreatitis. Computed tomography (CT) of the abdomen can identify pancreatic pseudocyst or pancreatic tumor that may have been overlooked, and it may help the clinician gauge the severity and progress of the disease (Figs. 63-2 and 63-3). Gallbladder evaluation with radionuclides is indicated if gallstones are a possible cause of chronic pancreatitis. Arterial blood gases can identify respiratory failure and metabolic acidosis.

DIFFERENTIAL DIAGNOSIS

The differential diagnosis includes perforated peptic ulcer, acute cholecystitis, bowel obstruction, renal calculi, myocardial infarction, mesenteric infarction, diabetic ketoacidosis, and pneumonia. Rarely, the collagen vascular diseases, including systemic lupus erythematosus and polyarteritis nodosa, may mimic chronic pancreatitis. Because the pain of acute herpes zoster may precede the rash by 3 to 7 days, it may erroneously be attributed to chronic pancreatitis in patients who have had previous bouts of the disease. In addition, the clinician should always consider the possibility of pancreatic malignancy.

TREATMENT

The initial management of chronic pancreatitis focuses on alleviating pain and treating malabsorption. As with acute pancreatitis, the pancreas is allowed to rest by giving the patient nothing by mouth to decrease serum gastrin secretion and, if ileus is present, instituting nasogastric suction. Short-acting opioid analgesics such as

hydrocodone are a reasonable next step if conservative measures do not control the patient's pain. If ileus is present, a parenteral narcotic such as meperidine is a good alternative. Because the opioid analgesics have the potential to suppress the cough reflex and respiration, the patient must be closely monitored and instructed in pulmonary toilet techniques. The use of opioid analgesics must be monitored carefully, because the potential for misuse and dependence is high.

If symptoms persist, CT-guided celiac plexus block with local anesthetic and steroid is indicated and may decrease the mortality and morbidity associated with this disease (Fig. 63-4). If the relief from this technique is short-lived, neurolytic CT-guided celiac plexus block with alcohol or phenol is a reasonable next step. Alternatively, continuous thoracic epidural block with local anesthetic, opioid, or both may provide adequate pain control and allow the patient to avoid the respiratory depression associated with systemic opioid analgesics.

Hypovolemia should be treated aggressively with crystalloid and colloid infusions. For prolonged cases of chronic pancreatitis, parenteral nutrition is indicated to avoid malnutrition. Surgical drainage and removal of necrotic tissue may be required if severe necrotizing pancreatitis fails to respond to these treatment modalities.

COMPLICATIONS AND PITFALLS

The major pitfall is failure to recognize the severity of the patient's condition and to identify and aggressively treat the extrapancreatic manifestations of chronic pancreatitis. Hypovolemia, hypocalcemia, and renal and respiratory failure occur with sufficient frequency that the clinician must actively seek these potentially fatal complications and treat them aggressively. If opioids are

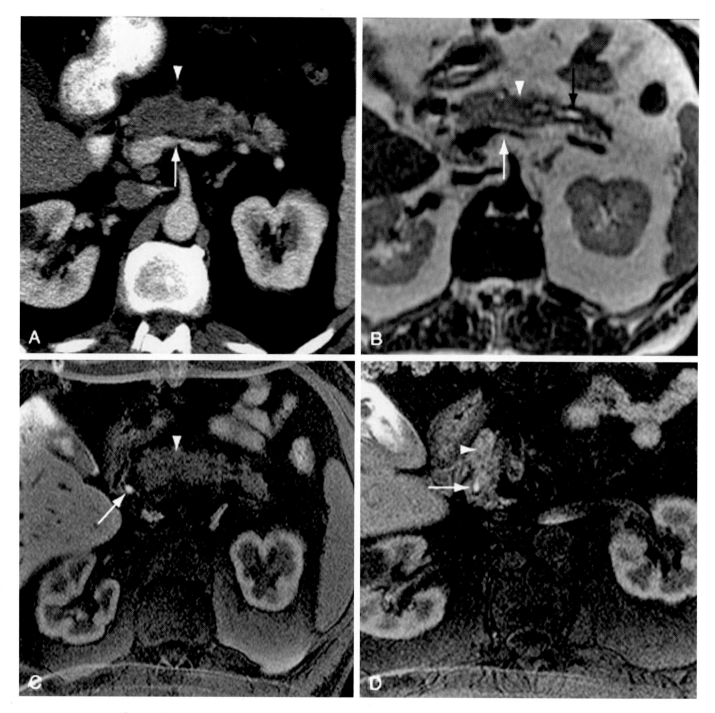

Figure 63–3. Pancreatic cancer. **A,** Axial contrast-enhanced computed tomography scan shows a large pancreatic body mass *(white arrowhead)* with distal ductal dilation *(black arrow)*. The splenic vein *(white arrow)* is not involved. **B,** Axial T1-weighted magnetic resonance image shows similar findings: pancreatic body mass *(arrowhead)*, distal ductal dilation *(black arrow)*, and a clear fat plane from the splenic vein *(white arrow)*. **C** and **D,** Postmanganese T1-weighted fat-saturated magnetic resonance images. The pancreatic mass does not enhance *(arrowhead)*. The common bile duct is enhanced and is seen as a high-signal structure *(arrow)*. (From Edelman RR, Hessellink JR, Zlatkin MB, Crues JV: Clinical Magnetic Resonance Imaging, 3rd ed. Philadelphia, Saunders, 2006, p 2672.)

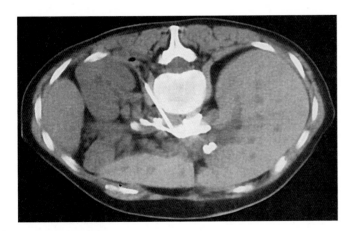

Figure 63–4. Computed tomography–guided celiac plexus block. (From Waldman SD: Atlas of Interventional Pain Management, 2nd ed. Philadelphia, Saunders, 2004, p 288.)

used, the clinician must constantly watch for overuse and dependence, especially if the underlying cause of the chronic pancreatitis is alcohol abuse.

Clinical Pearls

Chronic pancreatitis is a common cause of abdominal pain. Correct diagnosis is necessary to properly treat this painful condition and to avoid overlooking serious extrapancreatic complications. The judicious use of opioid analgesics is usually adequate to control the pain of acute exacerbations. If necessary, celiac plexus block and thoracic epidural block are straightforward techniques that can produce dramatic pain relief.

Chapter **64**

Ilioinguinal Neuralgia

ICD-9 CODE 355.8

THE CLINICAL SYNDROME

Ilioinguinal neuralgia is one of the most common causes of lower abdominal and pelvic pain encountered in clinical practice. Ilioinguinal neuralgia is caused by compression of the ilioinguinal nerve, and the most common causes of compression are traumatic injury to the nerve, including direct blunt trauma and damage during inguinal herniorrhaphy and pelvic surgery. Rarely, ilioinguinal neuralgia occurs spontaneously.

The ilioinguinal nerve is a branch of the L1 nerve root, with a contribution from T12 in some patients. The nerve follows a curvilinear course that takes it from its origin at the L1 (or occasionally T12) somatic nerves to inside the concavity of the ileum. The ilioinguinal nerve continues anteriorly to perforate the transverse abdominal muscle at the level of the anterior superior iliac spine. The nerve may interconnect with the iliohypogastric nerve as it continues to pass along its course medially and inferiorly, where it accompanies the spermatic cord through the inguinal ring and into the inguinal canal. The distribution of the sensory innervation of the ilioinguinal nerves varies from patient to patient, and there may be considerable overlap with the iliohypogastric nerve. In general, the ilioinguinal nerve provides sensory innervation to the skin of the upper inner thigh and the root of the penis and upper scrotum in men or the mons pubis and lateral labia in women.

SIGNS AND SYMPTOMS

Ilioinguinal neuralgia presents as paresthesias, burning pain, and occasionally numbness over the lower abdomen that radiates into the scrotum or labia and occasionally into the upper inner thigh; pain does not radiate below the knee. The pain of ilioinguinal neuralgia is made worse by extension of the lumbar spine, which puts traction on the nerve; thus, patients often assume a bent-forward, novice skier's position (Fig. 64-1). If the condition remains untreated, progressive motor deficit,

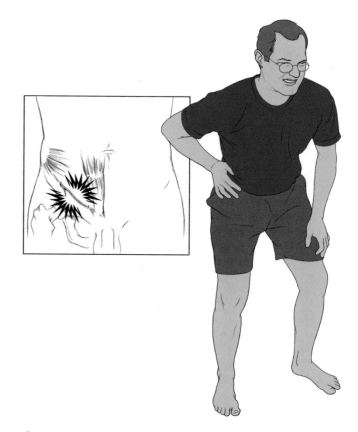

Figure 64–1. Patients suffering from ilioinguinal neuralgia often bend forward in the novice skier's position to relieve the pain.

consisting of bulging of the anterior abdominal wall muscles, may occur. This bulging may be confused with inguinal hernia.

Physical findings include sensory deficit in the inner thigh, scrotum, or labia in the distribution of the ilioinguinal nerve. Weakness of the anterior abdominal wall musculature may be present. Tinel's sign may be elicited by tapping over the ilioinguinal nerve at the point where it pierces the transverse abdominal muscle.

TESTING

Electromyography can distinguish ilioinguinal nerve entrapment from lumbar plexopathy, lumbar radiculopathy, and diabetic polyneuropathy. Plain radiographs of the hip and pelvis are indicated in all patients who present with ilioinguinal neuralgia to rule out occult bony pathology. Based on the patient's clinical presentation, additional testing may be warranted, including a complete blood count, uric acid level, erythrocyte sedimentation rate, and antinuclear antibody testing. Magnetic resonance imaging of the lumbar plexus is indicated if tumor or hematoma is suspected. The injection technique described later serves as both a diagnostic and a therapeutic maneuver.

DIFFERENTIAL DIAGNOSIS

Lesions of the lumbar plexus caused by trauma, hematoma, tumor, diabetic neuropathy, or inflammation can mimic the pain, numbness, and weakness of ilioinguinal neuralgia and must be ruled out. Further, there is significant variability in the anatomy of the ilioinguinal nerve, which can result in significant variation in the clinical presentation.

TREATMENT

Initial treatment of ilioinguinal neuralgia consists of simple analgesics, nonsteroidal anti-inflammatory drugs, or cyclooxygenase-2 inhibitors. Avoidance of repetitive activities thought to exacerbate the pain (e.g., squatting or sitting for prolonged periods) may also ameliorate the patient's symptoms. Pharmacologic treatment is usually disappointing, however, in which case ilioinguinal nerve block with local anesthetic and steroid is required.

Ilioinguinal nerve block is performed with the patient in the supine position; a pillow can be placed under the patient's knees if lying with the legs extended increases the pain due to traction on the nerve. The anterior superior iliac spine is identified by palpation, and a point 2 inches medial and 2 inches inferior to it is identified and prepared with antiseptic solution. A 1½-inch, 25-gauge needle is advanced at an oblique angle toward the pubic symphysis (Fig. 64-2). A total of 5 to 7 mL of 1% preservative-free lidocaine in solution with 40 mg methylprednisolone is injected in a fanlike manner as the needle pierces the fascia of the external oblique muscle. Care must be taken not to insert the needle too deeply, which risks entering the peritoneal cavity and perforating the abdominal viscera. Because of the overlapping innervation of the ilioinguinal and iliohypogastric nerves, it is usually not necessary to block branches of each nerve. After injection of the solution, pressure is applied to the injection site to decrease the incidence of ecchymosis and hematoma formation, which can be quite dramatic, especially in anticoagulated patients.

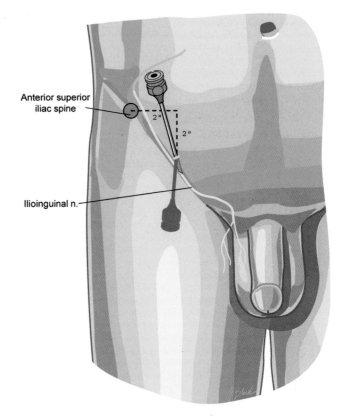

Figure 64–2. Correct needle placement for ilioinguinal nerve block. (From Waldman SD: Atlas of Interventional Pain Management. Philadelphia, Saunders, 1998.)

For patients who do not rapidly respond to ilioinguinal nerve block, consideration should be given to epidural steroid injection of the T12-L1 segments.

COMPLICATIONS AND PITFALLS

Owing to the anatomy of the ilioinguinal nerve, damage to or entrapment of the nerve anywhere along its course can produce a similar clinical syndrome. Therefore, a careful search for pathology at the T12-L1 spinal segments and along the path of the nerve in the pelvis is mandatory in all patients who present with ilioinguinal neuralgia without a history of inguinal surgery or trauma to the region.

The major complication of ilioinguinal nerve block is ecchymosis and hematoma formation. If the needle is too deep and enters the peritoneal cavity, perforation of the colon may result in the formation of an intra-abdominal abscess and fistula. Early detection of infection is crucial to avoid potentially life-threatening sequelae.

Clinical Pearls

Ilioinguinal neuralgia is a common cause of lower abdominal and pelvic pain, and ilioinguinal nerve block is a simple technique that can produce dramatic pain relief. If a patient presents with pain suggestive of ilioinguinal neuralgia and does not respond to ilioinguinal nerve block, a lesion more proximal in the lumbar plexus or an L1 radiculopathy should be considered. Such patients often respond to epidural steroid blocks. Electromyography and magnetic resonance imaging of the lumbar plexus are indicated in this patient population to rule out other causes of ilioinguinal pain, including malignancy invading the lumbar plexus or epidural or vertebral metastatic disease at T12-L1.

Chapter 65

Genitofemoral Neuralgia

ICD-9 CODE 355.8

THE CLINICAL SYNDROME

Genitofemoral neuralgia is one of the most common causes of lower abdominal and pelvic pain encountered in clinical practice. It may be caused by compression of or damage to the genitofemoral nerve anywhere along its path. The most common causes of genitofemoral neuralgia involve traumatic injury to the nerve, including direct blunt trauma and damage during inguinal herniorrhaphy and pelvic surgery. Rarely, genitofemoral neuralgia occurs spontaneously.

The genitofemoral nerve arises from fibers of the L1 and L2 nerve roots and passes through the substance of the psoas muscle, where it divides into a genital and a femoral branch. The femoral branch passes beneath the inguinal ligament, along with the femoral artery, and provides sensory innervation to a small area of skin on the inner thigh. The genital branch passes through the inguinal canal to provide innervation to the round ligament of the uterus and labia majora in women. In men, the genital branch passes with the spermatic cord to innervate the cremasteric muscles and provide sensory innervation to the bottom of the scrotum.

SIGNS AND SYMPTOMS

Genitofemoral neuralgia presents as paresthesias, burning pain, and occasionally numbness over the lower abdomen that radiates to the inner thigh in both men and women and into the labia majora in women and the bottom of the scrotum and cremasteric muscles in men (Fig. 65-1); the pain does not radiate below the knee. The pain of genitofemoral neuralgia is made worse by extension of the lumbar spine, which puts traction on the nerve. Therefore, patients with genitofemoral neuralgia often assume a bent-forward, novice skier's position (see Fig. 65-1).

Physical findings include sensory deficit in the inner thigh, base of the scrotum, or labia majora in the distribution of the genitofemoral nerve. Weakness of the anterior abdominal wall musculature may be present. Tinel's

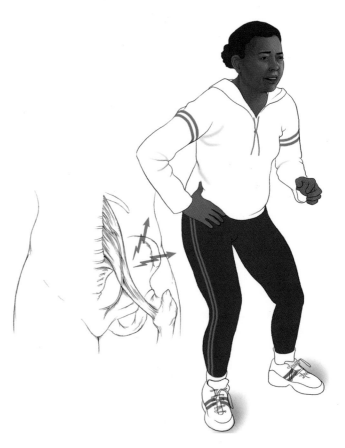

Figure 65–1. The pain of genitofemoral neuralgia radiates into the inner thigh of men and women and into the labia majora in women and the inferior scrotum in men.

sign may be elicited by tapping over the genitofemoral nerve at the point where it passes beneath the inguinal ligament.

TESTING

Electromyography can distinguish genitofemoral nerve entrapment from lumbar plexopathy, lumbar radiculopathy, and diabetic polyneuropathy. Plain radiographs of the hip and pelvis are indicated in all patients who present with genitofemoral neuralgia to rule out occult bony pathology. Based on the patient's clinical presentation, additional testing may be warranted, including a complete blood count, uric acid level, erythrocyte sedimentation rate, and antinuclear antibody testing. Magnetic resonance imaging of the lumbar plexus is indicated if tumor or hematoma is suspected. The injection technique described later serves as both a diagnostic and a therapeutic maneuver.

DIFFERENTIAL DIAGNOSIS

Lesions of the lumbar plexus caused by trauma, hematoma, tumor, diabetic neuropathy, or inflammation can mimic the pain, numbness, and weakness of genitofemoral neuralgia and must be ruled out. Further, there is significant variability in the anatomy of the genitofemoral nerve, which can result in significant variation in the clinical presentation.

TREATMENT

Initial treatment of genitofemoral neuralgia consists of simple analgesics, nonsteroidal anti-inflammatory drugs, or cyclooxygenase-2 inhibitors. Avoidance of repetitive activities thought to exacerbate the pain (e.g., squatting or sitting for prolonged periods) may also ameliorate the patient's symptoms. Pharmacologic treatment is usually disappointing, however, in which case genitofemoral nerve block with local anesthetic and steroid is required.

Genitofemoral nerve block is performed with the patient in the supine position; a pillow can be placed under the patient's knees if lying with the legs extended increases the pain due to traction on the nerve. The genital branch of the genitofemoral nerve is blocked as follows: The pubic tubercle is identified by palpation, and a point just lateral to it is identified and prepared with antiseptic solution. A 1½-inch, 25-gauge needle is advanced at an oblique angle toward the pubic symphysis (Fig. 65-2). A total of 3 to 5 mL of 1% preservative-free lidocaine in solution with 80 mg methylprednisolone is injected in a fanlike manner as the needle pierces the inguinal ligament. Care must be taken not to insert the needle deep enough to enter the peritoneal cavity and perforate the abdominal viscera.

The femoral branch of the genitofemoral nerve is blocked by identifying the middle third of the inguinal ligament. After preparation of the skin with antiseptic solution, 3 to 5 mL of 1% lidocaine is infiltrated subcutaneously just below the ligament (see Fig. 65-2). Care must be taken not to enter the femoral artery or vein or to inadvertently block the femoral nerve. The needle must be kept subcutaneous to avoid entering the peritoneal cavity and perforating the abdominal viscera. If there is an inflammatory component to the pain, the local anesthetic is combined with 80 mg methylprednis-

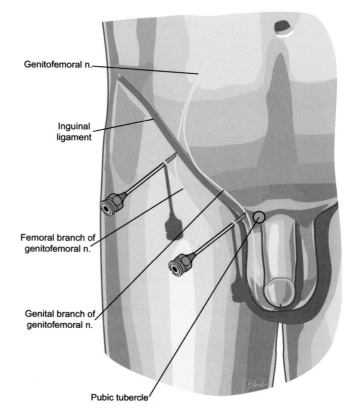

Figure 65–2. Correct needle placement for genitofemoral nerve block. (From Waldman SD: Atlas of Interventional Pain Management. Philadelphia, Saunders, 1998, p 365.)

olone and injected in incremental doses. Subsequent daily nerve blocks are carried out in a similar manner, substituting 40 mg methylprednisolone for the initial 80-mg dose. Because of overlapping innervation of the ilioinguinal and iliohypogastric nerves, it is usually not necessary to block branches of each nerve when performing genitofemoral nerve block. After injection of the solution, pressure is applied to the injection site to decrease the incidence of ecchymosis and hematoma formation, which can be quite dramatic, especially in anticoagulated patients.

For patients who do not rapidly respond to genitofemoral nerve block, consideration should be given to epidural steroid injection of the L1-2 segments.

COMPLICATIONS AND PITFALLS

Owing to the anatomy of the genitofemoral nerve, damage to or entrapment of the nerve anywhere along its course can produce a similar clinical syndrome. Therefore, a careful search for pathology at the L1-2 spinal segments and along the path of the nerve in the pelvis is mandatory in all patients who present with genitofemoral neuralgia without a history of inguinal surgery or trauma to the region.

The major complication of genitofemoral nerve block is ecchymosis and hematoma formation. If the needle is too deep and enters the peritoneal cavity, perforation of the colon may result in the formation of an intra-abdominal abscess and fistula. Early detection of infection is crucial to avoid potentially life-threatening sequelae.

Clinical Pearls

Genitofemoral neuralgia is a common cause of lower abdominal and pelvic pain, and genitofemoral nerve block is a simple technique that can produce dramatic pain relief. If a patient presents with pain suggestive of genitofemoral neuralgia and does not respond to genitofemoral nerve block, lesions more proximal in the lumbar plexus or an L1 radiculopathy should be considered. Such patients often respond to epidural steroid blocks. Electromyography and magnetic resonance imaging of the lumbar plexus are indicated in this patient population to rule out other causes of genitofemoral pain, including malignancy invading the lumbar plexus or epidural or vertebral metastatic disease at T12-L1.

Section 11

Pain Syndromes of the Lumbar Spine and Sacroiliac Joint

Chapter 66

Lumbar Radiculopathy

ICD-9 CODE 724.4

THE CLINICAL SYNDROME

Lumbar radiculopathy is a constellation of symptoms including neurogenic back and lower extremity pain emanating from the lumbar nerve roots. In addition to pain, patients may experience numbness, weakness, and loss of reflexes. The causes of lumbar radiculopathy include herniated disk, foraminal stenosis, tumor, osteophyte formation, and, rarely, infection. Many patients and their physicians refer to lumbar radiculopathy as *sciatica.*

SIGNS AND SYMPTOMS

Patients suffering from lumbar radiculopathy complain of pain, numbness, tingling, and paresthesias in the distribution of the affected nerve root or roots (Table 66-1). Patients may also note weakness and lack of coordination in the affected extremity. Muscle spasms and back pain, as well as pain referred into the buttocks, are common. Decreased sensation, weakness, and reflex changes are demonstrated on physical examination. Patients with lumbar radiculopathy commonly experience a reflex shifting of the trunk to one side, called *list* (Fig. 66-1). Lasègue's straight leg raising sign is almost always positive in patients with lumbar radiculopathy (Figs. 66-2 and 66-3). Occasionally, patients suffering from lumbar radiculopathy experience compression of the lumbar spinal nerve roots and cauda equina, resulting in lumbar myelopathy or cauda equina syndrome; if so, they experience varying degrees of lower extremity

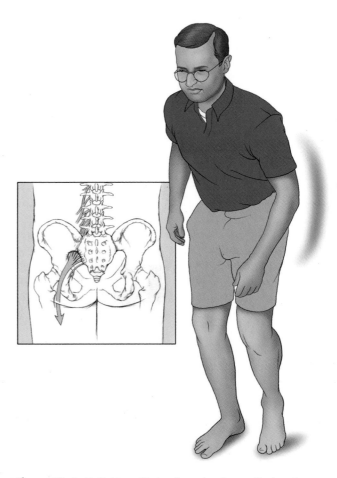

Figure 66–1. Patients suffering from lumbar radiculopathy often assume an unnatural posture in an attempt to take pressure off the affected nerve root and relieve pain.

Table 66–1. Clinical Features of Lumbar Radiculopathy

Lumbar Root	Pain	Sensory Changes	Weakness	Reflex Changes
L4	Back, shin, thigh, and leg	Shin numbness	Ankle dorsiflexors	Knee jerk
L5	Back, posterior thigh, and leg	Numbness of top of foot and first web space	Extensor hallucis longus	None
S1	Back, posterior calf, and leg	Numbness of lateral foot	Gastrocnemius and soleus	Ankle jerk

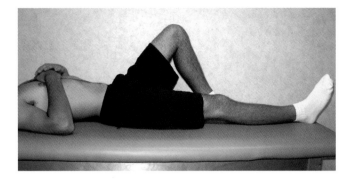

Figure 66–2. Lasègue's straight leg raising test: With the patient in the supine position, the unaffected leg is flexed 45 degrees at the knee and the affected leg is placed flat against the table. (From Waldman SD: Physical Diagnosis of Pain: An Atlas of Signs and Symptoms. Philadelphia, Saunders, 2006, p 243.)

weakness and bowel and bladder symptoms. This represents a neurosurgical emergency and should be treated as such.

TESTING

Magnetic resonance imaging (MRI) provides the best information about the lumbar spine and its contents and should be performed in all patients suspected of suffering from lumbar radiculopathy (Fig. 66-4). MRI is highly accurate and can identify abnormalities that may put the patient at risk for the development of lumbar myelopa-

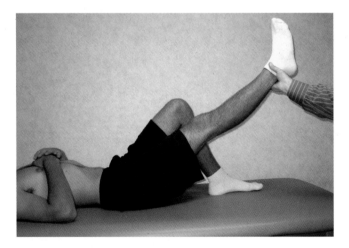

Figure 66–3. Lasègue's straight leg raising test: With the ankle of the affected leg placed at 90 degrees of flexion, the affected leg is slowly raised toward the ceiling while the knee is kept fully extended. (From Waldman SD: Physical Diagnosis of Pain: An Atlas of Signs and Symptoms. Philadelphia, Saunders, 2006, p 244.)

thy. In patients who cannot undergo MRI (e.g., those with pacemakers), computed tomography (CT) or myelography is a reasonable alternative. Radionuclide bone scanning and plain radiography are indicated if fracture or a bony abnormality, such as metastatic disease, is being considered.

Although MRI, CT, and myelography can supply useful neuroanatomic information, electromyography and nerve conduction velocity testing provide neurophysiologic information about the actual status of each individual nerve root and the lumbar plexus. Electromyography can also distinguish plexopathy from radiculopathy and identify a coexistent entrapment neuropathy, such as tarsal tunnel syndrome, which may confuse the diagnosis.

If the diagnosis of lumbar radiculopathy is in question, laboratory testing consisting of a complete blood count, erythrocyte sedimentation rate, antinuclear antibody testing, HLA B-27 antigen screening, and automated blood chemistry should be performed to rule out other causes of the patient's pain.

DIFFERENTIAL DIAGNOSIS

Lumbar radiculopathy is a clinical diagnosis supported by a combination of clinical history, physical examination, radiography, and MRI. Pain syndromes that may mimic lumbar radiculopathy include low back strain, lumbar bursitis, lumbar fibromyositis, inflammatory arthritis, and disorders of the lumbar spinal cord, roots, plexus, and nerves.

TREATMENT

Lumbar radiculopathy is best treated with a multimodality approach. Physical therapy, including heat modalities and deep sedative massage, combined with nonsteroidal anti-inflammatory drugs and skeletal muscle relaxants is a good starting point. If necessary, caudal or lumbar epidural nerve blocks can be added; nerve blocks with local anesthetic and steroid are extremely effective in the treatment of lumbar radiculopathy. Underlying sleep disturbance and depression are best treated with a tricyclic antidepressant such as nortriptyline, which can be started at a single bedtime dose of 25 mg.

COMPLICATIONS AND PITFALLS

Failure to accurately diagnosis lumbar radiculopathy may put the patient at risk for the development of lumbar myelopathy, which, if untreated, may progress to paraparesis or paraplegia.

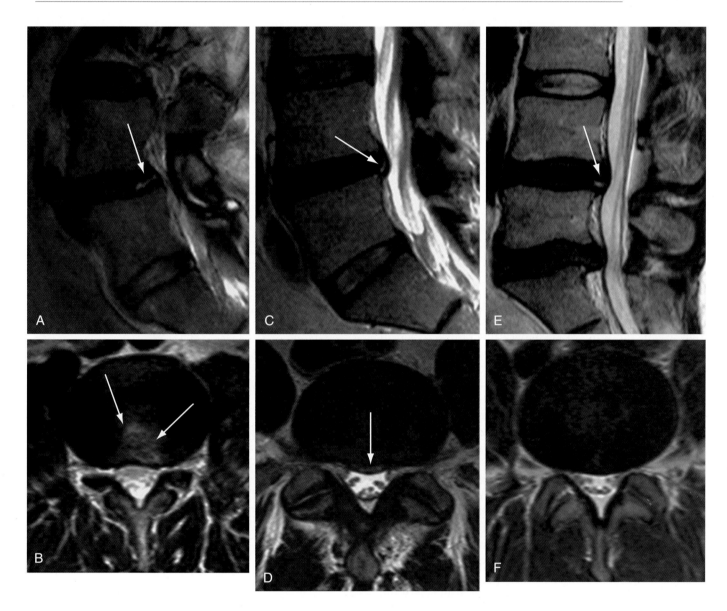

Radial   Concentric   Transverse

Figure 66–4. Magnetic resonance appearance of annular tears on sagittal **(A, C, E)** and axial **(B, D, F)** T2-weighted scans. **A** and **B,** Radial tear *(arrows)*. **C** and **D,** Concentric tear *(arrows)*. **E** and **F,** Transverse tear, visible only on the sagittal image *(arrow)*. (From Edelman RR, Hessellink JR, Zlatkin MB, Crues JV: Clinical Magnetic Resonance Imaging, 3rd ed. Philadelphia, Saunders, 2006, p 2203.)

Clinical Pearls

Tarsal tunnel syndrome must be differentiated from lumbar radiculopathy involving the lumbar nerve roots, which may also mimic tibial nerve compression. Further, it should be remembered that lumbar radiculopathy and tibial nerve entrapment may coexist in the "double crush" syndrome.

Chapter 67

Latissimus Dorsi Syndrome

ICD-9 CODE 729.1

THE CLINICAL SYNDROME

The latissimus dorsi muscle is a broad, sheetlike muscle whose primary function is to extend, adduct, and medially rotate the arm; its secondary function is to aid in deep inspiration and expiration. The latissimus dorsi muscle originates on the spine of T7; the spinous processes and supraspinous ligaments of all lower thoracic, lumbar, and sacral vertebrae; the lumbar fascia; the posterior third iliac crest; the last four ribs; and the inferior angle of the scapula. The muscle inserts on the bicipital groove of the humerus and is innervated by the thoracodorsal nerve.

The latissimus dorsi muscle is susceptible to myofascial pain syndrome, which most often results from repetitive microtrauma to the muscle during such activities as vigorous use of exercise equipment or tasks that require reaching in a forward and upward motion (Fig. 67-1). Blunt trauma to the muscle may also incite latissimus dorsi myofascial pain syndrome.

Myofascial pain syndrome is a chronic pain syndrome that affects a focal or regional portion of the body. The sine qua non of myofascial pain syndrome is the finding of myofascial trigger points on physical examination. Although these trigger points are generally localized to the part of the body affected, the pain is often referred to other areas. This referred pain may be misdiagnosed or attributed to other organ systems, leading to extensive evaluation and ineffective treatment.

The trigger point is pathognomonic of myofascial pain syndrome and is characterized by a local point of exquisite tenderness in the affected muscle. Mechanical stimulation of the trigger point by palpation or stretching produces not only intense local pain but referred pain as well. In addition, there is often an involuntary withdrawal of the stimulated muscle, called a "jump sign," which is also characteristic of myofascial pain syndrome.

Taut bands of muscle fibers are often identified when myofascial trigger points are palpated. In spite of this

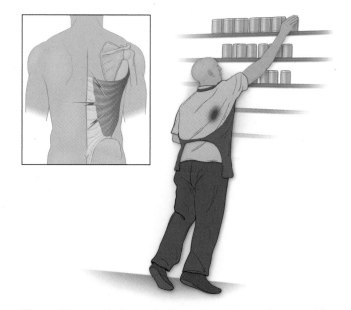

Figure 67–1. Latissimus dorsi syndrome is usually caused by repetitive microtrauma to the muscle during such activities as vigorous use of exercise equipment or tasks that require reaching forward and up.

consistent physical finding, the pathophysiology of the myofascial trigger point remains elusive, although it is believed that trigger points are the result of microtrauma to the affected muscle. This may result from a single injury, repetitive microtrauma, or chronic deconditioning of the agonist and antagonist muscle unit.

In addition to muscle trauma, a variety of other factors seems to predispose patients to develop myofascial pain syndrome. For instance, a weekend athlete who subjects his or her body to unaccustomed physical activity may develop myofascial pain syndrome. Poor posture while sitting at a computer or while watching television has also been implicated as a predisposing factor. Previous injuries may result in abnormal muscle function and lead to the development of myofascial pain syndrome. All these predisposing factors may be intensified if the patient also suffers from poor nutritional status or coexisting psychological or behavioral abnormalities, including chronic stress and depression. The latissimus dorsi muscle seems to be particularly susceptible to stress-induced myofascial pain syndrome.

Stiffness and fatigue often coexist with pain, increasing the functional disability associated with this disease and complicating its treatment. Myofascial pain syndrome may occur as a primary disease state or in conjunction with other painful conditions, including radiculopathy and chronic regional pain syndromes. Psychological or behavioral abnormalities, including depression, frequently coexist with the muscle abnormalities, and management of these psychological disorders is an integral part of any successful treatment plan.

SIGNS AND SYMPTOMS

The trigger point is the pathologic lesion of latissimus dorsi syndrome, and it is characterized by a local point of exquisite tenderness at the inferior angle of the scapula; this pain is referred to the axilla and the back of the ipsilateral upper extremity into the doral aspect of the ring and little fingers (Fig. 67-2). Mechanical stimulation of the trigger point by palpation or stretching produces both intense local pain and referred pain. In addition, the jump sign is often present.

TESTING

Biopsies of clinically identified trigger points have not revealed consistently abnormal histology. The muscle hosting the trigger points has been described either as "moth eaten" or as containing "waxy degeneration." Increased plasma myoglobin has been reported in some patients with latissimus dorsi syndrome, but this finding has not been corroborated by other investigators. Electrodiagnostic testing has revealed an increase in muscle tension in some patients, but again, this finding has not been reproducible. Because of the lack of objective diagnostic testing, the clinician must rule out other coexisting disease processes that may mimic latissimus dorsi syndrome (see Differential Diagnosis).

DIFFERENTIAL DIAGNOSIS

The diagnosis of latissimus dorsi syndrome is based on clinical findings rather than specific laboratory, electrodiagnostic, or radiographic testing. For this reason, a targeted history and physical examination, with a systematic search for trigger points and identification of a positive jump sign, must be carried out in every patient suspected of suffering from latissimus dorsi syndrome. It is incumbent on the clinician to rule out other coexisting disease processes that may mimic latissimus dorsi syndrome, including primary inflammatory muscle disease, multiple sclerosis, and collagen vascular disease. The use of electrodiagnostic and radiographic testing can identify coexisting pathology such as subscapular bursitis, cervi-

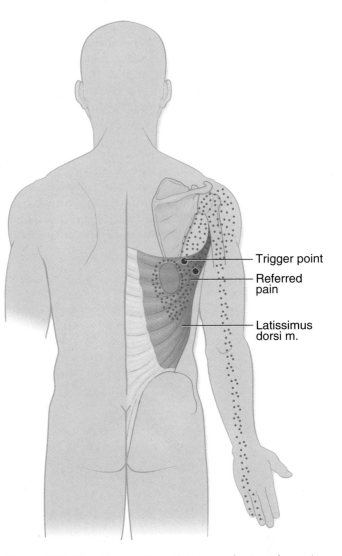

Figure 67–2. The trigger point of latissimus dorsi syndrome is at the inferior angle of the scapula, with pain referred to the axilla and the back of the ipsilateral upper extremity into the dorsal aspect of the ring and little fingers. (From Waldman SD: Atlas of Pain Management Injection Techniques, 2nd ed. Philadelphia, Saunders, 2007, p 299.)

cal radiculopathy, herniated nucleus pulposus, and rotator cuff tear. The clinician must also identify coexisting psychological and behavioral abnormalities that may mask or exacerbate the symptoms of latissimus dorsi syndrome.

TREATMENT

Treatment is focused on eliminating the myofascial trigger and achieving relaxation of the affected muscle. It is hoped that interrupting the pain cycle in this way will allow the patient to obtain prolonged pain relief. The mechanism of action of the treatment modalities used is poorly understood, so an element of trial and error is involved in developing a treatment plan.

Conservative therapy consisting of trigger point injection with local anesthetic or saline is the initial treatment of latissimus dorsi syndrome. Because underlying depression and anxiety are present in many patients, antidepressants are an integral part of most treatment plans. Other therapies, including transcutaneous nerve stimulation and electrical stimulation, may be helpful on a case-by-case basis. For patients who do not respond to these traditional measures, consideration should be given to the use of botulinum toxin type A; although not currently approved by the Food and Drug Administration for this indication, the injection of minute quantities of botulinum toxin type A directly into trigger points has been successful in the treatment of persistent latissimus dorsi syndrome.

COMPLICATIONS AND PITFALLS

Trigger point injections are extremely safe if careful attention is paid to the clinically relevant anatomy. Sterile technique must be used to avoid infection, along with universal precautions to minimize any risk to the operator. Most complications of trigger point injection are related to needle-induced trauma at the injection site and in underlying tissues. The incidence of ecchymosis and hematoma formation can be decreased if pressure is applied to the injection site immediately after injection. The avoidance of overly long needles can decrease the incidence of trauma to underlying structures. Special care must be taken to avoid pneumothorax when injecting trigger points in proximity to the underlying pleural space.

Clinical Pearls

Although latissimus dorsi syndrome is a common disorder, it is often misdiagnosed. Therefore, in patients suspected of suffering from latissimus dorsi syndrome, a careful evaluation to identify underlying disease processes is mandatory. Latissimus dorsi syndrome often coexists with a variety of somatic and psychological disorders.

Chapter 68

Spinal Stenosis

ICD-9 CODE 724.02

THE CLINICAL SYNDROME

Spinal stenosis is the result of congenital or acquired narrowing of the spinal canal. Clinically, spinal stenosis usually presents in a characteristic manner as pain and weakness in the legs when walking. This neurogenic pain is called *pseudoclaudication* or *neurogenic claudication* (Fig. 68-1). These symptoms are usually accompanied by lower extremity pain emanating from the lumbar nerve roots. In addition, patients with spinal stenosis may experience numbness, weakness, and loss of reflexes. The causes of spinal stenosis include bulging or herniated disk, facet arthropathy, and thickening and buckling of the interlaminar ligaments. All these inciting factors tend to worsen with age.

SIGNS AND SYMPTOMS

Patients suffering from spinal stenosis complain of calf and leg pain and fatigue when walking, standing, or lying supine. These symptoms disappear if they flex the lumbar spine or assume the sitting position. Frequently, patients suffering from spinal stenosis exhibit a simian posture, with a forward-flexed trunk and slightly bent knees when walking, to decrease the symptoms of pseudoclaudication (Fig. 68-2). Extension of the spine may cause an increase in symptoms. Patients also complain of pain, numbness, tingling, and paresthesias in the distribution of the affected nerve root or roots. Weakness and lack of coordination in the affected extremity may be noted. A positive stoop test for spinal stenosis is often present (Fig. 68-3). Muscle spasms and back pain, as well as pain referred to the trapezius and interscapular region, are common. Decreased sensation, weakness, and reflex changes are demonstrated on physical examination.

Occasionally, patients suffering from spinal stenosis experience compression of the lumbar spinal nerve roots and cauda equina, resulting in lumbar myelopathy or cauda equina syndrome. These patients experience varying degrees of lower extremity weakness and bowel and bladder symptoms. This represents a neurosurgical emergency and should be treated as such, although the onset of symptoms is often insidious.

TESTING

Magnetic resonance imaging (MRI) provides the best information about the lumbar spine and its contents and should be performed in all patients suspected of having spinal stenosis. MRI is highly accurate and can identify abnormalities that may put the patient at risk for lumbar myelopathy (Fig. 68-4). In patients who cannot undergo MRI (e.g., those with pacemakers), computed

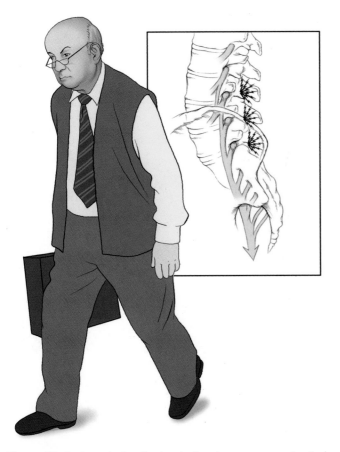

Figure 68–1. Pseudoclaudication is the sine qua non of spinal stenosis.

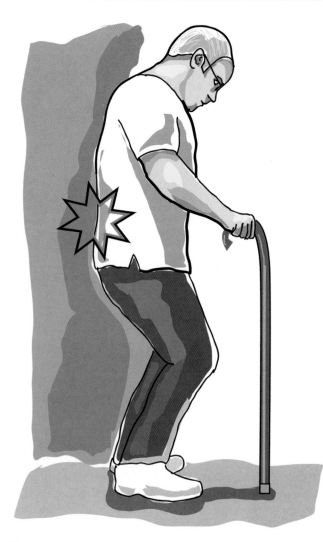

Figure 68–2. Patients suffering from spinal stenosis often assume a simian posture, with a forward-flexed trunk and slightly bent knees when walking, to decrease the symptoms of pseudoclaudication. (From Waldman SD: Physical Diagnosis of Pain: An Atlas of Signs and Symptoms. Philadelphia, Saunders, 2006, p 260.)

tomography (CT) or myelography is a reasonable alternative. Radionuclide bone scanning and plain radiography are indicated if a coexistent fracture or bony abnormality, such as metastatic disease, is being considered.

Although MRI, CT, and myelography can supply useful neuroanatomic information, electromyography and nerve conduction velocity testing provide neurophysiologic information about the actual status of each individual nerve root and the lumbar plexus. Electromyography can also distinguish plexopathy from radiculopathy and identify a coexistent entrapment neuropathy that may confuse the diagnosis.

If the diagnosis is in question, laboratory tests consisting of a complete blood count, erythrocyte sedimentation rate, antinuclear antibody testing, HLA B-27 antigen screening, and automated blood chemistry should be performed to rule out other causes of the patient's pain.

DIFFERENTIAL DIAGNOSIS

Spinal stenosis is a clinical diagnosis supported by a combination of clinical history, physical examination, radiography, and MRI. Pain syndromes that may mimic spinal stenosis include low back strain, lumbar bursitis, lumbar fibromyositis, inflammatory arthritis, and disorders of the lumbar spinal cord, roots, plexus, and nerves, including diabetic femoral neuropathy.

TREATMENT

Spinal stenosis is best treated with a multimodality approach. Physical therapy, including heat modalities and deep sedative massage, combined with nonsteroidal anti-inflammatory drugs and skeletal muscle relaxants is a reasonable starting point. If necessary, caudal or lumbar epidural nerve blocks can be added. Caudal epidural blocks with local anesthetic and steroid are extremely effective in the treatment of spinal stenosis. Underlying sleep disturbance and depression are best treated with a tricyclic antidepressant such as nortriptyline, which can be started at a single bedtime dose of 25 mg.

COMPLICATIONS AND PITFALLS

Failure to accurately diagnose spinal stenosis may put the patient at risk for the development of lumbar myelopathy or cauda equina syndrome, which, if untreated, may progress to paraparesis or paraplegia.

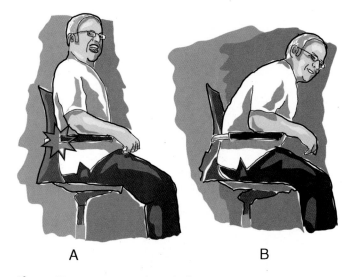

A   B

Figure 68–3. Stoop test for spinal stenosis. **A,** Extension of the lumbar spine exacerbates the pain of spinal stenosis. **B,** Flexion of the lumbar spine will relieve the pain of spinal stenosis. (From Waldman SD: Physical Diagnosis of Pain: An Atlas of Signs and Symptoms. Philadelphia, Saunders, 2006, p 261.)

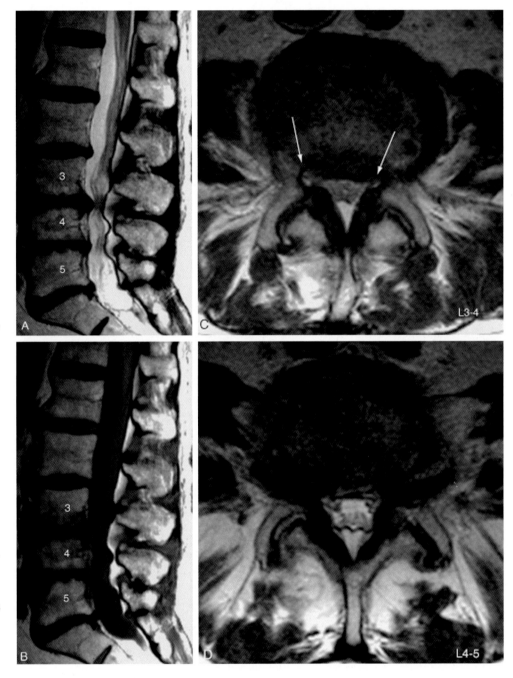

Figure 68–4. Acquired degenerative spinal stenosis. **A** and **B,** Sagittal T2- and T1-weighted images demonstrate severe disk degeneration at L3-4 and L4-5, with disk desiccation, disk space narrowing, irregularity of the adjacent vertebral end plates, and posterior bulging disks. The nerve roots of the cauda equina have an undulating or wavy appearance because of the marked constriction at L3-4. **C** and **D,** On axial T2-weighted scans, the combination of posterior bulging disks, facet hypertrophy, and thickened ligamenta flava causes severe spinal canal stenosis at L3-4 and moderate stenosis at L4-5. Also note severe compromise of the lateral recesses at L3-4 bilaterally. (From Edelman RR, Hessellink JR, Zlatkin MB, Crues JV: Clinical Magnetic Resonance Imaging, 3rd ed. Philadelphia, Saunders, 2006, p 2228.)

Clinical Pearls

Spinal stenosis is a common cause of back and lower extremity pain, and the finding of pseudoclaudication should point the clinician toward this diagnosis. It should be remembered that this syndrome tends to worsen with age. The onset of lumbar myelopathy or cauda equina syndrome may be insidious, so careful questioning and physical examination are required to avoid missing these complications.

Chapter 69

Arachnoiditis

ICD-9 CODE 322.9

THE CLINICAL SYNDROME

Arachnoiditis consists of thickening, scarring, and inflammation of the arachnoid membrane. These abnormalities may be self-limited or may lead to compression of the nerve roots and spinal cord. In addition to pain, patients with arachnoiditis may experience numbness, weakness, loss of reflexes, and bowel and bladder symptoms. The exact cause of arachnoiditis is unknown, but it may be related to herniated disk, infection, tumor, myelography, spinal surgery, or intrathecal administration of drugs. Anecdotal reports of arachnoiditis after epidural and subarachnoid administration of methylprednisolone have surfaced.

SIGNS AND SYMPTOMS

Patients suffering from arachnoiditis complain of pain, numbness, tingling, and paresthesias in the distribution of the affected nerve root or roots (Table 69-1). Weakness and lack of coordination in the affected extremity may be noted; muscle spasms, back pain, and pain referred to the buttocks are common. Decreased sensation, weakness, and reflex changes are demonstrated on physical examination. Occasionally, patients with arachnoiditis experience compression of the lumbar spinal cord, nerve roots, and cauda equina, resulting in lumbar myelopathy or cauda equina syndrome (Fig. 69-1). These patients experience varying degrees of lower extremity weakness and bowel and bladder symptoms.

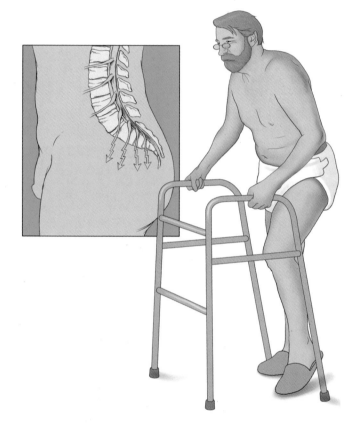

Figure 69–1. Arachnoiditis may result in lumbar myelopathy or cauda equina syndrome.

Table 69–1. Clinical Features of Arachnoiditis

Lumbar Root	Pain	Sensory Changes	Weakness	Reflex Changes
L4	Back, shin, thigh, and leg	Shin numbness	Ankle dorsiflexors	Knee jerk
L5	Back, posterior thigh, and leg	Numbness of top of foot and first web space	Extensor hallucis longus	None
S1	Back, posterior calf, and leg	Numbness of lateral foot	Gastrocnemius and soleus	Ankle jerk

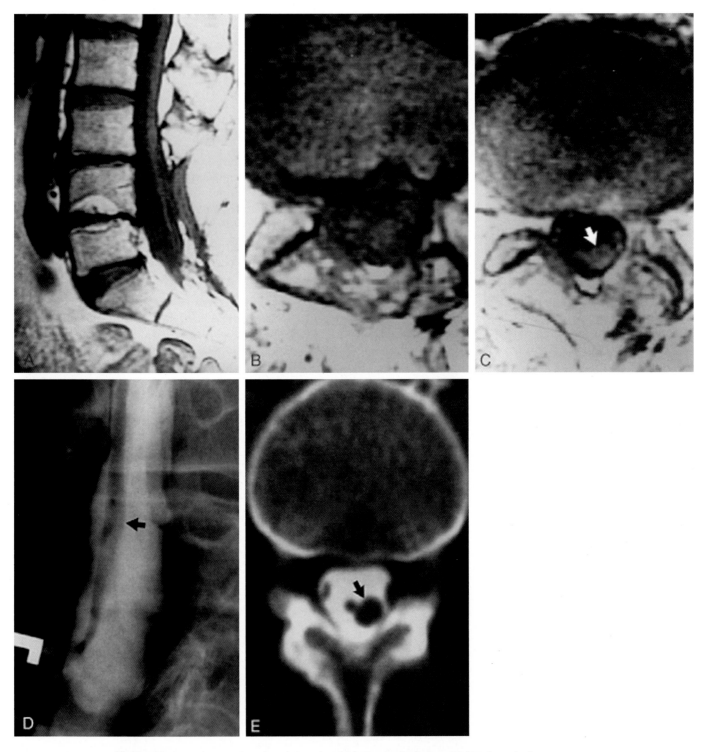

Figure 69–2. Postoperative chronic arachnoiditis. **A,** Sagittal short TR/TE (600/15) conventional spin echo image demonstrates degeneration of the L4-5 intervertebral disk. **B,** Axial short TR/TE (600/15) conventional spin echo image at the level of L3 demonstrates spondylosis with no associated abnormality. **C,** Axial short TR/TE (600/15) conventional spin echo image after gadolinium administration shows enhancement of matted nerve roots forming a thickened cord *(arrow)*, indicating the presence of adhesive arachnoiditis. **D,** Oblique view from a water-soluble contrast myelogram shows the partially empty sac and the cordlike matting of the nerve roots *(arrow)*. **E,** Axial computed tomography scan obtained through L3 shows matting of the nerve roots into a cordlike structure *(arrow)*. (From Edelman RR, Hesselink JR, Zlatkin MB, Crues JV: Clinical Magnetic Resonance Imaging, 3rd ed. Philadelphia, Saunders, 2006, p 2274.)

TESTING

Magnetic resonance imaging (MRI) provides the best information about the lumbar spine and its contents and should be performed in all patients suspected of suffering from arachnoiditis. MRI is highly accurate and can identify abnormalities that may put the patient at risk for the development of lumbar myelopathy or cauda equina syndrome. In patients who cannot undergo MRI (e.g., those with pacemakers), computed tomography (CT) or myelography is a reasonable alternative (Fig. 69-3). Radionuclide bone scanning and plain radiography are indicated if a fracture or bony abnormality, such as metastatic disease, is being considered.

Although MRI, CT, and myelography can supply useful neuroanatomic information, electromyography and nerve conduction velocity testing provide neurophysiologic information about the actual status of each individual nerve root and the lumbar plexus. Electromyography can also distinguish plexopathy from arachnoiditis and identify a coexistent entrapment neuropathy that may confuse the diagnosis.

If the diagnosis is in question, laboratory tests consisting of a complete blood count, erythrocyte sedimentation rate, antinuclear antibody testing, HLA B-27 antigen screening, and automated blood chemistry should be performed to rule out other causes of the patient's pain.

DIFFERENTIAL DIAGNOSIS

Arachnoiditis is a clinical diagnosis supported by a combination of clinical history, physical examination, radiography, and MRI. Conditions that may mimic arachnoiditis include tumor, infection, and disorders of the lumbar spinal cord, roots, plexus, and nerves.

TREATMENT

There is little consensus on the best treatment of arachnoiditis; most efforts are aimed at decompressing the nerve roots and spinal cord and treating the inflammatory component of the disease. Epidural neurolysis or the caudal administration of steroids may decompress the

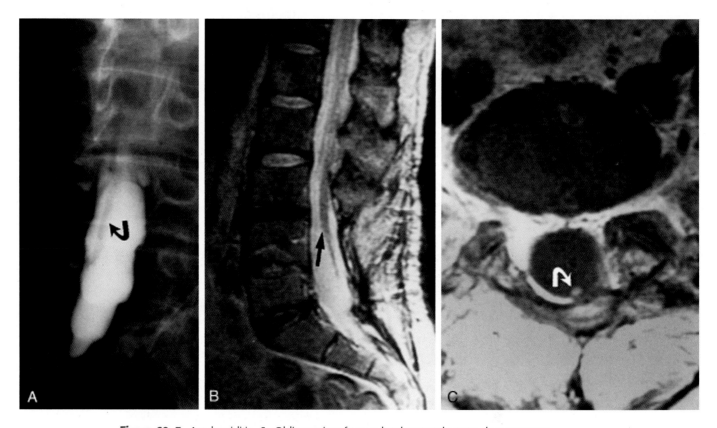

Figure 69–3. Arachnoiditis. **A,** Oblique view from a lumbar myelogram demonstrates nonfilling of the root sleeves, as well as thickened nerve roots *(arrow)*. **B,** Sagittal T2-weighted image shows clumped, thickened nerve roots *(arrow)*. **C,** Axial T1-weighted image after contrast administration reveals a nearly empty sac with a single thickened, slightly enhanced nerve root *(arrow)* adherent to the dorsal aspect of the dura. (From Edelman RR, Hessellink JR, Zlatkin MB, Crues JV: Clinical Magnetic Resonance Imaging, 3rd ed. Philadelphia, Saunders, 2006, p 2186.)

nerve roots if the pathology is localized. More generalized arachnoiditis often requires surgical decompressive laminectomy. The results of these treatment modalities are disappointing at best.

Underlying sleep disturbance and depression are treated with a tricyclic antidepressant such as nortriptyline, which can be started at a single bedtime does of 25 mg. Neuropathic pain associated with arachnoiditis may respond to gabapentin. Spinal cord stimulation may also provide symptomatic relief. Opioid analgesics should be used with caution, if at all.

COMPLICATIONS AND PITFALLS

Failure to accurately diagnosis arachnoiditis may put the patient at risk for the development of lumbar myelopathy or cauda equina syndrome, which, if untreated, may progress to paraparesis or paraplegia.

Clinical Pearls

Arachnoiditis is a potentially devastating disease that may erroneously be attributed to the clinician's efforts to diagnose and treat low back and lower extremity pain. For this reason, MRI and electromyography should be obtained early in patients with no clear cause of their symptoms.

Chapter 70

Sacroiliac Joint Pain

ICD-9 CODE 724.6

THE CLINICAL SYNDROME

Pain from the sacroiliac joint commonly occurs when lifting in an awkward position, putting strain on the joint, its supporting ligaments, and soft tissues. The sacroiliac joint is also susceptible to the development of arthritis from a variety of conditions that can damage the joint cartilage. Osteoarthritis is the most common form of arthritis that results in sacroiliac joint pain; rheumatoid arthritis and post-traumatic arthritis are also common causes of sacroiliac joint pain. Less common causes include the collagen vascular diseases, such as ankylosing spondylitis; infection; and Lyme disease. Collagen vascular disease generally presents as a polyarthropathy rather than a monoarthropathy limited to the sacroiliac joint, although sacroiliac pain secondary to ankylosing spondylitis responds exceedingly well to the intra-articular injection technique described later. Occasionally, patients present with iatrogenically induced sacroiliac joint dysfunction due to overaggressive bone graft harvesting for spinal fusion.

SIGNS AND SYMPTOMS

The majority of patients presenting with sacroiliac joint pain secondary to strain or arthritis complain of pain localized around the sacroiliac joint and upper leg that radiates into the posterior buttocks and backs of the legs (Fig. 70-1); the pain does not radiate below the knees. Activity makes the pain worse, whereas rest and heat provide some relief. The pain is constant and characterized as aching in nature; it may interfere with sleep. On physical examination, the affected sacroiliac joint is tender to palpation. The patient often favors the affected leg and lists toward the unaffected side. Spasm of the lumbar paraspinal musculature is often present, as is limited range of motion of the lumbar spine in the erect position; this improves in the sitting position owing to relaxation of the hamstring muscles.

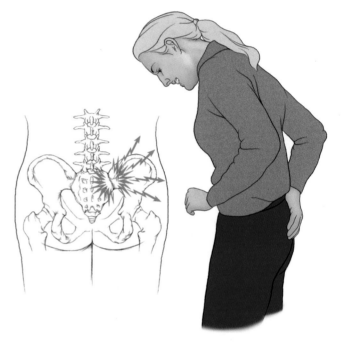

Figure 70–1. Sacroiliac joint pain radiates into the buttock and upper leg.

Patients with pain emanating from the sacroiliac joint exhibit a positive pelvic rock test. This test is performed by placing the examiner's hands on the iliac crests and the thumbs on the anterior superior iliac spines and then forcibly compressing the pelvis toward the midline. A positive test is indicated by the production of pain around the sacroiliac joint.

TESTING

Plain radiography is indicated in all patients who present with sacroiliac joint pain. Because the sacrum is susceptible to stress fractures and to the development of both primary and secondary tumors, magnetic resonance imaging of the distal lumbar spine and sacrum is indicated if the cause of the patient's pain is in question (Fig. 70-2). Radionuclide bone scanning should also be considered in such patients to rule out tumor and

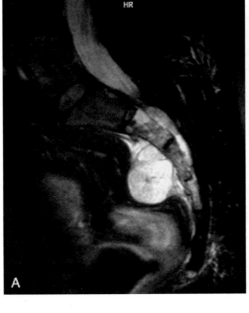
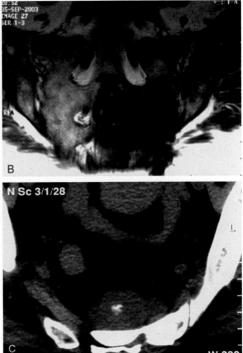
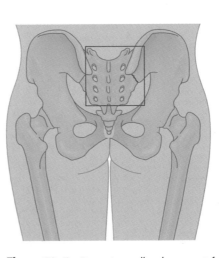

Figure 70–2. Sacral chordoma. Sagittal, fast spin echo, T2-weighted **(A)** and axial T1-weighted **(B)** images show a large soft tissue mass arising from the sacrum, with bony destruction. The bulk of the tumor is presacral. Axial computed tomography scan **(C)** demonstrates bony involvement of the left half of the sacrum by a large, midline, presacral mass with calcification. (From Edelman RR, Hessellink JR, Zlatkin MB, Crues JV: Clinical Magnetic Resonance Imaging, 3rd ed. Philadelphia, Saunders, 2006, p 2333.)

insufficiency fractures that may be missed on conventional radiographs. Based on the patient's clinical presentation, additional testing may be warranted, including a complete blood count, erythrocyte sedimentation rate, HLA B-27 antigen screening, antinuclear antibody testing, and automated blood chemistry.

DIFFERENTIAL DIAGNOSIS

Pain emanating from the sacroiliac joint can be confused with low back strain, lumbar bursitis, lumbar fibromyositis, inflammatory arthritis, and disorders of the lumbar spinal cord, roots, plexus, and nerves.

TREATMENT

Initial treatment of the pain and functional disability of sacroiliac joint pain includes a combination of nonsteroidal anti-inflammatory drugs or cyclooxygenase-2 inhibitors and physical therapy. The local application of heat and cold may also be beneficial. For patients who do not respond to these treatment modalities, injection with local anesthetic and steroid is a reasonable next step.

Injection of the sacroiliac joint is carried out by placing the patient in the supine position and preparing the skin overlying the affected sacroiliac joint space with antiseptic solution. A sterile syringe containing 4 mL of 0.25% preservative-free bupivacaine and 40 mg methylprednisolone is attached to a 25-gauge needle using strict aseptic technique. The posterior superior spine of the ilium is identified. At this point, the needle is carefully advanced

through the skin and subcutaneous tissues at a 45-degree angle toward the affected sacroiliac joint (Fig. 70-3). If bone is encountered, the needle is withdrawn into the subcutaneous tissues and redirected superiorly and slightly more laterally. After the joint space is entered, the contents of the syringe are gently injected. There should be little resistance to injection. If resistance is encountered, the needle is probably in a ligament and should be advanced slightly into the joint space until the

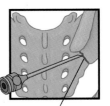

Arthritic and inflamed sacroiliac joint

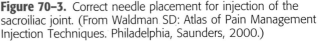

Figure 70–3. Correct needle placement for injection of the sacroiliac joint. (From Waldman SD: Atlas of Pain Management Injection Techniques. Philadelphia, Saunders, 2000.)

injection can proceed without significant resistance. The needle is then removed, and a sterile pressure dressing and ice pack are applied to the injection site.

Physical modalities, including local heat and gentle range-of-motion exercises, should be introduced several days after the patient undergoes injection for sacroiliac pain. Vigorous exercises should be avoided, because they will exacerbate the patient's symptoms.

COMPLICATIONS AND PITFALLS

The injection technique is safe if careful attention is paid to the clinically relevant anatomy. For instance, if the needle is inserted too laterally, it may traumatize the sciatic nerve. The major complication of intra-articular injection of the sacroiliac joint is infection, although it should be exceedingly rare if strict aseptic technique is followed, as well as universal precautions to minimize any risk to the operator. The incidence of ecchymosis and hematoma formation can be decreased if pressure is applied to the injection site immediately after injection. Approximately 25% of patients complain of a transient increase in pain after intra-articular injection, and they should be warned of this possibility.

Clinical Pearls

Disorders of the sacroiliac joint can be distinguished from those of the lumbar spine by having the patient bend forward while seated. Patients with sacroiliac pain can bend forward with relative ease owing to relaxation of the hamstring muscles in this position. In contrast, patients with lumbar spine pain experience an exacerbation of symptoms when bending forward while seated.

The injection technique described is extremely effective in the treatment of sacroiliac joint pain. Coexistent bursitis and tendinitis may contribute to sacroiliac pain, necessitating additional treatment with more localized injection of local anesthetic and methylprednisolone.

Section 12

Pain Syndromes of the Pelvis

Chapter 71

Osteitis Pubis

ICD-9 CODE 733.5

THE CLINICAL SYNDROME

Osteitis pubis causes localized tenderness over the symphysis pubis, pain radiating into the inner thigh, and a waddling gait. Radiographic changes consisting of erosion, sclerosis, and widening of the symphysis pubis are pathognomonic for osteitis pubis (Fig. 71-1). This is a disease of the second through fourth decades, and females are affected more frequently than males. Osteitis pubis occurs most commonly after bladder, inguinal, or prostate surgery and is thought to be due to the hematogenous spread of infection to the relatively avascular symphysis pubis. Osteitis pubis can also occur without an obvious inciting factor or infection.

SIGNS AND SYMPTOMS

On physical examination, patients exhibit point tenderness over the symphysis pubis, and the pain may radiate into the inner thigh with palpation of the symphysis pubis. There may also be tenderness over the anterior pelvis. Patients often adopt a waddling gait to avoid movement of the symphysis pubis (Fig. 71-2). This dysfunctional gait may result in lower extremity bursitis and tendinitis, which can confuse the clinical picture and add to the patient's pain and disability.

TESTING

Plain radiography is indicated in all patients who present with pain thought to be emanating from the symphysis pubis to rule out occult bony pathology and tumor. Based on the patient's clinical presentation, additional testing may be warranted, including a complete blood count, prostate-specific antigen level, erythrocyte sedimentation rate, serum protein electrophoresis, and antinuclear antibody testing. Magnetic resonance imaging of

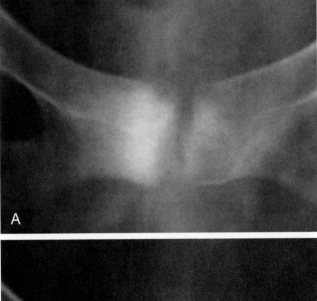

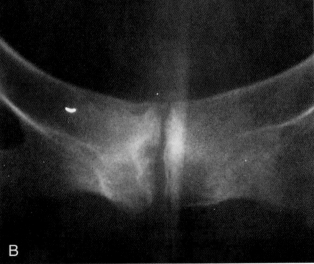

Figure 71–1. This 26-year-old woman developed pain and tenderness about the symphysis pubis during the third trimester of pregnancy. Radiographs obtained 2 years apart (**A** and **B**) reveal partial resolution of the abnormalities of osteitis pubis. (From Resnick D: Diagnosis of Bone and Joint Disorders, 4th ed. Philadelphia, Saunders, 2002, p 2133.)

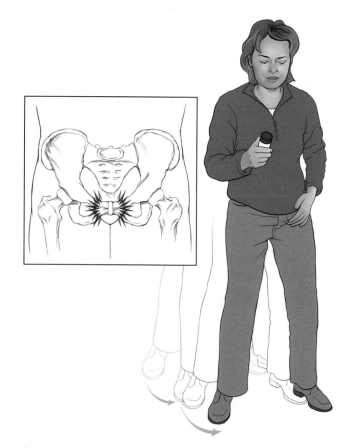

Figure 71–2. Patients with osteitis pubis often develop a waddling gait.

the pelvis is indicated if occult mass or tumor is suspected (Fig. 71-3). Radionuclide bone scanning may be useful to rule out stress fractures not visible on plain radiographs. The injection technique described later serves as both a diagnostic and a therapeutic maneuver.

DIFFERENTIAL DIAGNOSIS

A pain syndrome that is clinically similar to osteitis pubis may occur in patients with rheumatoid arthritis or ankylosing spondylitis; however, the characteristic radiographic changes of osteitis pubis are lacking. Multiple myeloma and metastatic tumor may also mimic the pain and radiographic changes of osteitis pubis. Insufficiency fractures of the pubic rami should be considered if generalized osteoporosis is present.

TREATMENT

Initial treatment of the pain and functional disability associated with osteitis pubis includes a combination of nonsteroidal anti-inflammatory drugs or cyclooxygenase-2 inhibitors and physical therapy. The local application of heat and cold may also be beneficial. For patients who do not respond to these treatment modalities, injection with local anesthetic and steroid is a reasonable next step.

Injection for osteitis pubis is carried out by placing the patient in the supine position. The midpoints of the pubic bones and the symphysis pubis are identified by palpation, and the overlying skin is prepared with antiseptic solution. A syringe containing 2 mL of 0.25% preservative-free bupivacaine and 40 mg methylprednisolone is attached to a 3½-inch, 25-gauge needle. The needle is advanced very slowly through the previously identified point at a right angle to the skin, directly toward the center of the symphysis pubis. Once the needle impinges on the fibroelastic cartilage of the joint, it is withdrawn slightly out of the joint. After careful aspiration for blood, and if no paresthesia is present, the contents of the syringe are gently injected. There should be minimal resistance to injection.

Physical modalities, including local heat and gentle stretching exercises, should be introduced several days after the patient undergoes injection. Vigorous exercises should be avoided, because they will exacerbate the patient's symptoms. Simple analgesics, nonsteroidal anti-inflammatory drugs, and antimyotonic agents such as tizanidine may be used concurrently with this injection technique.

COMPLICATIONS AND PITFALLS

The injection technique is safe if careful attention is paid to the clinically relevant anatomy. The proximity to the pelvic contents makes it imperative that injection for osteitis pubis be performed only by those familiar with the regional anatomy and experienced in such techniques. Reactivation of latent infection, though rare, can occur; therefore, strict attention to sterile technique is mandatory, along with universal precautions to minimize any risk to the operator. Most complications of the injection technique are related to needle-induced trauma at the injection site and in underlying tissues. The incidence of ecchymosis and hematoma formation can be decreased if pressure is applied to the injection site immediately after injection. Many patients complain of a transient increase in pain after injection, and they should be warned of this possibility.

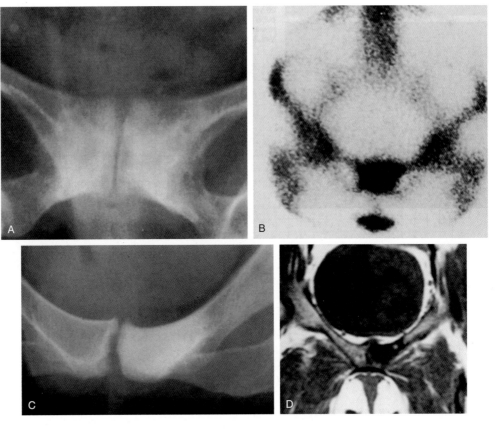

Figure 71–3. A and **B,** In this 61-year-old woman with osteitis pubis, local pain and tenderness about the symphysis pubis were the major clinical abnormalities. The radiograph **(A)** reveals considerable bone sclerosis on both sides of the symphysis, with narrowing of the joint space. A marked increase in the accumulation of a bone-seeking radiopharmaceutical agent is observed **(B). C** and **D,** In this 34-year-old woman, a routine radiograph **(C)** shows unilateral osteitis pubis. A coronal T1-weighted spin echo magnetic resonance image **(D)** shows low signal intensity in the involved bone. (From Resnick D: Diagnosis of Bone and Joint Disorders, 4th ed. Philadelphia, Saunders, 2002, p 2132.)

Clinical Pearls

Osteitis pubis should be suspected in patients presenting with pain over the symphysis pubis in the absence of trauma. The injection technique described is an extremely effective treatment.

Chapter 72

Gluteus Maximus Syndrome

ICD-9 CODE 729.1

THE CLINICAL SYNDROME

The gluteus maximus muscle's primary function is hip extension. It originates at the posterior aspect of the dorsal ilium, the posterior superior iliac crest, the posterior inferior aspect of the sacrum and coccyx, and the sacrotuberous ligament. The muscle inserts on the fascia lata at the iliotibial band and the gluteal tuberosity on the femur. The muscle is innervated by the inferior gluteal nerve.

The gluteus maximus muscle is susceptible to trauma and to wear and tear from overuse and misuse and to the development of myofascial pain syndrome, which may also be associated with gluteal bursitis. Such pain is usually the result of repetitive microtrauma to the muscle during such activities as running on soft surfaces, overuse of exercise equipment, or other repetitive activities that require hip extension (Fig. 72-1). Blunt trauma to the muscle may also incite gluteus maximus myofascial pain syndrome.

Myofascial pain syndrome is a chronic pain syndrome that affects a focal or regional portion of the body. The sine qua non of myofascial pain syndrome is the finding of myofascial trigger points on physical examination. Although these trigger points are generally localized to the part of the body affected, the pain is often referred to other areas. This referred pain may be misdiagnosed or attributed to other organ systems, leading to extensive evaluation and ineffective treatment. Patients with myofascial pain syndrome involving the gluteus maximus have primary pain in the medial and lower aspects of the muscle that is referred across the buttocks and into the coccygeal area (Fig. 72-2).

The trigger point is pathognomonic of myofascial pain syndrome and is characterized by a local point of exquisite tenderness in the affected muscle. Mechanical stimulation of the trigger point by palpation or stretching produces not only intense local pain but referred pain as well. In addition, there is often an involuntary withdrawal of the stimulated muscle, called a "jump sign,"

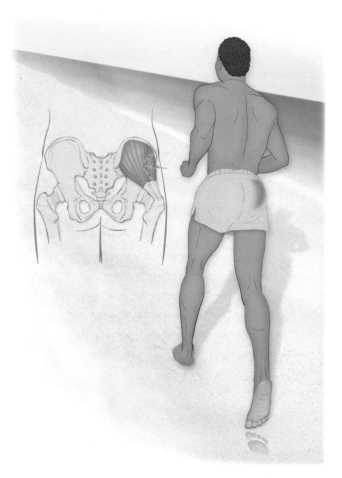

Figure 72–1. Gluteus maximus syndrome usually results from repetitive microtrauma to the muscle during such activities as running on soft surfaces, overuse of exercise equipment, or other repetitive activities that require hip extension.

which is also characteristic of myofascial pain syndrome. Patients with gluteus maximus syndrome have a trigger point over the upper, medial, and lower aspects of the muscle (see Fig. 72-1).

Taut bands of muscle fibers are often identified when myofascial trigger points are palpated. In spite of this consistent physical finding, the pathophysiology of the myofascial trigger point remains elusive, although it is believed that trigger points are the result of microtrauma

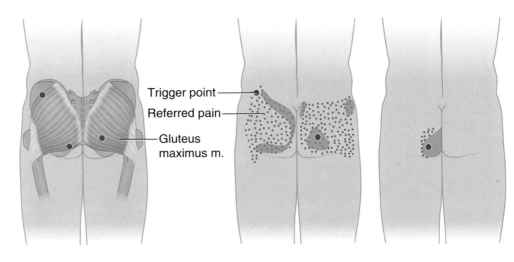

Figure 72–2. Patients with myofascial pain syndrome involving the gluteus maximus have primary pain in the medial and lower aspects of the muscle that is referred across the buttocks and into the coccygeal area. (From Waldman SD: Atlas of Pain Management Injection Techniques, 2nd ed. Philadelphia, Saunders, 2007, p 379.)

to the affected muscle. This may result from a single injury, repetitive microtrauma, or chronic deconditioning of the agonist and antagonist muscle unit.

In addition to muscle trauma, a variety of other factors seems to predispose patients to develop myofascial pain syndrome. For instance, a weekend athlete who subjects his or her body to unaccustomed physical activity may develop myofascial pain syndrome. Poor posture while sitting at a computer or while watching television has also been implicated as a predisposing factor. Previous injuries may result in abnormal muscle function and lead to the development of myofascial pain syndrome. All these predisposing factors may be intensified if the patient also suffers from poor nutritional status or coexisting psychological or behavioral abnormalities, including chronic stress and depression. The gluteus maximus muscle seems to be particularly susceptible to stress-induced myofascial pain syndrome.

Stiffness and fatigue often coexist with pain, increasing the functional disability associated with this disease and complicating its treatment. Myofascial pain syndrome may occur as a primary disease state or in conjunction with other painful conditions, including radiculopathy and chronic regional pain syndromes. Psychological or behavioral abnormalities, including depression, frequently coexist with the muscle abnormalities, and management of these psychological disorders is an integral part of any successful treatment plan.

SIGNS AND SYMPTOMS

The trigger point is the pathologic lesion of gluteus maximus syndrome, and it is characterized by a local point of exquisite tenderness in gluteus maximus muscle. Mechanical stimulation of the trigger point by palpation or stretching produces both intense local pain in the medial and lower aspects of the muscle and referred pain

across the buttocks and into the coccygeal area (see Fig. 72-2). In addition, the jump sign is often present.

TESTING

Biopsies of clinically identified trigger points have not revealed consistently abnormal histology. The muscle hosting the trigger points has been described either as "moth eaten" or as containing "waxy degeneration." Increased plasma myoglobin has been reported in some patients with gluteus maximus syndrome, but this finding has not been corroborated by other investigators. Electrodiagnostic testing has revealed an increase in muscle tension in some patients, but again, this finding has not been reproducible. Because of the lack of objective diagnostic testing, the clinician must rule out other coexisting disease processes that may mimic gluteus maximus syndrome (see Differential Diagnosis).

DIFFERENTIAL DIAGNOSIS

The diagnosis of gluteus maximus syndrome is based on clinical findings rather than specific laboratory, electrodiagnostic, or radiographic testing. For this reason, a targeted history and physical examination, with a systematic search for trigger points and identification of a positive jump sign, must be carried out in every patient suspected of suffering from gluteus maximus syndrome. It is incumbent on the clinician to rule out other coexisting disease processes that may mimic gluteus maximus syndrome, including primary inflammatory muscle disease, primary hip pathology, gluteal bursitis, and gluteal nerve entrapment (Fig. 72-3). The use of electrodiagnostic and radiographic testing can identify coexisting pathology such as rectal or pelvic tumors or lumbosacral nerve lesions. The clinician must also identify coexisting psychological and behavioral abnormalities that may mask or exacerbate the symptoms associated with gluteus maximus syndrome.

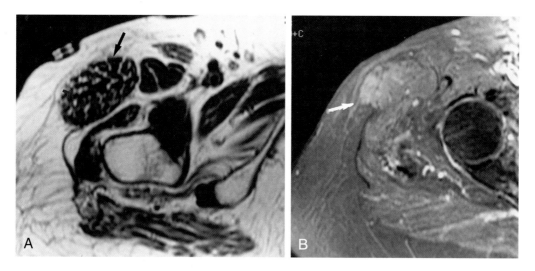

Figure 72–3. Possible entrapment of the superior gluteal nerve. **A,** Transverse, T1-weighted, spin echo magnetic resonance image shows denervation hypertrophy of the tensor fasciae latae muscle *(arrow)*. **B,** Similar hypertrophy and high signal intensity are seen in the muscle *(arrow)* on a transverse, fat-suppressed, T1-weighted, spin echo magnetic resonance image obtained after intravenous gadolinium administration. (From Resnick D: Diagnosis of Bone and Joint Disorders, 4th ed. Philadelphia, Saunders, 2002, p 3551.)

TREATMENT

Treatment is focused on eliminating the myofascial trigger and achieving relaxation of the affected muscle. It is hoped that interrupting the pain cycle in this way will allow the patient to obtain prolonged pain relief. The mechanism of action of the treatment modalities used is poorly understood, so an element of trial and error is involved in developing a treatment plan.

Conservative therapy consisting of trigger point injection with local anesthetic or saline is the initial treatment of gluteus maximus syndrome. Because underlying depression and anxiety are present in many patients, antidepressants are an integral part of most treatment plans. Other methods, including physical therapy, therapeutic heat and cold, transcutaneous nerve stimulation, and electrical stimulation, may be helpful on a case-by-case basis. For patients who do not respond to these traditional measures, consideration should be given to the use of botulinum toxin type A; although not currently approved by the Food and Drug Administration for this indication, the injection of minute quantities of botulinum toxin type A directly into trigger points has been successful in the treatment of persistent gluteus maximus syndrome.

COMPLICATIONS AND PITFALLS

Trigger point injections are extremely safe if careful attention is paid to the clinically relevant anatomy. Sterile technique must be used to avoid infection, along with universal precautions to minimize any risk to the operator. Most complications of trigger point injection are related to needle-induced trauma at the injection site and in underlying tissues. The incidence of ecchymosis and hematoma formation can be decreased if pressure is applied to the injection site immediately after injection. The avoidance of overly long needles can decrease the incidence of trauma to underlying structures. Special care must be taken to avoid trauma to the sciatic nerve.

Clinical Pearls

Although gluteus maximus syndrome is a common disorder, it is often misdiagnosed. Therefore, in patients suspected of suffering from gluteus maximus syndrome, a careful evaluation to identify underlying disease processes is mandatory. Gluteus maximus syndrome often coexists with a variety of somatic and psychological disorders.

Chapter 73

Piriformis Syndrome

ICD-9 CODE 355.0

THE CLINICAL SYNDROME

Piriformis syndrome is an entrapment neuropathy that presents as pain, numbness, paresthesias, and weakness in the distribution of the sciatic nerve. It is caused by compression of the sciatic nerve by the piriformis muscle as it passes through the sciatic notch (Fig. 73-1). The piriformis muscle's primary function is to externally rotate the femur at the hip joint; it is innervated by the sacral plexus. With internal rotation of the femur, the tendinous insertion and belly of the muscle can com-press the sciatic nerve; if this persists, it can cause entrapment of the nerve.

The symptoms of piriformis syndrome usually begin after direct trauma to the sacroiliac and gluteal region. Occasionally, the syndrome is the result of repetitive hip and lower extremity motions or repeated pressure on the piriformis muscle and underlying sciatic nerve.

SIGNS AND SYMPTOMS

Initial symptoms include severe pain in the buttocks that may radiate into the lower extremity and foot. Patients suffering from piriformis syndrome may develop an altered gait, leading to coexistent sacroiliac, back, and hip pain that confuses the clinical picture. Physical

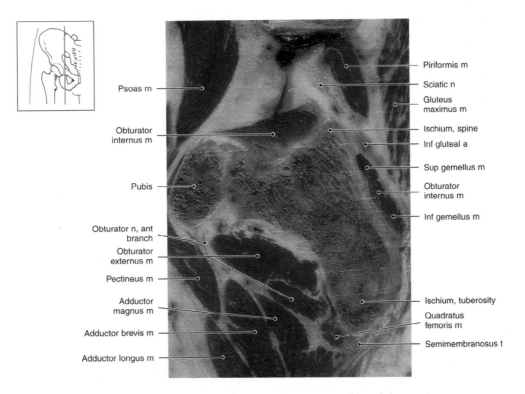

Psoas m
Obturator internus m
Pubis
Obturator n, ant branch
Obturator externus m
Pectineus m
Adductor magnus m
Adductor brevis m
Adductor longus m

Piriformis m
Sciatic n
Gluteus maximus m
Ischium, spine
Inf gluteal a
Sup gemellus m
Obturator internus m
Inf gemellus m
Ischium, tuberosity
Quadratus femoris m
Semimembranosus t

Figure 73–1. Anatomic relationship between the piriformis muscle and the sciatic nerve. (From Kang HS, Ahn JM, Resnick D: MRI of the Extremities: An Anatomic Atlas, 2nd ed. Philadelphia, Saunders, 2002, p 251.)

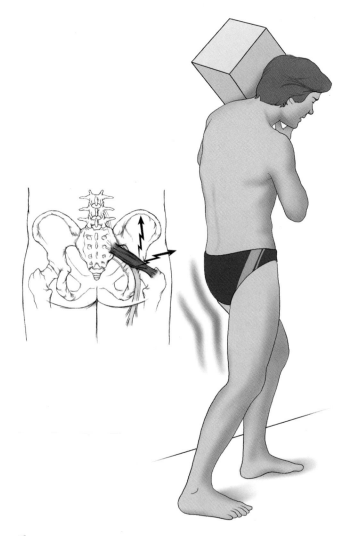

Figure 73–2. The pain of piriformis syndrome can be exacerbated by lifting.

findings include tenderness over the sciatic notch. Palpation of the piriformis muscle reveals tenderness and a swollen, indurated muscle belly. A positive Tinel's sign over the sciatic nerve as it passes beneath the piriformis muscle is often present. A positive straight leg raising test is suggestive of sciatic nerve entrapment. Lifting or bending at the waist and hips increases the pain in most patients suffering from piriformis syndrome (Fig. 73-2). Weakness of the affected gluteal muscles and lower extremity and, ultimately, muscle wasting are seen in advanced, untreated cases of piriformis syndrome.

TESTING

Electromyography can distinguish lumbar radiculopathy from piriformis syndrome. Plain radiographs of the back, hip, and pelvis are indicated in all patients who present with piriformis syndrome to rule out occult bony pathology. Based on the patient's clinical presentation, addi-

tional testing may be warranted, including a complete blood count, uric acid level, erythrocyte sedimentation rate, and antinuclear antibody testing. Magnetic resonance imaging of the back is indicated if herniated disk, spinal stenosis, or space-occupying lesion is suspected. Magnetic resonance imaging of the hip may elucidate the cause of compression of the sciatic nerve (Fig. 73-3). Injection in the region of the sciatic nerve at this level serves as both a diagnostic and a therapeutic maneuver.

DIFFERENTIAL DIAGNOSIS

Piriformis syndrome is often misdiagnosed as lumbar radiculopathy or primary hip pathology; radiographs of the hip and electromyography can make the distinction. In addition, most patients with lumbar radiculopathy have back pain associated with reflex, motor, and sensory changes, whereas patients with piriformis syndrome have only secondary back pain and no reflex changes. The motor and sensory changes of piriformis syndrome are limited to the distribution of the sciatic nerve below the sciatic notch. It should be remembered that lumbar

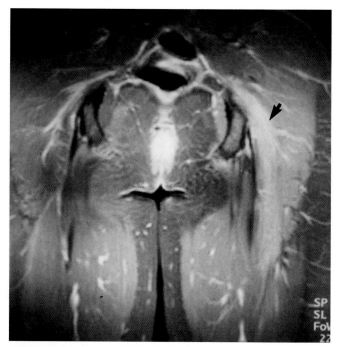

Figure 73–3. Coronal, fat-suppressed, T1-weighted, spin echo magnetic resonance image obtained after intravenous gadolinium administration shows gross enlargement of and enhancement of signal intensity in the left sciatic nerve *(arrow)*. Transverse magnetic resonance images (not shown) suggested the presence of a fibrolipomatous hamartoma, although a plexiform neurofibroma was also considered. (From Resnick D: Diagnosis of Bone and Joint Disorders, 4th ed. Philadelphia, Saunders, 2002, p 3550.)

radiculopathy and sciatic nerve entrapment may coexist as the "double crush" syndrome.

TREATMENT

Initial treatment of the pain and functional disability associated with piriformis syndrome includes a combination of nonsteroidal anti-inflammatory drugs or cyclooxygenase-2 inhibitors and physical therapy. The local application of heat and cold may also be beneficial. Any repetitive activity that may exacerbate the patient's symptoms should be avoided. If the patient sleeps on his or her side, placing a pillow between the legs may be helpful. If the patient is suffering from significant paresthesias, gabapentin may be added. For patients who do not respond to these treatment modalities, injection of local anesthetic and methlyprednisolone in the region of the sciatic nerve at the level of the piriformis muscle is a reasonable next step. Rarely, surgical release of the entrapment is required to obtain relief.

COMPLICATIONS AND PITFALLS

The main complications of injection in the region of the sciatic nerve are ecchymosis and hematoma. Because a paresthesia is elicited with the injection technique, needle-induced trauma to the sciatic nerve is a possibility. By advancing the needle slowly and withdrawing the needle slightly away from the nerve, injury to the sciatic nerve can be avoided.

Clinical Pearls

Because patients suffering from piriformis syndrome may develop an altered gait, resulting in coexistent sacroiliac, back, and hip pain, careful physical examination and appropriate testing are required to sort out the diagnostic possibilities.

Chapter 74

Ischiogluteal Bursitis

ICD-9 CODE 726.5

THE CLINICAL SYNDROME

The ischial bursa lies between the gluteus maximus muscle and the bone of the ischial tuberosity. It may exist as a single bursal sac or, in some patients, as a multisegmented series of loculated sacs. The ischial bursa is vulnerable to injury from both acute trauma and repeated microtrauma. Acute injuries are often caused by direct trauma to the bursa from falls onto the buttocks or by overuse, such as prolonged riding of horses or bicycles. Running on uneven or soft surfaces such as sand may also cause ischiogluteal bursitis (Fig. 74-1). If inflammation of the ischial bursa becomes chronic, calcification may occur.

SIGNS AND SYMPTOMS

Patients suffering from ischiogluteal bursitis frequently complain of pain at the base of the buttock with resisted extension of the lower extremity. The pain is localized to the area over the ischial tuberosity; referred pain is noted in the hamstring muscle, which may develop coexistent tendinitis. Patients are often unable to sleep on the affected hip and may complain of a sharp, catching sensation when extending and flexing the hip, especially on first awakening. Physical examination may reveal point tenderness over the ischial tuberosity. Passive straight leg raising and active resisted extension of the affected lower extremity reproduce the pain (Fig. 74-2). Sudden release of resistance during this maneuver causes a marked increase in pain.

TESTING

Plain radiographs of the hip may reveal calcification of the bursa and associated structures, consistent with chronic inflammation. Magnetic resonance imaging is indicated if disruption of the hamstring musculotendinous unit is suspected. The injection technique described later serves as both a diagnostic and a therapeutic maneu-

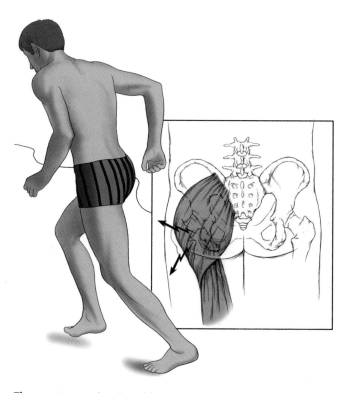

Figure 74–1. Ischiogluteal bursitis can be caused by running on soft, uneven surfaces. It presents clinically as point tenderness over the ischial tuberosity.

ver and is also used to treat hamstring tendinitis. Laboratory tests, including a complete blood count, erythrocyte sedimentation rate, and antinuclear antibody testing, are indicated if collagen vascular disease is suspected. Plain radiography and radionuclide bone scanning are indicated in the presence of trauma or if tumor is a possibility.

DIFFERENTIAL DIAGNOSIS

Although the diagnosis of ischiogluteal bursitis is usually straightforward, this painful condition is occasionally confused with sciatica, primary pathology of the hip, insufficiency fractures of the pelvis, and tendinitis of the hamstrings. Tumors of the hip and pelvis should also be

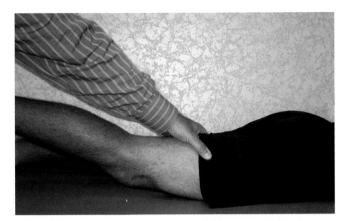

Figure 74–2. Resisted hip extension test for ischiogluteal bursitis. (From Waldman SD: Physical Diagnosis of Pain: An Atlas of Signs and Symptoms. Philadelphia, Saunders, 2006, p 309.)

considered in the differential diagnosis of ischiogluteal bursitis.

TREATMENT

Initial treatment of the pain and functional disability associated with ischiogluteal bursitis includes a combination of nonsteroidal anti-inflammatory drugs or cyclooxygenase-2 inhibitors and physical therapy. The local application of heat and cold may also be beneficial. Any repetitive activity that may exacerbate the patient's symptoms should be avoided. For patients who do not respond to these treatment modalities, injection with local anesthetic and steroid is a reasonable next step.

To inject the ischiogluteal bursa, the patient is placed in the lateral position with the affected side up and the affected leg flexed at the knee. The skin overlying the ischial tuberosity is prepared with antiseptic solution. A syringe containing 4 mL of 0.25% preservative-free bupivacaine and 40 mg methylprednisolone is attached to a 1½-inch, 25-gauge needle. The ischial tuberosity is identified with a sterilely gloved finger. Before needle placement, the patient should be instructed to say "There!" immediately if he or she feels a paresthesia in the lower extremity, indicating that the needle has impinged on the sciatic nerve. Should a paresthesia occur, the needle is immediately withdrawn and repositioned more medially. The needle is then carefully advanced at that point through the skin, subcutaneous tissues, muscle, and tendon until it impinges on the bone of the ischial tuberosity. Care must be taken to keep the needle in the midline and not to advance it laterally, to avoid contacting the sciatic nerve. After careful aspiration, and if no paresthesia is present, the contents of the syringe are gently injected into the bursa.

Physical modalities, including local heat and gentle stretching exercises, should be introduced several days after the patient undergoes injection. Vigorous exercises should be avoided, because they will exacerbate the patient's symptoms. Simple analgesics, nonsteroidal anti-inflammatory drugs, and antimyotonic agents such as tizanidine may be used concurrently with this injection technique.

COMPLICATIONS AND PITFALLS

The injection technique is safe if careful attention is paid to the clinically relevant anatomy. Because of the proximity to the sciatic nerve, injection for ischiogluteal bursitis should be performed only by those familiar with the regional anatomy and experienced in the technique. Many patients complain of a transient increase in pain after injection of the affected bursa and tendons, and they should be warned of this possibility. If patients continue to engage in the repetitive activities responsible for ischiogluteal bursitis, improvement will be limited.

Clinical Pearls

To distinguish ischiogluteal bursitis from hamstring tendinitis, remember that ischiogluteal bursitis presents with point tenderness over the ischial bursa, whereas the tenderness of hamstring tendinitis is more diffuse over the upper muscle and tendons. The treatment, however, is the same. Injection is extremely effective in relieving the pain of both ischiogluteal bursitis and hamstring tendinitis.

Chapter 75

Levator Ani Syndrome

ICD-9 CODE **729.1**

THE CLINICAL SYNDROME

The levator ani muscle is susceptible to the development of myofascial pain syndrome. Such pain is often the result of repetitive microtrauma to the muscle during such activities as mountain biking and horseback riding (Fig. 75-1). Injury to the muscle during childbirth or blunt trauma to the muscle may also incite levator ani myofascial pain syndrome.

Myofascial pain syndrome is a chronic pain syndrome that affects a focal or regional portion of the body. The sine qua non of myofascial pain syndrome is the finding of myofascial trigger points on physical examination. Although these trigger points are generally localized to the part of the body affected, the pain is often referred to other areas. This referred pain may be misdiagnosed or attributed to other organ systems, leading to extensive evaluation and ineffective treatment. Patients with myofascial pain syndrome involving the levator ani have primary pain in the pelvic floor that may be referred to the posterior buttocks and posterior lower extremity (Fig. 75-2).

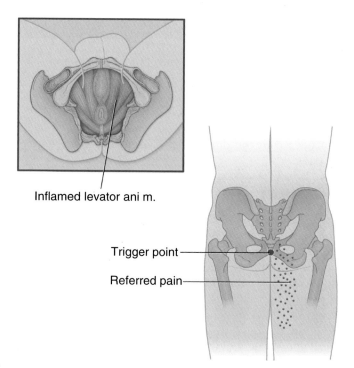

Inflamed levator ani m.

Trigger point

Referred pain

Figure 75–2. Patients with myofascial pain syndrome involving the levator ani have primary pain in the pelvic floor that may be referred to the posterior buttocks and posterior lower extremity. (From Waldman SD: Atlas of Pain Management Injection Techniques, 2nd ed. Philadelphia, Saunders, 2007, p 385.)

The trigger point is pathognomonic of myofascial pain syndrome and is characterized by a local point of exquisite tenderness in the affected muscle. Mechanical stimulation of the trigger point by palpation or stretching produces not only intense local pain but referred pain as well. In addition, there is often an involuntary withdrawal of the stimulated muscle, called a "jump sign," which is also characteristic of myofascial pain syndrome. Patients with levator ani syndrome have a trigger point along the rectum or perineum.

Taut bands of muscle fibers are often identified when myofascial trigger points are palpated. In spite of this consistent physical finding, the pathophysiology of the myofascial trigger point remains elusive, although it is

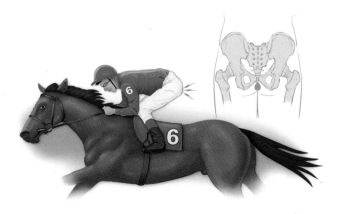

Figure 75–1. Levator ani syndrome may be caused by repetitive microtrauma to the muscle during such activities as mountain biking and horseback riding.

believed that trigger points are the result of microtrauma to the affected muscle. This may result from a single injury, repetitive microtrauma, or chronic deconditioning of the agonist and antagonist muscle unit.

In addition to muscle trauma, a variety of other factors seem to predispose patients to develop myofascial pain syndrome. For instance, a weekend athlete who subjects his or her body to unaccustomed physical activity may develop myofascial pain syndrome. Poor posture while sitting at a computer or while watching television has also been implicated as a predisposing factor. Previous injuries may result in abnormal muscle function and lead to the development of myofascial pain syndrome. All these predisposing factors may be intensified if the patient also suffers from poor nutritional status or coexisting psychological or behavioral abnormalities, including chronic stress and depression. The levator ani muscle seems to be particularly susceptible to stress-induced myofascial pain syndrome.

Stiffness and fatigue often coexist with pain, increasing the functional disability associated with this disease and complicating its treatment. Myofascial pain syndrome may occur as a primary disease state or in conjunction with other painful conditions, including radiculopathy and chronic regional pain syndromes. Psychological or behavioral abnormalities, including depression, frequently coexist with the muscle abnormalities, and management of these psychological disorders is an integral part of any successful treatment plan.

SIGNS AND SYMPTOMS

The trigger point is the pathologic lesion of levator ani syndrome, and it is characterized by a local point of exquisite tenderness in the levator ani muscle. Mechanical stimulation of the trigger point by palpation or stretching produces primary pain in the pelvic floor and referred pain in the posterior buttocks and posterior lower extremity (see Fig. 75-2). In addition, the jump sign is often present.

TESTING

Biopsies of clinically identified trigger points have not revealed consistently abnormal histology. The muscle hosting the trigger points has been described either as "moth eaten" or as containing "waxy degeneration." Increased plasma myoglobin has been reported in some patients with levator ani syndrome, but this finding has not been corroborated by other investigators. Electrodiagnostic testing has revealed an increase in muscle tension in some patients, but again, this finding has not been reproducible. Because of the lack of objective diagnostic testing, the clinician must rule out other coexisting disease processes that may mimic levator ani syndrome (see Differential Diagnosis).

DIFFERENTIAL DIAGNOSIS

The diagnosis of levator ani syndrome is based on clinical findings rather than specific laboratory, electrodiagnostic, or radiographic testing. For this reason, a targeted history and physical examination, with a systematic search for trigger points and identification of a positive jump sign, must be carried out in every patient suspected of suffering from levator ani syndrome. It is incumbent on the clinician to rule out other coexisting disease processes that may mimic levator ani syndrome, including primary inflammatory muscle disease, primary hip pathology, rectal and pelvic tumors, gluteal bursitis, and gluteal nerve entrapment (Fig. 75-3). The use of electrodiagnostic and radiographic testing can identify coexisting pathology such as rectal and pelvic tumors and lumbosacral nerve lesions. The clinician must also identify coexisting psychological and behavioral abnormalities that may mask or exacerbate the symptoms of levator ani syndrome.

TREATMENT

Treatment is focused on eliminating the myofascial trigger and achieving relaxation of the affected muscle. It is hoped that interrupting the pain cycle in this way will allow the patient to obtain prolonged pain relief. The mechanism of action of the treatment modalities used is poorly understood, so an element of trial and error is involved in developing a treatment plan.

Conservative therapy consisting of trigger point injection with local anesthetic or saline is the initial treatment of levator ani syndrome. Because underlying depression and anxiety are present in many patients, antidepressants are an integral part of most treatment plans. Other methods, including physical therapy, therapeutic heat and cold, transcutaneous nerve stimulation, and electrical stimulation, may be helpful on a case-by-case basis. For patients who do not respond to these traditional measures, consideration should be given to the use of botulinum toxin type A; although not currently approved by the Food and Drug Administration for this indication, the injection of minute quantities of botulinum toxin type A directly into trigger points has been successful in the treatment of persistent levator ani syndrome.

COMPLICATIONS AND PITFALLS

Trigger point injections are extremely safe if careful attention is paid to the clinically relevant anatomy. Sterile technique must be used to avoid infection, along with universal precautions to minimize any risk to the

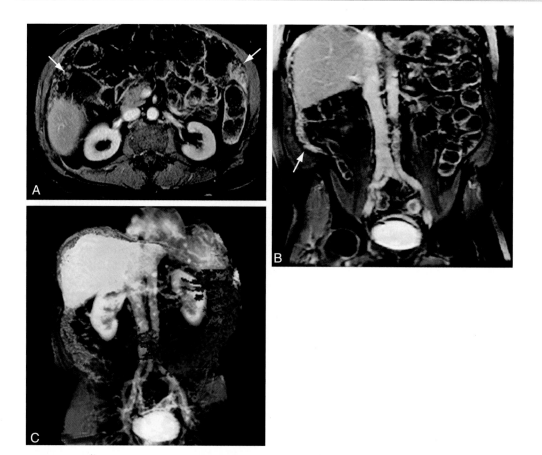

Figure 75–3. Recurrent rectal cancer with carcinomatosis. Axial **(A)** and coronal **(B)** gadolinium-enhanced spoiled gradient echo magnetic resonance images show heterogeneously enhancing peritoneal and omental metastases *(arrows)* from recurrent rectal cancer. **C,** Three-dimensional color model generated from the coronal gadolinium-enhanced images shows the distribution of the peritoneal and omental tumor in purple. (From Edelman RR, Hessellink JR, Zlatkin MB, Crues JV: Clinical Magnetic Resonance Imaging, 3rd ed. Philadelphia, Saunders, 2006, p 2780.)

operator. Most complications of trigger point injection are related to needle-induced trauma at the injection site and in underlying tissues. The incidence of ecchymosis and hematoma formation can be decreased if pressure is applied to the injection site immediately after injection. The avoidance of overly long needles can decrease the incidence of trauma to underlying structures. Special care must be taken to avoid trauma to the sciatic nerve.

Clinical Pearls

Although levator ani syndrome is a common disorder, it is often misdiagnosed. Therefore, in patients suspected of suffering from levator ani syndrome, a careful evaluation to identify underlying disease processes is mandatory. Levator ani syndrome often coexists with a variety of somatic and psychological disorders.

Chapter 76

Coccydynia

ICD-9 CODE **724.79**

THE CLINICAL SYNDROME

Coccydynia is a common syndrome characterized by pain localized to the tailbone that radiates into the lower sacrum and perineum. Coccydynia affects females more frequently than males. It occurs most commonly after direct trauma from a kick or a fall directly onto the coccyx. Coccydynia can also occur after a difficult vaginal delivery. The pain of coccydynia is thought to be the result of strain of the sacrococcygeal ligament or, occasionally, fracture of the coccyx. Less commonly, arthritis of the sacrococcygeal joint can result in coccydynia.

SIGNS AND SYMPTOMS

On physical examination, patients exhibit point tenderness over the coccyx; the pain increases with movement of the coccyx. Movement of the coccyx may also cause sharp paresthesias into the rectum, which patients find quite distressing. On rectal examination, the levator ani, piriformis, and coccygeus muscles may feel indurated, and palpation of these muscles may induce severe spasm. Sitting exacerbates the pain of coccydynia, and patients often attempt to sit on one buttock to avoid pressure on the coccyx (Fig. 76-1).

TESTING

Plain radiography is indicated in all patients who present with pain thought to be emanating from the coccyx to rule out occult bony pathology and tumor. Based on the patient's clinical presentation, additional testing may be warranted, including a complete blood count, prostate-specific antigen level, erythrocyte sedimentation rate, and antinuclear antibody testing. Magnetic resonance imaging of the pelvis is indicated if occult mass or tumor is suspected. Radionuclide bone scanning may be useful to rule out stress fractures not visible on plain radiographs. The injection technique described later serves as both a diagnostic and a therapeutic maneuver.

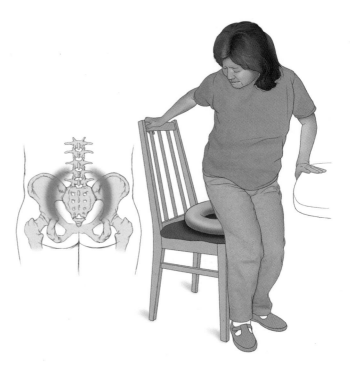

Figure 76–1. The pain of coccydynia is localized to the coccyx and is made worse by sitting.

DIFFERENTIAL DIAGNOSIS

Primary pathology of the rectum and anus is occasionally confused with the pain of coccydynia. Primary tumors or metastatic lesions of the sacrum or coccyx may also present as coccydynia (Fig. 76-2). Proctalgia fugax can be distinguished from coccydynia because movement of the coccyx does not reproduce the pain. Insufficiency fractures of the pelvis or sacrum and pathology of the sacroiliac joints may on occasion mimic coccydynia.

TREATMENT

A short course of conservative therapy consisting of simple analgesics, nonsteroidal anti-inflammatory drugs or cyclooxygenase-2 inhibitors, and a foam donut to prevent further irritation to the sacrococcygeal ligament

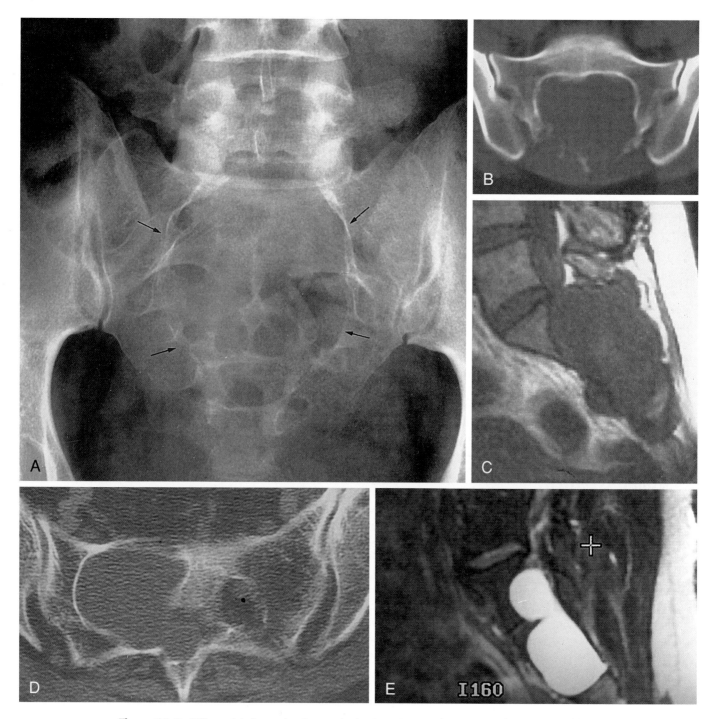

Figure 76–2. Differential diagnosis of coccydynia. **A** to **C,** Ependymoma. In this 28-year-old woman with low back pain of several years' duration and a normal neurologic examination, routine radiography **(A)** reveals an osteolytic lesion *(arrows)* in the sacrum. Transaxial computed tomography scan **(B)** confirms its central location and posterior extension. Sagittal, T1-weighted, spin echo magnetic resonance image **(C)** shows its large size, posterior extension, and low signal intensity. The tumor was of high signal intensity on T2-weighted spin echo magnetic resonance images (not shown). Histologic analysis confirmed a myxopapillary ependymoma that did not communicate with the dural sac. **D** and **E,** Meningocele. Transaxial computed tomography scan **(D)** shows a right-sided sacral lesion distorting the neural foramen. It is sharply delineated, with a sclerotic margin. Sagittal fast spin echo magnetic resonance image **(E)** reveals a lesion of high signal intensity with bone erosion. (From Resnick D: Diagnosis of Bone and Joint Disorders, 4th ed. Philadelphia, Saunders, 2002, p 4018.)

is a reasonable first step in the treatment of coccydynia. If the patient does not experience rapid improvement, injection is a reasonable next step.

To treat the pain of coccydynia, the patient is placed in the prone position. The legs and heels are abducted to prevent tightening of the gluteal muscles, which can make identification of the sacrococcygeal joint difficult. A wide area of skin is prepared with antiseptic solution so that all the landmarks can be palpated aseptically. A fenestrated sterile drape is placed to avoid contamination of the palpating finger. The middle finger of the operator's nondominant hand is placed over the sterile drape into the natal cleft, with the fingertip palpating the sacrococcygeal joint at the base of the sacrum. After locating the sacrococcygeal joint, a 1½-inch, 25-gauge needle is inserted through the skin at a 45-degree angle into the region of the sacrococcygeal joint and ligament. If the ligament is penetrated, a "pop" will be felt, and the needle should be withdrawn through the ligament. If contact with the bony wall of the sacrum occurs, the needle should be withdrawn slightly to disengage the needle tip from the periosteum. When the needle is satisfactorily positioned, a syringe containing 5 mL of 1% preservative-free lidocaine and 40 mg methylprednisolone is attached to the needle. Gentle aspiration is carried out to identify cerebrospinal fluid or blood. If the aspiration test is negative, the contents of the syringe are slowly injected. There should be little resistance to injection. Any significant pain or sudden increase in resistance during injection suggests incorrect needle placement, and the clinician should stop injecting immediately and reassess the needle position. After injection, the needle is removed, and a sterile pressure dressing and ice pack are applied to the injection site.

Physical modalities, including local heat, gentle range-of-motion exercises, and rectal massage of the affected muscles, should be introduced several days after the patient undergoes injection for coccygeal pain. Vigorous exercises should be avoided, because they will exacerbate the patient's symptoms. Simple analgesics and nonsteroidal anti-inflammatory drugs can be used concurrently with the injection technique.

COMPLICATIONS AND PITFALLS

Coccydynia should be considered a diagnosis of exclusion in the absence of trauma to the coccyx and its ligaments, because failure to diagnose underlying tumor can have disastrous consequences. The injection technique is safe if careful attention is paid to clinically relevant anatomy. The major complication of injection is infection, owing to the proximity to the rectum. This complication should be exceedingly rare if strict aseptic technique is followed, as well as universal precautions to minimize any risk to the operator. The incidence of ecchymosis and hematoma formation can be decreased if pressure is applied to the injection site immediately after injection. Approximately 25% of patients complain of a transient increase in pain after injection, and they should be warned of this possibility.

Clinical Pearls

The use of a foam donut when sitting, along with the other treatment modalities discussed, may provide symptomatic relief and allow the sacrococcygeal ligament to heal. The injection technique described is extremely effective in the treatment of coccydynia. Coexistent sacroiliitis may contribute to coccygeal pain, necessitating additional treatment with more localized injection of local anesthetic and methylprednisolone.

Section 13

Pain Syndromes of the Hip and Lower Extremity

Chapter 77

Arthritis Pain of the Hip

ICD-9 CODE **715.95**

THE CLINICAL SYNDROME

Arthritis of the hip is commonly encountered in clinical practice. The hip joint is susceptible to the development of arthritis from a variety of conditions that have the ability to damage the joint cartilage. Osteoarthritis is the most common form of arthritis that results in hip joint pain; rheumatoid arthritis and post-traumatic arthritis are also common causes of hip pain. Less common causes of arthritis-induced hip pain include the collagen vascular diseases, infection, villonodular synovitis, and Lyme disease. Acute infectious arthritis is usually accompanied by significant systemic symptoms, including fever and malaise, and should be easily recognized; it is treated with culture and antibiotics rather than injection therapy. Collagen vascular disease generally presents as a polyarthropathy rather than a monoarthropathy limited to the hip joint, although hip pain secondary to collagen vascular disease responds exceedingly well to the treatment modalities described here.

SIGNS AND SYMPTOMS

The majority of patients presenting with hip pain secondary to arthritis complain of pain localized around the hip and upper leg (Fig. 77-1). Most patients with intrinsic hip pathology have a positive Patrick-FABERE (flexion, abduction, external rotation, extension) test (Fig. 77-2). Patients may initially present with ill-defined pain in the groin; occasionally, the pain is localized to the buttocks. Activity makes the pain worse, whereas rest and heat provide some relief. The pain is constant and is characterized as aching in nature; it may interfere with sleep. Some patients complain of a grating or popping sensation with use of the joint, and crepitus may be present on physical examination.

In addition to pain, patients often experience a gradual decrease in functional ability caused by reduced hip range of motion, making simple everyday tasks such as walking, climbing stairs, and getting in and out of a car

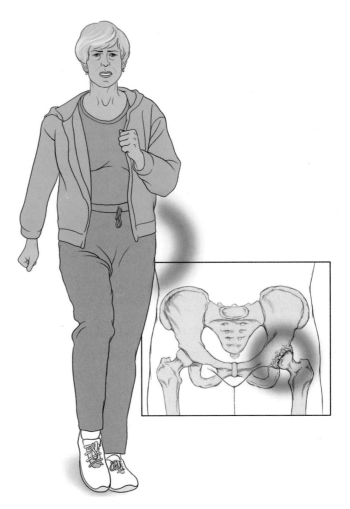

Figure 77–1. The pain of arthritis of the hip is localized to the hip, groin, and upper leg; it is made worse by weight-bearing exercise.

quite difficult. With continued disuse, muscle wasting may occur, and a frozen hip due to adhesive capsulitis may develop.

TESTING

Plain radiography is indicated in all patients who present with hip pain. Based on the patient's clinical presentation, additional testing may be warranted, including a

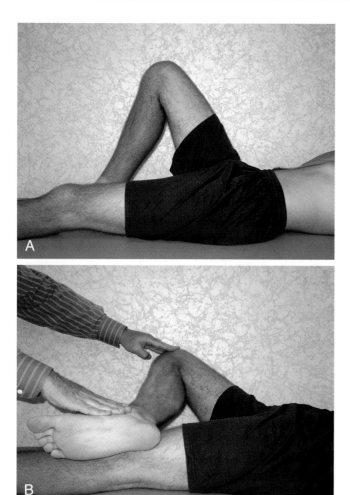

Figure 77–2. A and **B,** Performing the Patrick-FABERE test. (From Waldman SD: Physical Diagnosis of Pain: An Atlas of Signs and Symptoms. Philadelphia, Saunders, 2006, p 304.)

complete blood count, erythrocyte sedimentation rate, and antinuclear antibody testing. Magnetic resonance imaging of the hip is indicated if aseptic necrosis or occult mass or tumor is suspected or if the diagnosis is in question (Fig. 77-3).

DIFFERENTIAL DIAGNOSIS

Many diseases can cause hip pain (Table 77-1). Lumbar radiculopathy may mimic the pain and disability associated with arthritis of the hip; however, in such patients, the hip examination should be negative. Entrapment neuropathies, such as meralgia paresthetica, and trochanteric bursitis may confuse the diagnosis; both these conditions can coexist with arthritis of the hip. Primary and metastatic tumors of the hip and spine may also present similarly to arthritis of the hip.

TREATMENT

Initial treatment of the pain and functional disability of arthritis of the hip includes a combination of nonsteroidal anti-inflammatory drugs or cyclooxygenase-2 inhibitors and physical therapy. The local application of heat and cold may also be beneficial. For patients who do not respond to these treatment modalities, intra-articular injection of local anesthetic and steroid is a reasonable next step.

Intra-articular injection of the hip is performed by placing the patient in the supine position. The skin overlying the hip, subacromial region, and joint space is prepared with antiseptic solution. A sterile syringe containing 4 mL of 0.25% preservative-free bupivacaine and 40 mg methylprednisolone is attached to a 2-inch, 25-gauge needle using strict aseptic technique. The femoral artery

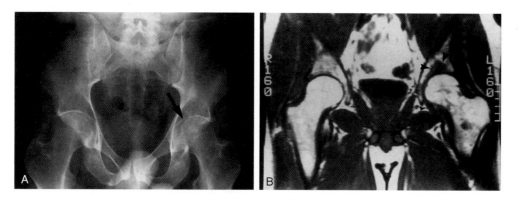

Figure 77–3. Monoarticular left hip pain of 6 months' duration in a 29-year-old man. **A,** Radiograph of the pelvis shows mild axial narrowing of the hip without erosions *(large arrow).* **B,** Coronal T1-weighted magnetic resonance image shows soft tissue thickening (synovitis) of intermediate density about the hip *(small arrowheads)* and acetabular erosion *(large arrowheads).* (From Haaga JR, Lanzieri CF, Gilkeson RC [eds]: CT and MR Imaging of the Whole Body, 4th ed. Philadelphia, Mosby, 2003, p 1913.)

Table 77-1. Causes of Hip Pain and Dysfunction

Localized Bony or Joint Space Pathology	Periarticular Pathology	Systemic Disease	Sympathetically Mediated Pain	Referred from Other Body Areas	Vascular Disease
Fracture	Bursitis	Rheumatoid arthritis	Causalgia	Lumbar plexopathy	Aortoiliac
Primary bone tumor	Tendinitis	Collagen vascular disease	Reflex sympathetic	Lumbar radiculopathy	atherosclerosis
Primary synovial tissue tumor	Adhesive capsulitis	Reiter's syndrome	dystrophy	Lumbar spondylosis	Internal iliac artery
Joint instability	Joint instability	Gout		Fibromyalgia	occlusion
Localized arthritis	Muscle strain	Other crystal arthropathies		Myofascial pain syndromes	
Osteophyte formation	Muscle sprain	Charcot's neuropathic arthritis		Inguinal hernia	
Osteonecrosis of femoral head	Periarticular infection not involving joint space			Entrapment neuropathies	
Joint space infection				Intrapelvic tumors	
Hemarthrosis				Retroperitoneal tumors	
Villonodular synovitis					
Intra-articular foreign body					
Slipped capital femoral epiphysis (Legg's disease)					
Chronic hip dislocation					

From Waldman SD: Physical Diagnosis of Pain: An Atlas of Signs and Symptoms. Philadelphia, Saunders, 2006.

is identified; then, at a point approximately 2 inches lateral to the femoral artery, just below the inguinal ligament, the hip joint space is identified. The needle is carefully advanced through the skin and subcutaneous tissues through the joint capsule into the joint. If bone is encountered, the needle is withdrawn into the subcutaneous tissues and redirected superiorly and slightly more medially. After the joint space is entered, the contents of the syringe are gently injected. There should be little resistance to injection. If resistance is encountered, the needle is probably in a ligament or tendon and should be advanced slightly into the joint space until the injection can proceed without significant resistance. The needle is removed, and a sterile pressure dressing and ice pack are applied to the injection site.

Physical modalities, including local heat and gentle range-of-motion exercises, should be introduced several days after the patient undergoes injection for hip pain. Vigorous exercises should be avoided, because they will exacerbate the patient's symptoms.

COMPLICATIONS AND PITFALLS

Failure to identify a primary or metastatic tumor of the hip or spine that is causing the patient's pain can be disastrous. The injection technique is safe if careful attention is paid to the clinically relevant anatomy. The major complication of intra-articular injection of the hip is infection; however, it should be exceedingly rare if strict aseptic technique is followed, along with universal precautions to minimize any risk to the operator. The incidence of ecchymosis and hematoma formation can be decreased if pressure is applied to the injection site immediately after injection. Approximately 25% of patients complain of a transient increase in pain after intra-articular injection of the hip joint, and they should be warned of this possibility.

Clinical Pearls

Coexistent bursitis and tendinitis may contribute to hip pain, necessitating additional treatment with more localized injection of local anesthetic and methylprednisolone. The injection technique described is extremely effective in the treatment of pain secondary to arthritis of the hip joint.

Chapter 78

Snapping Hip Syndrome

ICD-9 CODE 727.09

THE CLINICAL SYNDROME

Patients with snapping hip syndrome experience a snapping sensation in the lateral hip associated with sudden, sharp pain in the area of the greater trochanter. The snapping sensation and pain are the result of the iliopsoas tendon subluxating over the greater trochanter or iliopectineal eminence (Fig. 78-1). The trochanteric bursa lies between the greater trochanter and the tendon of the gluteus medius and the iliotibial tract. The gluteus medius muscle originates from the outer surface of the ilium, and its fibers pass downward and laterally to attach on the lateral surface of the greater trochanter. The gluteus medius muscle locks the pelvis in place during walking and running; it is innervated by the superior gluteal nerve. The iliopectineal eminence is the point at which the ilium and the pubis bone merge. The psoas and iliacus muscles join at the lateral side of the psoas, and the combined fibers are referred to as the iliopsoas muscle (Fig. 78-2). Like the psoas muscle, the iliacus flexes the thigh on the trunk or, if the thigh is fixed, flexes the trunk on the thigh, such as when moving from a supine to a sitting position.

The symptoms of snapping hip syndrome occur most commonly when rising from a sitting to a standing position or when walking briskly (Fig. 78-3). Often, trochanteric bursitis coexists with snapping hip syndrome, increasing the patient's pain and disability.

SIGNS AND SYMPTOMS

Physical examination reveals that patients can re-create the snapping and pain by moving from a sitting to a standing position and adducting the hip. This positive snap sign is considered diagnostic for snapping hip syndrome (Fig. 78-4). Point tenderness over the trochanteric bursa, indicative of trochanteric bursitis, is often present.

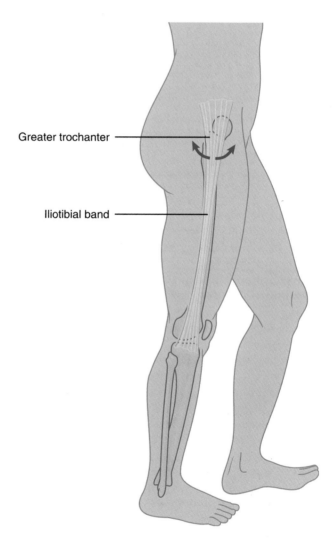

Greater trochanter

Iliotibial band

Figure 78–1. The snapping sensation and pain are the result of the iliopsoas tendon subluxating over the greater trochanter or iliopectineal eminence. (From Waldman SD: Atlas of Pain Management Injection Techniques, 2nd ed. Philadelphia, Saunders, 2007, p 368.)

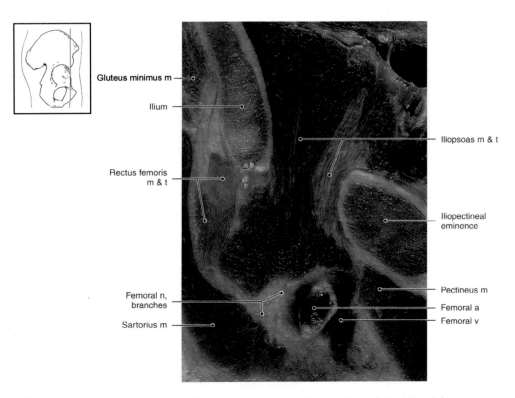

Figure 78–2. Coronal view of the hip. (From Kang HS, Ahn JM, Resnick D: MRI of the Extremities: An Anatomic Atlas, 2nd ed. Philadelphia, Saunders, 2002, p 233.)

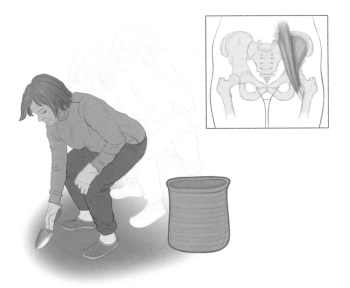

Figure 78–3. The symptoms of snapping hip syndrome commonly occur when rising from a sitting to a standing position or when walking briskly.

TESTING

Plain radiographs are indicated in all patients who present with pain thought to be emanating from the hip to rule out occult bony pathology and tumor. Based on the patient's clinical presentation, additional testing may be warranted, including a complete blood count, prostate-specific antigen level, erythrocyte sedimentation rate, and antinuclear antibody testing. Magnetic resonance imaging of the affected hip is indicated if occult mass or aseptic necrosis is suspected. Electrodiagnostic and radiographic testing can identify coexisting pathology such as internal derangement of the hip joint and lumbosacral nerve lesions. The injection technique described later serves as both a diagnostic and a therapeutic maneuver.

DIFFERENTIAL DIAGNOSIS

The diagnosis of snapping hip syndrome is based on clinical findings rather than specific laboratory, electrodiagnostic, or radiographic testing. For this reason, a targeted history and physical examination, with a

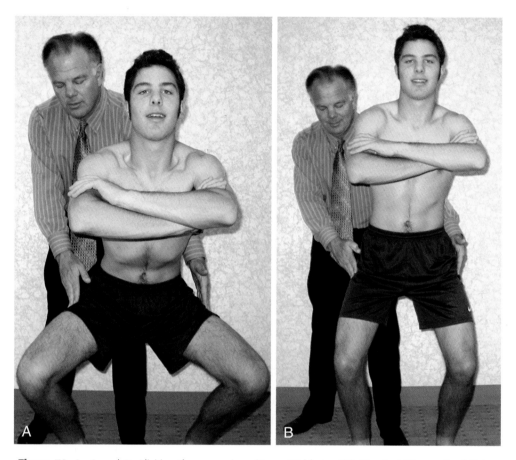

Figure 78–4. A and **B,** Eliciting the snap sign. (From Waldman SD: Physical Diagnosis of Pain: An Atlas of Signs and Symptoms. Philadelphia, Saunders, 2006, p 320.)

systematic search for other causes of hip pain, should be carried out. It is incumbent on the clinician to rule out other coexisting disease processes that may mimic snapping hip syndrome, including primary inflammatory muscle disease, primary hip pathology, and rectal and pelvic tumors.

TREATMENT

Initial treatment of the pain and functional disability associated with snapping hip syndrome includes a combination of nonsteroidal anti-inflammatory drugs or cyclooxygenase-2 inhibitors and physical therapy. The local application of heat and cold may also be beneficial. For patients who do not respond to these treatment modalities, injection with local anesthetic and steroid is a reasonable next step.

To perform the injection, the patient is placed in the lateral decubitus position with the affected side up. The midpoint of the greater trochanter is identified, and the skin overlying this point is prepared with antiseptic solution. A syringe containing 2 mL of 0.25% preserva-

tive-free bupivacaine and 40 mg methylprednisolone is attached to a 3½-inch, 25-gauge needle. Before needle placement, the patient should be instructed to say "There!" as soon as a paresthesia is felt in the lower extremity, indicating that the needle has impinged on the sciatic nerve. Should a paresthesia occur, the needle is immediately withdrawn and repositioned more laterally. The needle is slowly advanced through the previously identified point at a right angle to the skin, directly toward the center of the greater trochanter, until it hits bone; the needle is then withdrawn out of the periosteum. After careful aspiration for blood, and if no paresthesia is present, the contents of the syringe are gently injected. There should be minimal resistance to injection.

COMPLICATIONS AND PITFALLS

The injection technique is safe if careful attention is paid to the clinically relevant anatomy, particularly the sciatic nerve. The proximity to the sciatic nerve makes it imperative that this procedure be performed only by those familiar with the regional anatomy and experienced in the technique. Although infection is rare, sterile technique must be used, along with universal precautions to minimize any risk to the operator. Most complications of the injection technique are related to needle-induced trauma at the injection site and in the underlying tissues. The incidence of ecchymosis and hematoma formation can be decreased if pressure is applied to the injection site immediately after injection. Many patients complain of a transient increase in pain after injection, and they should be warned of this possibility.

Clinical Pearls

Snapping hip syndrome is a common disorder that often coexists with trochanteric bursitis. Because snapping hip syndrome is often misdiagnosed, a careful evaluation to identify underlying disease processes is mandatory. The injection technique described is extremely effective in the treatment of snapping hip syndrome.

Chapter 79

Iliopectineal Bursitis

ICD-9 CODE 726.5

THE CLINICAL SYNDROME

Bursae are formed from synovial sacs, whose purpose is to allow the easy sliding of muscles and tendons across one another at areas of repetitive movement. Lining these synovial sacs is a synovial membrane invested with a network of blood vessels that secrete synovial fluid. With overuse or misuse, the bursa may become inflamed or, rarely, infected; inflammation of the bursa results in an increase in the production of synovial fluid, causing swelling of the bursal sac. Although there is significant interpatient variability in the number, size, and location of bursae, the iliopectineal bursa generally lies between the psoas and iliacus muscles and the iliopectineal eminence (Fig. 79-1). This bursa may exist as a single bursal sac or, in some patients, a multisegmented series of loculated sacs.

The iliopectineal bursa is vulnerable to injury from both acute trauma and repeated microtrauma. Acute injuries often involve direct trauma to the bursa via hip

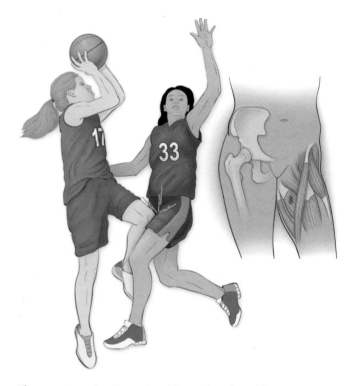

Figure 79–2. The iliopectineal bursa is vulnerable to injury from both acute trauma and repeated microtrauma. Acute injuries may be caused by direct trauma to the bursa via hip injuries.

injuries (Fig. 79-2); overuse injuries may also occur, such as the use of exercise equipment for lower extremity strengthening. If inflammation of the iliopectineal bursa becomes chronic, calcification may occur.

SIGNS AND SYMPTOMS

Patients with iliopectineal bursitis frequently complain of pain in the anterior hip and groin. The pain is localized to the area just below the crease of the groin anteriorly, with referred pain noted in the hip joint and anterior pelvis. Often, patients are unable to sleep on the affected hip and may complain of a sharp "catching" sensation with range of motion of the hip. Iliopectineal bursitis often coexists with arthritis of the hip joint.

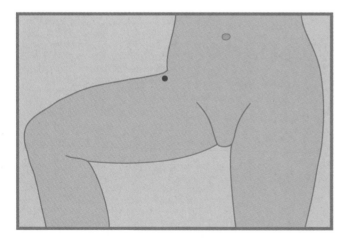

Figure 79–1. The iliopectineal bursa lies between the psoas and iliacus muscles and the iliopectineal eminence. (From Waldman SD: Atlas of Pain Management Injection Techniques, 2nd ed. Philadelphia, Saunders, 2007, p 359.)

Physical examination may reveal point tenderness in the upper thigh just below the crease of the groin. Passive flexion, adduction, and abduction, as well as active resisted flexion and adduction of the affected lower extremity, can reproduce the pain. Sudden release of resistance during this maneuver causes a marked increase in pain.

TESTING

Plain radiographs and/or CT scanning may reveal calcification of the bursa and associated structures, consistent with chronic inflammation (Fig. 79-3). Magnetic resonance imaging of the hip and pelvis is indicated if tendinitis, partial disruption of the ligaments, stress fracture, internal derangement of the hip, or pelvic mass is suspected. Radionuclide bone scanning is indicated if occult fracture, metastatic disease, or primary tumor involving the hip or pelvis is being considered. Based on the patient's clinical presentation, additional testing may be warranted, including a complete blood count, erythrocyte sedimentation rate, and antinuclear antibody testing. The injection technique described later serves as both a diagnostic and a therapeutic maneuver.

DIFFERENTIAL DIAGNOSIS

Iliopectineal bursitis is a common causes of hip and groin pain. Osteoarthritis, rheumatoid arthritis, post-traumatic arthritis, and, less commonly, aseptic necrosis of the femoral head are also common causes of hip and groin pain that may coexist with iliopectineal bursitis. Less common causes of arthritis-induced pain include the collagen vascular diseases, infection, villonodular synovitis, and Lyme disease. Acute infectious arthritis is usually accompanied by significant systemic symptoms, including fever and malaise, and should be easily recognized; it is treated with culture and antibiotics rather than injection therapy. Collagen vascular disease generally presents as a polyarthropathy rather than a monoarthropathy limited to the hip joint, although pain secondary to collagen vascular disease responds exceedingly well to the injection technique described here.

TREATMENT

Initial treatment of the pain and functional disability associated with iliopectineal bursitis includes a combination of nonsteroidal anti-inflammatory drugs or cyclooxygenase-2 inhibitors and physical therapy. The local application of heat and cold may also be beneficial. For patients who do not respond to these treatment modalities, injection of local anesthetic and steroid into the iliopectineal bursa is a reasonable next step.

Injection into the iliopectineal bursa is performed with the patient in the supine position. The pulsation of the femoral artery at the midpoint of the inguinal ligament is identified. At a point 2½ inches below and 3½ inches lateral to this pulsation lies the entry point of the needle; this point should be at the lateral edge of the sartorius muscle. The skin overlying this point is prepared with antiseptic solution. A syringe containing 9 mL of 0.25% preservative-free bupivacaine and 40 mg methylprednisolone is attached to a 3½-inch, 25-gauge needle. Before needle placement, the patient should be instructed to say "There!" as soon as a paresthesia is felt in the lower extremity, indicating that the needle has impinged on the femoral nerve. Should a paresthesia occur, the needle is immediately withdrawn and repositioned more

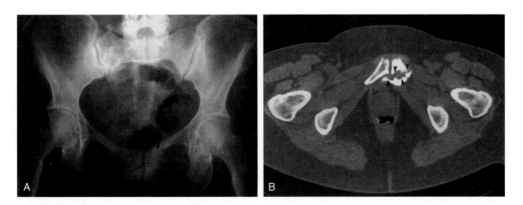

Figure 79–3. Pubic insufficiency fracture simulating a neoplasm in a 61-year-old woman. **A,** Pelvic radiograph shows changes in the symphysis on the left with sclerosis, suggesting a chondroid- or osteoid-producing lesion *(arrows)*. **B,** Computed tomography reveals a linear fracture plane and surrounding callus *(arrowheads)* resulting from a healing fracture; there is no evidence of a soft tissue mass. (From Haaga JR, Lanzieri CF, Gilkeson RC [eds]: CT and MR Imaging of the Whole Body, 4th ed. Philadelphia, Mosby, 2003, p 1924.)

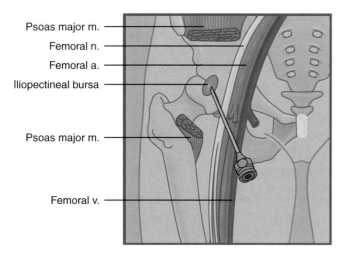

Psoas major m.
Femoral n.
Femoral a.
Iliopectineal bursa
Psoas major m.
Femoral v.

Figure 79–4. Correct needle placement for injection of the iliopectineal bursa. (From Waldman SD: Atlas of Pain Management Injection Techniques, 2nd ed. Philadelphia, Saunders, 2007, p 359.)

laterally. The needle is then carefully advanced through the previously identified point at a 45-degree angle cephalad, to allow the needle to safely pass beneath the femoral artery, vein, and nerve. The needle is advanced very slowly to avoid trauma to the femoral nerve until it hits bone at the point where the ilium and pubic bones merge (Fig. 79-4); the needle is then withdrawn out of the periosteum. After careful aspiration for blood, and if no paresthesia is present, the contents of the syringe are gently injected into the bursa. There should be minimal resistance to injection.

Physical modalities, including local heat and gentle stretching exercises, should be introduced several days after the patient undergoes injection. Vigorous exercises should be avoided, because they will exacerbate the patient's symptoms. Simple analgesics and nonsteroidal anti-inflammatory agents can be used concurrently with this injection technique.

COMPLICATIONS AND PITFALLS

The injection technique is safe if careful attention is paid to the clinically relevant anatomy. Specifically, care must be taken to avoid trauma to the femoral nerve. The major complication of injection of the iliopectineal bursa is infection, although it should be exceedingly rare if strict aseptic technique is followed, along with universal precautions to minimize any risk to the operator. Other complications are related to needle-induced trauma at the injection site and in the underlying tissues. The incidence of ecchymosis and hematoma formation can be decreased if pressure is applied to the injection site immediately after injection. Approximately 25% of patients complain of a transient increase in pain after injection, and they should be warned of this possibility.

Clinical Pearls

The injection technique described is extremely effective in the treatment of iliopectineal bursitis. Iliopectineal bursitis frequently coexists with arthritis of the hip, which may require specific treatment to achieve pain relief and return of function.

Chapter 80

Ischial Bursitis

ICD-9 CODE 726.5

THE CLINICAL SYNDROME

Bursae are formed from synovial sacs, whose purpose is to allow the easy sliding of muscles and tendons across one another at areas of repetitive movement. Lining these synovial sacs is a synovial membrane invested with a network of blood vessels that secrete synovial fluid. With overuse or misuse, the bursa may become inflamed or, rarely, infected; inflammation of the bursa results in an increase in the production of synovial fluid, causing swelling of the bursal sac. Although there is significant interpatient variability in the number, size, and location of bursae, the ischial bursa generally lies between the gluteus maximus muscle and the bone of the ischial tuberosity. It may exist as a single bursal sac or, in some patients, as a multisegmented series of loculated sacs.

The ischial bursa is vulnerable to injury from both acute trauma and repeated microtrauma. Acute injuries are often caused by direct trauma to the bursa from falls onto the buttocks and from overuse, such as prolonged riding of horses or bicycles (Fig. 80-1). Running on uneven or soft surfaces such as sand also may cause ischial bursitis. If inflammation of the ischial bursa becomes chronic, calcification may occur.

SIGNS AND SYMPTOMS

Patients suffering from ischial bursitis frequently complain of pain at the base of the buttock with resisted extension of the lower extremity (Fig. 80-2). The pain is localized to the area over the ischial tuberosity; referred pain is noted in the hamstring muscle, which may develop coexistent tendinitis. Often, patients are unable to sleep on the affected hip and may complain of a sharp "catching" sensation when extending and flexing the hip, especially on first awakening. Physical examination may reveal point tenderness over the ischial tuberosity. Passive straight leg raising and active resisted extension of the affected lower extremity reproduce the pain. Sudden release of resistance during this maneuver causes

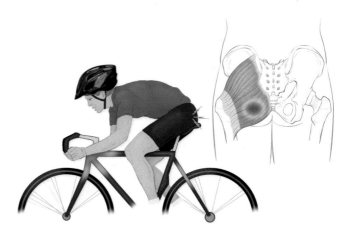

Figure 80–1. The ischial bursa is vulnerable to injury from both acute trauma and repeated microtrauma. Acute injuries are caused by direct trauma to the bursa from falls onto the buttocks and from overuse, such as prolonged riding of horses or bicycles.

a marked increase in pain; this increase in pain is considered a positive resisted hip extension test, supporting the diagnosis of ischial bursitis (Fig. 80-3).

TESTING

Plain radiographs may reveal calcification of the bursa and associated structures, consistent with chronic inflammation. Magnetic resonance imaging of the hip and

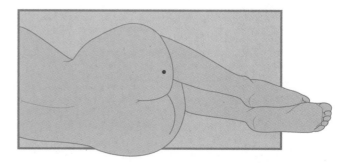

Figure 80–2. The ischial bursa lies between the gluteus maximus muscle and the ischial tuberosity. (From Waldman SD: Atlas of Pain Management Injection Techniques, 2nd ed. Philadelphia, Saunders, 2007.)

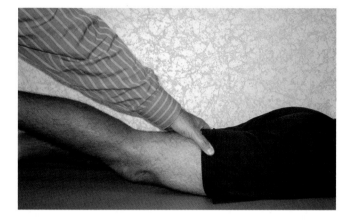

Figure 80-3. The resisted hip extension test for ischial bursitis. (From Waldman SD: Physical Diagnosis of Pain: An Atlas of Signs and Symptoms. Philadelphia, Saunders, 2006, p 309.)

pelvis is indicated if tendinitis, partial disruption of the ligaments, stress fracture, internal derangement of the hip, or hip or pelvic mass is suspected (Fig. 80-4). Radionuclide bone scanning is indicated if occult fracture, metastatic disease, or primary tumor involving the hip or pelvis is being considered. Based on the patient's clinical presentation, additional testing may be warranted, including a complete blood count, erythrocyte sedimentation rate, and antinuclear antibody testing. The injection technique described later serves as both a diagnostic and a therapeutic maneuver.

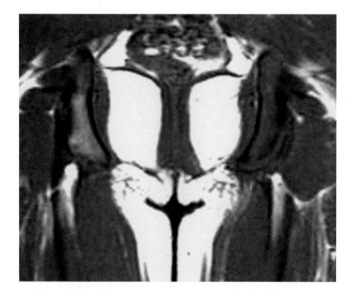

Figure 80-4. Ischial stress injury in a 16-year-old female athlete. Coronal T1-weighted image shows asymmetrical decreased marrow signal intensity involving the left ischium. (From Edelman RR, Hessellink JR, Zlatkin MB, Crues JV: Clinical Magnetic Resonance Imaging, 3rd ed. Philadelphia, Saunders, 2006, p 3385.)

DIFFERENTIAL DIAGNOSIS

Ischial bursitis is a common cause of hip and groin pain. Osteoarthritis, rheumatoid arthritis, post-traumatic arthritis, and, less commonly, aseptic necrosis of the femoral head are also common causes of hip and groin pain that may coexist with ischial bursitis. Hamstring tendinitis or tears of the hamstring muscles may also be present. Less common causes of arthritis-induced pain include the collagen vascular diseases, infection, villonodular synovitis, and Lyme disease. Acute infectious arthritis is usually accompanied by significant systemic symptoms, including fever and malaise, and should be easily recognized; it is treated with culture and antibiotics rather than injection therapy. Collagen vascular disease generally presents as a polyarthropathy rather than a monoarthropathy limited to the hip joint, although pain secondary to collagen vascular disease responds exceedingly well to the injection technique described here.

TREATMENT

Initial treatment of the pain and functional disability associated with ischial bursitis includes a combination of nonsteroidal anti-inflammatory drugs or cyclooxygenase-2 inhibitors and physical therapy. The local application of heat and cold may also be beneficial. For patients who do not respond to these treatment modalities, injection of local anesthetic and steroid into the ischial bursa is a reasonable next step.

To inject the ischial bursa, the patient is placed in the lateral position with the affected side up and the affected leg flexed at the knee. The skin overlying the ischial tuberosity is prepared with antiseptic solution. A syringe containing 4 mL of 0.25% preservative-free bupivacaine and 40 mg methylprednisolone is attached to a 1½-inch, 25-gauge needle. The ischial tuberosity is identified with a sterilely gloved finger. Before needle placement, the patient should be instructed to say "There!" as soon as a paresthesia is felt in the lower extremity, indicating that the needle has impinged on the sciatic nerve. Should a paresthesia occur, the needle is immediately withdrawn and repositioned more medially. The needle is then carefully advanced through the skin, subcutaneous tissues, muscle, and tendon until it impinges on the bone of the ischial tuberosity (Fig. 80-5). Care must be taken to keep the needle in the midline and not to advance it laterally, or it could contact the sciatic nerve. After careful aspiration, and if no paresthesia is present, the contents of the syringe is gently injected into the bursa.

Physical modalities, including local heat and gentle stretching exercises, should be introduced several days after the patient undergoes injection. Vigorous exercises should be avoided, because they will exacerbate the patient's symptoms. Simple analgesics and nonsteroidal

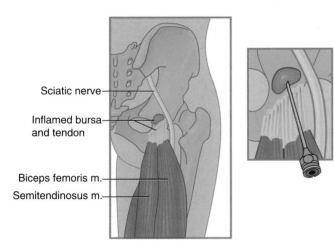

Sciatic nerve

Inflamed bursa
and tendon

Biceps femoris m.

Semitendinosus m.

Figure 80–5. Correct needle placement for injection of the ischial bursa. (From Waldman SD: Atlas of Pain Management Injection Techniques, 2nd ed. Philadelphia, Saunders, 2007.)

anti-inflammatory agents can be used concurrently with this injection technique.

COMPLICATIONS AND PITFALLS

The injection technique is safe if careful attention is paid to the clinically relevant anatomy. Special care must be taken to avoid trauma to the sciatic nerve. The major complication of injection of the ischial bursa is infection, although it should be exceedingly rare if strict aseptic technique is followed, along with universal precautions to minimize any risk to the operator. Other complications are related to needle-induced trauma at the injection site and in the underlying tissues. The incidence of ecchymosis and hematoma formation can be decreased if pressure is applied to the injection site immediately after injection. Approximately 25% of patients complain of a transient increase in pain after injection, and they should be warned of this possibility.

Clinical Pearls
The injection technique described is extremely effective in the treatment of ischial bursitis. Ischial bursitis frequently coexists with arthritis of the hip, which may require specific treatment to achieve pain relief and return of function.

Chapter 81

Meralgia Paresthetica

ICD-9 CODE 355.1

THE CLINICAL SYNDROME

Meralgia paresthetica is caused by compression of the lateral femoral cutaneous nerve by the inguinal ligament. This entrapment neuropathy presents as pain, numbness, and dysesthesias in the distribution of the lateral femoral cutaneous nerve. The symptoms often begin as a burning pain in the lateral thigh, with associated cutaneous sensitivity. Patients suffering from meralgia paresthetica note that sitting, squatting, or wearing wide belts causes the symptoms to worsen (Fig. 81-1). Although traumatic lesions to the lateral femoral cutaneous nerve have been implicated in meralgia paresthetica, in most patients, no obvious antecedent trauma can be identified.

SIGNS AND SYMPTOMS

Physical findings include tenderness over the lateral femoral cutaneous nerve at the origin of the inguinal ligament at the anterior superior iliac spine. A positive Tinel's sign over the lateral femoral cutaneous nerve as it passes beneath the inguinal ligament may be present. Patients may complain of burning dysesthesias in the nerve's distribution (Fig. 81-2). Careful sensory examination of the lateral thigh reveals a sensory deficit in the distribution of the lateral femoral cutaneous nerve; no motor deficit should be present. Sitting or the wearing of tight waistbands or wide belts can compress the nerve and exacerbate the symptoms of meralgia paresthetica.

TESTING

Electromyography can distinguish lumbar radiculopathy and diabetic femoral neuropathy from meralgia paresthetica. Plain radiographs of the back, hip, and pelvis are indicated in all patients who present with meralgia paresthetica to rule out occult bony pathology. Based on the patient's clinical presentation, additional testing may be warranted, including a complete blood count, uric acid level, erythrocyte sedimentation rate, and antinu-

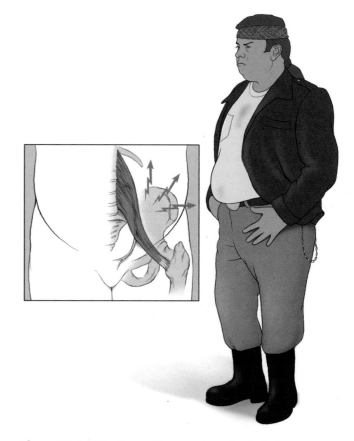

Figure 81–1. Obesity and the wearing of wide belts may compress the lateral femoral cutaneous nerve, resulting in meralgia paresthetica.

clear antibody testing. Magnetic resonance imaging of the back is indicated if herniated disk, spinal stenosis, or space-occupying lesion is suspected. The injection technique described later serves as both a diagnostic and a therapeutic maneuver.

DIFFERENTIAL DIAGNOSIS

Meralgia paresthetica is often misdiagnosed as lumbar radiculopathy, trochanteric bursitis, or primary hip pathology. Radiographs of the hip and electromyography can distinguish meralgia paresthetica from radicu-

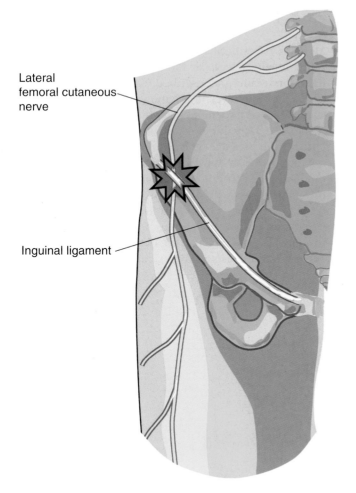

Lateral
femoral cutaneous
nerve

Inguinal ligament

Figure 81–2. Burning pain in the lateral thigh is indicative of meralgia paresthetica. (From Waldman SD: Physical Diagnosis of Pain: An Atlas of Signs and Symptoms. Philadelphia, Saunders, 2006, p 279.)

TREATMENT

Patients suffering from meralgia paresthetica should be instructed in avoidance techniques to reduce the symptoms and pain associated with this entrapment neuropathy. A short course of conservative therapy consisting of simple analgesics, nonsteroidal anti-inflammatory drugs, or cyclooxygenase-2 inhibitors is a reasonable first step in the treatment of meralgia paresthetica. If patients do not experience rapid improvement, injection is the next step.

To treat the pain of meralgia paresthetica, the patient is placed in the supine position with a pillow under the knees if lying with the legs extended increases the pain due to traction on the nerve. The anterior superior iliac spine is identified by palpation. A point 1 inch medial to the anterior superior iliac spine and just inferior to the inguinal ligament is identified and prepared with antiseptic solution. A 1½-inch, 25-gauge needle is slowly advanced perpendicular to the skin until the needle is felt to pop through the fascia. A paresthesia is often elicited. After careful aspiration, a solution of 5 to 7 mL of 1% preservative-free lidocaine and 40 mg methylprednisolone is injected in a fanlike pattern as the needle pierces the fascia of the external oblique muscle. Care must be taken not to place the needle deep enough to enter the peritoneal cavity and perforate the abdominal viscera (Fig. 81-3). After injection of the solution, pressure is applied to the injection site to decrease the incidence of ecchymosis and hematoma formation, which can be quite dramatic, especially in anticoagulated patients.

lopathy or pain emanating from the hip. In addition, most patients suffering from lumbar radiculopathy have back pain associated with reflex, motor, and sensory changes, whereas patients with meralgia paresthetica have no back pain and no motor or reflex changes; the sensory changes of meralgia paresthetica are limited to the distribution of the lateral femoral cutaneous nerve and should not extend below the knee. It should be remembered that lumbar radiculopathy and lateral femoral cutaneous nerve entrapment may coexist as the "double crush" syndrome. Occasionally, diabetic femoral neuropathy produces anterior thigh pain, which may confuse the diagnosis.

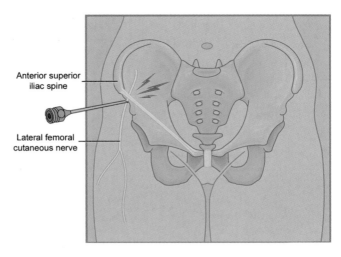

Anterior superior
iliac spine

Lateral femoral
cutaneous nerve

Figure 81–3. Correct needle placement for injection of the lateral femoral cutaneous nerve to treat meralgia paresthetica. (From Waldman SD: Atlas of Pain Management Injection Techniques. Philadelphia, Saunders, 2000.)

COMPLICATIONS AND PITFALLS

Care must be taken to rule out other conditions that may mimic the pain of meralgia paresthetica. The main complications of the injection technique are ecchymosis and hematoma. If the needle is placed too deep and it enters the peritoneal cavity, perforation of the colon may result in the formation of an intra-abdominal abscess and fistula. Early detection of infection is crucial to avoid potentially life-threatening sequelae. If the needle is placed too medially, blockade of the femoral nerve may occur, making ambulation difficult.

Clinical Pearls

Meralgia paresthetica is a common complaint that is often misdiagnosed as lumbar radiculopathy. The injection technique described can produce dramatic pain relief; however, if a patient presents with pain suggestive of meralgia paresthetica but does not respond to lateral femoral cutaneous nerve block, a lesion more proximal in the lumbar plexus or an L2-3 radiculopathy should be considered. Such patients often respond to epidural block with steroid. Electromyography and magnetic resonance imaging of the lumbar plexus are indicated in this patient population to rule out other causes of their pain, including malignancy invading the lumbar plexus or epidural or vertebral metastatic disease at L2-3.

Chapter 82

Phantom Limb Pain

ICD-9 CODE 353.6

THE CLINICAL SYNDROME

Almost all patients who undergo amputation experience the often painful and distressing sensation that the absent body part is still present (Fig. 82-1). The cause of this phenomenon is not fully understood, but it is thought to be mediated in large part at the spinal cord level. Congenitally absent limbs do not seem to be subject to the same phenomenon. Patients may be able to describe the limb in vivid detail, although it is often distorted or in an abnormal position. In many patients, the sensation of the phantom limb fades with time, but in some, phantom pain remains a distressing part of daily life. Phantom limb pain is often described as a constant, unpleasant, dysesthetic pain that may be exacerbated by movement or stimulation of the affected cutaneous regions; a sharp, shooting neuritic pain may be superimposed on the constant dysesthetic symptoms, and some patients also note a burning component reminiscent of reflex sympathetic dystrophy. Some investigators report that severe limb pain before amputation increases the incidence of phantom limb pain, but other investigators have failed to find this correlation.

SIGNS AND SYMPTOMS

Phantom limb pain can take multiple forms, but it usually consists of dysesthetic pain. Additionally, patients may experience abnormal kinesthetic sensations (i.e., that the limb is in an abnormal position) or abnormal kinetic sensations (i.e., that the limb is moving). It has been reported that many patients with phantom limb pain experience a telescoping phenomenon; for example, a patient may report that the phantom foot feels like it is attached directly to the proximal thigh. Phantom limb pain may fade over time, and younger patients are more likely to experience this diminution in symptoms. Owing to the unusual nature of phantom limb pain, a behavioral component is invariably present.

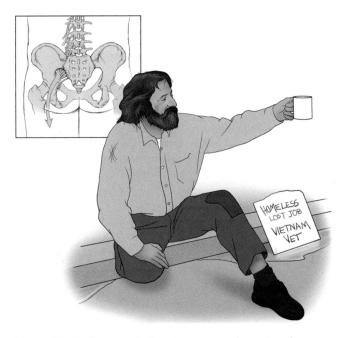

Figure 82–1. Phantom limb pain occurs with varying degrees of intensity in almost all patients who undergo amputation.

TESTING

In most cases, the diagnosis of phantom limb pain is easily made on clinical grounds. Testing is generally used to identify other treatable coexisting diseases, such as radiculopathy. Such testing includes basic laboratory tests; examination of the stump for neuroma, tumor, or occult infection; and plain radiographs and radionuclide bone scanning if fracture or osteomyelitis is suspected.

DIFFERENTIAL DIAGNOSIS

A careful initial evaluation, including a thorough history and physical examination, is indicated in all patients suffering from phantom limb pain if infection or fracture is a possibility. If the amputation was necessitated by malignancy, occult tumor must be ruled out. Other causes of pain in the distribution of the innervation of the affected

285

limb, including radiculopathy and peripheral neuropathy, should be considered.

TREATMENT

The first step is to reassure patients that phantom pain is normal after the loss of a limb and that these sensations are real, not imagined; this alone can reduce patients' anxiety and suffering. It is the consensus of many pain specialists that preemptive analgesia early in the natural course of a disease that may lead to amputation, such as peripheral vascular insufficiency, can reduce the likelihood that patients will develop phantom limb pain. The following treatments may be useful to relieve phantom limb pain.

Analgesics

The anticonvulsant gabapentin is a first-line treatment in the palliation of phantom limb pain. It should be administered early in the course of the pain syndrome and can be used concurrently with neural blockade, opioid analgesics, and other adjuvant analgesics, including antidepressants, if care is taken to avoid central nervous system side effects. Gabapentin is started at a bedtime dose of 300 mg and is titrated upward in 300-mg increments to a maximum of 3600 mg/day given in divided doses, as side effects allow.

Carbamazepine should be considered in patients with severe neuritic pain who do not respond to nerve block and gabapentin. If this drug is used, rigid monitoring of hematologic parameters is indicated, especially in patients receiving chemotherapy or radiation therapy. Phenytoin may also be beneficial in the treatment of neuritic pain, but it should not be used in patients with lymphoma; the drug may induce a pseudolymphoma-like state that is difficult to distinguish from the actual lymphoma.

Antidepressants

Antidepressants may be useful adjuncts in the initial treatment of phantom limb pain. On an acute basis, these drugs can alleviate the significant sleep disturbance that is common in this setting. In addition, antidepressants may be valuable in ameliorating the neuritic component of the pain, which is treated less effectively with narcotic analgesics. After several weeks of treatment, antidepressants may exert a mood-elevating effect, which may be desirable in some patients. Care must be taken to observe closely for central nervous system side effects in this patient population, and these drugs may cause urinary retention and constipation.

Nerve Block

Neural blockade with local anesthetic and steroid via either epidural nerve block or blockade of the sympathetic nerves subserving the painful area is a reasonable next step if the aforementioned pharmacologic modalities fail to control phantom limb pain. The exact mechanism by which neural blockade relieves phantom limb pain is unknown, but it may be related to the modulation of pain transmission at the spinal cord level. In general, neurodestructive procedures have a very low success rate and should be used only after all other treatments have failed, if at all.

Opioid Analgesics

Opioid analgesics have a limited role in the management of phantom limb pain, and they frequently do more harm than good. Careful administration of potent, long-acting narcotic analgesics (e.g., oral morphine elixir, methadone) on a time-contingent rather than as-needed basis may be a beneficial adjunct to sympathetic neural blockade. Because many patients suffering from phantom limb pain are elderly or have severe multisystem disease, close monitoring for the potential side effects of narcotic analgesics (e.g., confusion or dizziness, which may cause a patient to fall) is warranted. Daily dietary fiber supplementation and milk of magnesia should be started along with opioid analgesics to prevent constipation.

Adjunctive Treatments

The application of ice packs to the stump may provide relief in some patients with phantom limb pain. The application of heat increases pain in most patients, presumably because of increased conduction of small fibers, but it may be worth trying if the application of cold is ineffective. Transcutaneous electrical nerve stimulation and vibration may also be effective in a limited number of patients. The favorable risk-benefit ratio of these modalities makes them reasonable alternatives for patients who cannot or will not undergo sympathetic neural blockade or cannot tolerate pharmacologic treatment. The topical application of capsaicin may be beneficial in some patients suffering from phantom limb pain; however, the burning associated with application of this drug often limits its usefulness.

COMPLICATIONS AND PITFALLS

Although there are no complications associated with phantom limb pain itself, the consequences of unremitting pain can be devastating. Failure to aggressively treat phantom limb pain and the associated symptoms of sleep disturbance and depression can result in suicide.

Clinical Pearls

Because phantom limb pain can be so severe and have such devastating consequences, the clinician must treat it rapidly and aggressively. Special attention must be paid to the insidious onset of severe depression, which mandates hospitalization with suicide precautions.

Chapter 83

Trochanteric Bursitis

ICD-9 CODE 726.5

THE CLINICAL SYNDROME

Trochanteric bursitis is commonly encountered in clinical practice. Patients suffering from trochanteric bursitis frequently complain of pain in the lateral hip that radiates down the leg, mimicking sciatica (Fig. 83-1). The pain is localized to the area over the trochanter. Often, patients are unable to sleep on the affected hip and may complain of a sharp "catching" sensation with range of motion of the hip, especially on first arising. Patients may note that walking upstairs is becoming increasingly difficult. Trochanteric bursitis often coexists with arthritis of the hip, back and sacroiliac joint disease, and gait disturbance.

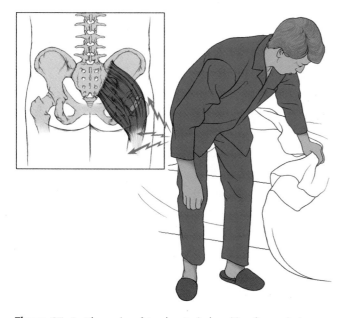

Figure 83–1. The pain of trochanteric bursitis often mimics that of sciatica.

The trochanteric bursa lies between the greater trochanter and the tendon of the gluteus medius and the iliotibial tract (Fig. 83-2). This bursa may exist as a single bursal sac or, in some patients, as a multisegmented series of loculated sacs. The trochanteric bursa is vulnerable to injury from both acute trauma and repeated microtrauma. Acute injuries may be caused by direct trauma to the bursa from falls onto the greater trochanter or previous hip surgery, as well as by overuse injuries, including running on soft or uneven surfaces. If inflammation of the trochanteric bursa becomes chronic, calcification may occur.

SIGNS AND SYMPTOMS

Physical examination reveals point tenderness in the lateral thigh just over the greater trochanter. Passive adduction and abduction, as well as active resisted abduction, of the affected lower extremity reproduce the pain. Sudden release of resistance during this maneuver causes a marked increase in pain (Fig. 83-3). There should be no sensory deficit in the distribution of the lateral femoral cutaneous nerve; this distinguishes trochanteric bursitis from meralgia paresthetica.

TESTING

Plain radiographs of the hip may reveal calcification of the bursa and associated structures, consistent with chronic inflammation. Magnetic resonance imaging is indicated if occult mass or tumor of the hip or groin is suspected or to confirm the diagnosis (Fig. 83-4). A complete blood count and erythrocyte sedimentation rate are useful if infection is suspected. Electromyography can distinguish trochanteric bursitis from meralgia paresthetica and sciatica. The injection technique described later serves as both a diagnostic and a therapeutic maneuver.

DIFFERENTIAL DIAGNOSIS

Trochanteric bursitis frequently coexists with arthritis of the hip. Occasionally, trochanteric bursitis can be con-

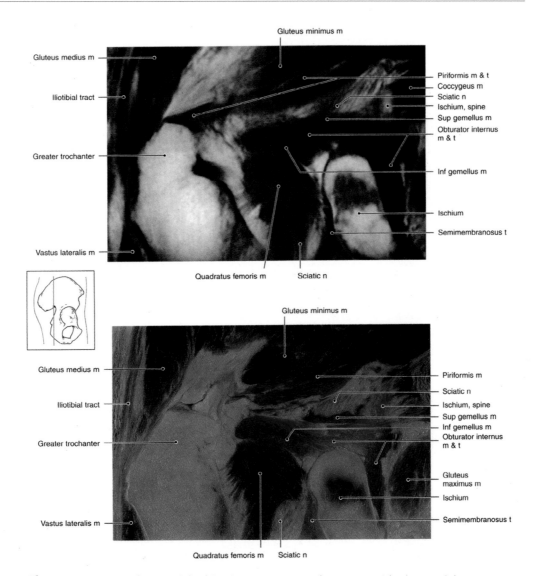

Figure 83–2. Coronal view of the hip. (From Kang HS, Ahn JM, Resnick D: MRI of the Extremities: An Anatomic Atlas, 2nd ed. Philadelphia, Saunders, 2002, p 221.)

fused with meralgia paresthetica, because both present with pain in the lateral thigh; however, in patients with meralgia paresthetica, palpation over the greater trochanter does not elicit pain. Electromyography can help sort out confusing clinical presentations. Primary or secondary tumors of the hip must also be considered in the differential diagnosis of trochanteric bursitis.

TREATMENT

A short course of conservative therapy consisting of simple analgesics, nonsteroidal anti-inflammatory drugs, or cyclooxygenase-2 inhibitors is a reasonable first step in the treatment of trochanteric bursitis. Patients should be instructed to avoid repetitive activities that may

be responsible for the development of trochanteric bursitis, such as running on sand. If patients do not experience rapid improvement, injection is a reasonable next step.

Injection of the trochanteric bursa is carried out by placing the patient in the lateral decubitus position with the affected side up. The midpoint of the greater trochanter is identified, and the skin overlying this point is prepared with antiseptic solution. A syringe containing 2 mL of 0.25% preservative-free bupivacaine and 40 mg methylprednisolone is attached to a 3½-inch, 25-gauge needle. Before needle placement, the patient should be instructed to say "There!" as soon as a paresthesia is felt in the lower extremity, indicating that the needle has impinged on the sciatic nerve. If a paresthesia occurs,

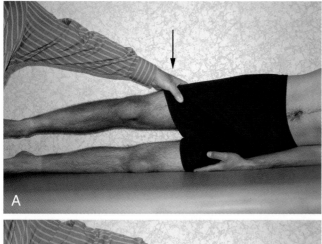

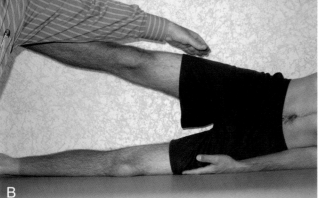

Figure 83-3. A and **B,** The resisted abduction release test. (From Waldman SD: Physical Diagnosis of Pain: An Atlas of Signs and Symptoms. Philadelphia, Saunders, 2006, p 316.)

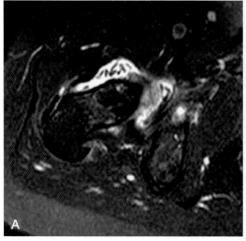

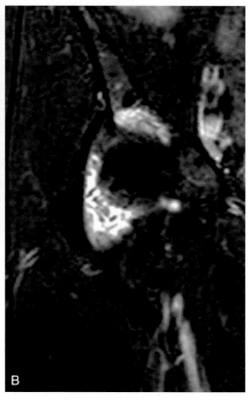

Figure 83-4. Synovial osteochondromatosis or chondromatosis. **A,** Axial, fat-saturated, T2-weighted image. **B,** Coronal, fat-saturated, T2-weighted image. (From Edelman RR, Hessellink JR, Zlatkin MB, Crues JV: Clinical Magnetic Resonance Imaging, 3rd ed. Philadelphia, Saunders, 2006, p 3392.)

the needle is immediately withdrawn and repositioned more laterally. The needle is then slowly advanced through the previously identified point at a right angle to the skin, directly toward the center of the greater trochanter (Fig. 83-5), until it hits bone; it is then withdrawn out of the periosteum. After careful aspiration for blood, and if no paresthesia is present, the contents of the syringe are gently injected into the bursa. There should be minimal resistance to injection.

Physical modalities, including local heat and gentle stretching exercises, should be introduced several days after the patient undergoes injection. Vigorous exercises should be avoided, because they will exacerbate the patient's symptoms. Simple analgesics, nonsteroidal anti-inflammatory drugs, and antimyotonic agents can be used concurrently with this injection technique.

COMPLICATIONS AND PITFALLS

Other conditions that may mimic the pain of trochanteric bursitis must be ruled out. The injection technique is safe if careful attention is paid to the clinically relevant anatomy. Special care must be taken to avoid trauma to the sciatic nerve, which makes it imperative that this procedure be performed only by those familiar with the regional anatomy and experienced in the technique. Most complications of the injection technique are related to needle-induced trauma at the injection site and in the underlying tissues. Infection, though rare, can occur, making careful attention to sterile technique mandatory. Many patients complain of a transient increase in pain after injection, and they should be warned of this possibility.

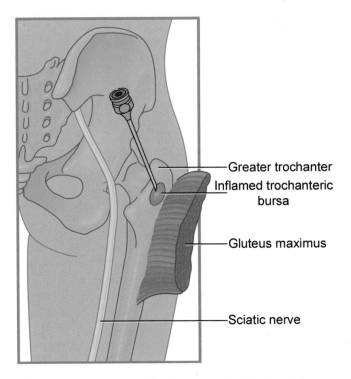

Greater trochanter
Inflamed trochanteric bursa
Gluteus maximus
Sciatic nerve

Figure 83–5. Correct needle placement for injection of the trochanteric bursa. (From Waldman SD: Atlas of Pain Management Injection Techniques. Philadelphia, Saunders, 2000.)

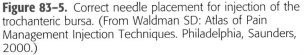

Clinical Pearls

Trochanteric bursitis frequently coexists with arthritis of the hip, which may require specific treatment to achieve pain relief and return of function. The injection technique described is extremely effective in the treatment of trochanteric bursitis.

Section 14

Pain Syndromes of the Knee

Chapter 84

Arthritis Pain of the Knee

ICD-9 CODE 715.96

THE CLINICAL SYNDROME

Arthritis of the knee is a common painful condition. The knee joint is susceptible to the development of arthritis from a variety of conditions that have the ability to damage the joint cartilage. Osteoarthritis is the most common form of arthritis that results in knee pain; rheumatoid arthritis and post-traumatic arthritis are also common causes of knee pain. Less common causes of arthritis-induced knee pain include the collagen vascular diseases, infection, villonodular synovitis, and Lyme disease. Acute infectious arthritis is usually accompanied by significant systemic symptoms, including fever and malaise, and should be easily recognized; it is treated with culture and antibiotics rather than injection therapy. Collagen vascular disease generally presents as a polyarthropathy rather than a monoarthropathy limited to the knee joint, although knee pain secondary to collagen vascular disease responds exceedingly well to the treatment modalities described here.

SIGNS AND SYMPTOMS

The majority of patients with osteoarthritis or post-traumatic arthritis of the knee complain of pain localized around the knee and distal femur. Activity makes the pain worse, whereas rest and heat provide some relief. The pain is constant and is characterized as aching in nature; it may interfere with sleep. Some patients complain of a grating or popping sensation with use of the joint, and crepitus may be present on the physical examination.

In addition to pain, patients often experience a gradual reduction in functional ability because of decreasing knee range of motion, making simple everyday tasks such as walking, climbing stairs, and getting in and out of a car quite difficult (Fig. 84-1). With continued disuse, muscle wasting may occur, and a frozen knee due to adhesive capsulitis may develop.

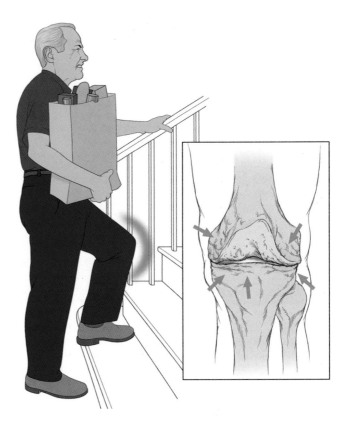

Figure 84–1. The pain of arthritis of the knee is made worse with weight-bearing activities.

TESTING

Plain radiographs or magnetic resonance imaging (MRI) is indicated in all patients who present with knee pain (Fig. 84-2). Based on the patient's clinical presentation, additional testing may be warranted, including a complete blood count, erythrocyte sedimentation rate, and antinuclear antibody testing. MRI of the knee is also indicated if the diagnosis is in question, if occult mass or tumor is suspected, or in the presence of trauma.

DIFFERENTIAL DIAGNOSIS

Lumbar radiculopathy may mimic the pain and disability associated with arthritis of the knee. In such patients,

For intra-articular injection of the knee, the patient is placed in the supine position with a rolled blanket underneath the knee to gently flex the joint. The skin overlying the medial joint is prepared with antiseptic solution. A sterile syringe containing 5 mL of 0.25% preservative-free bupivacaine and 40 mg methylprednisolone is attached to a 1½-inch, 25-gauge needle using strict aseptic technique. The joint space is identified, and the clinician places his or her thumb on the lateral margin of the patella and pushes it medially. At a point in the middle of the medial edge of the patella, the needle is inserted between the patella and the femoral condyles. The needle is then carefully advanced through the skin and subcutaneous tissues through the joint capsule and into the joint (Fig. 84-3). If bone is encountered, the needle is withdrawn into the subcutaneous tissues and redirected superiorly. After the joint space is entered, the contents of the syringe is gently injected. There should be little resistance to injection. If resistance is encountered, the needle is probably in a ligament or tendon and should be advanced slightly into the joint space until the injection can proceed without significant resistance. The needle is then removed, and a sterile pressure dressing and ice pack are applied to the injection site.

Physical modalities, including local heat and gentle range-of-motion exercises, should be introduced several days after the patient undergoes injection. Vigorous exercises should be avoided, because they will exacerbate the patient's symptoms.

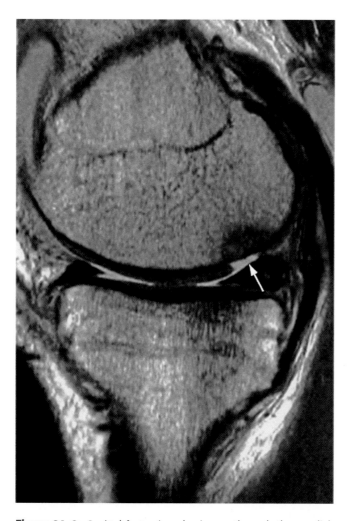

Figure 84–2. Sagittal fast spin echo image through the medial joint line demonstrates focal full-thickness chondral injury with associated subchondral osseous changes *(arrow)*. (From Edelman RR, Hessellink JR, Zlatkin MB, Crues JV: Clinical Magnetic Resonance Imaging, 3rd ed. Philadelphia, Saunders, 2006, p 3425.)

the knee examination should be negative. Bursitis of the knee and entrapment neuropathies such as meralgia paresthetica may also confuse the diagnosis; both these conditions may coexist with arthritis of the knee. Primary and metastatic tumors of the femur and spine may also present in a manner similar to arthritis of the knee.

TREATMENT

Initial treatment of the pain and functional disability associated with arthritis of the knee includes a combination of nonsteroidal anti-inflammatory drugs or cyclooxygenase-2 inhibitors and physical therapy. The local application of heat and cold may also be beneficial. For patients who do not respond to these treatment modalities, intra-articular injection of local anesthetic and steroid is a reasonable next step.

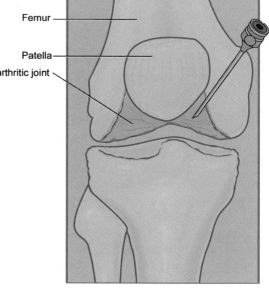

Femur
Patella
Inflamed, arthritic joint

Figure 84–3. Proper needle placement for intra-articular injection of the knee. (From Waldman SD: Atlas of Pain Management Injection Techniques. Philadelphia, WB Saunders, 2000.)

COMPLICATIONS AND PITFALLS

Failure to identify primary or metastatic tumor of the knee or spine that is causing the patient's pain can have disastrous results. The injection technique is safe if careful attention is paid to the clinically relevant anatomy. The major complication of intra-articular injection of the knee is infection, although it should be exceedingly rare if strict aseptic technique is followed, along with universal precautions to minimize any risk to the operator. The incidence of ecchymosis and hematoma formation can be decreased if pressure is applied to the injection site immediately after the injection. Approximately 25% of patients complain of a transient increase in pain after injection, and they should be warned of this possibility.

Clinical Pearls

Coexistent bursitis and tendinitis may contribute to knee pain, necessitating additional treatment with more localized injection of local anesthetic and methylprednisolone. The injection technique described is extremely effective in the treatment of pain secondary to arthritis of the knee.

Chapter 85

Medial Collateral Ligament Syndrome

ICD-9 CODE 717.82

THE CLINICAL SYNDROME

Medial collateral ligament syndrome is characterized by pain at the medial aspect of the knee joint. It is usually the result of trauma to the medial collateral ligament from falls with the leg in valgus and externally rotated, typically during snow skiing accidents or football clipping injuries (Fig. 85-1). The medial collateral ligament is a broad, flat, bandlike ligament that runs from the medial condyle of the femur to the medial aspect of the shaft of the tibia, where it attaches just above the groove where the semimembranosus muscle attaches. It also attaches to the edge of the medial semilunar cartilage. The ligament is susceptible to strain at the joint line or avulsion at its origin or insertion.

SIGNS AND SYMPTOMS

Patients with medial collateral ligament syndrome present with pain over the medial joint and increased pain on passive valgus and external rotation of the knee.

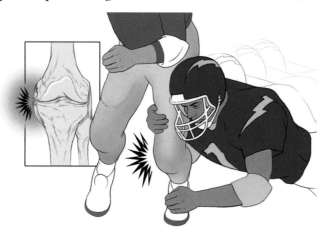

Figure 85–1. Medial collateral ligament syndrome is characterized by medial joint pain that is made worse with flexion or external rotation of the knee.

Activity, especially flexion and external rotation of the knee, makes the pain worse, whereas rest and heat provide some relief. The pain is constant and is characterized as aching in nature; it may interfere with sleep. Patients with injury to the medial collateral ligament may complain of locking or popping with flexion of the affected knee. Coexistent bursitis, tendinitis, arthritis, or internal derangement of the knee may confuse the clinical picture after trauma to the knee joint.

On physical examination, patients with injury to the medial collateral ligament exhibit tenderness along the course of the ligament from the medial femoral condyle to its tibial insertion. If the ligament is avulsed from its bony insertions, tenderness may be localized to the proximal or distal ligament, whereas patients suffering from strain of the ligament have more diffuse tenderness. Patients with severe injury to the ligament may exhibit joint laxity when valgus and varus stress is placed on the affected knee. Because pain may produce muscle guarding, magnetic resonance imaging (MRI) of the knee may be necessary to confirm the clinical impression. Joint effusion and swelling may be present with injury to the medial collateral ligament, but these findings are also suggestive of intra-articular damage. Again, MRI can confirm the diagnosis.

TESTING

MRI is indicated in all patients who present with medial collateral ligament pain, particularly if internal derangement or occult mass or tumor is suspected (Fig. 85-2). In addition, MRI should be performed in all patients with injury to the medial collateral ligament who fail to respond to conservative therapy or who exhibit joint instability on clinical examination. Bone scan may be useful to identify occult stress fractures involving the joint, especially if trauma has occurred. Based on the patient's clinical presentation, additional testing may be warranted, including a complete blood count, erythrocyte sedimentation rate, and antinuclear antibody testing.

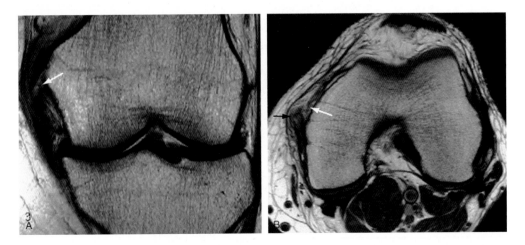

Figure 85–2. A, Coronal fast spin echo magnetic resonance image demonstrates a high-grade proximal medial collateral ligament tear *(arrow)*. **B,** Axial fast spin echo image in the same patient demonstrates a tear of the medial collateral ligament from the femur. (From Edelman RR, Hessellink JR, Zlatkin MB, Crues JV: Clinical Magnetic Resonance Imaging, 3rd ed. Philadelphia, Saunders, 2006, p 3407.)

DIFFERENTIAL DIAGNOSIS

Any condition affecting the medial compartment of the knee joint may mimic the pain of medial collateral ligament syndrome. Bursitis, arthritis, and entrapment neuropathies may also confuse the diagnosis, as may primary tumors of the knee and spine.

TREATMENT

Initial treatment of the pain and functional disability associated with injury to the medial collateral ligament includes a combination of nonsteroidal anti-inflammatory drugs or cyclooxygenase-2 inhibitors and physical therapy. The local application of heat and cold may also be beneficial. Any repetitive activity that exacerbates the patient's symptoms should be avoided. For patients who do not respond to these treatment modalities and do not have lesions that require surgical repair, injection is a reasonable next step.

Injection of the medial collateral ligament is carried out with the patient in the supine position with a rolled blanket underneath the knee to gently flex the joint. The skin overlying the lateral aspect of the knee joint is prepared with antiseptic solution. A sterile syringe containing 2 mL of 0.25% preservative-free bupivacaine and 40 mg methylprednisolone is attached to a 1½-inch, 25-gauge needle using strict aseptic technique. The most tender portion of the ligament is identified, and the needle is inserted at this point at a 45-degree angle to the skin. The needle is carefully advanced through the skin and subcutaneous tissues into proximity with the medial collateral ligament. If bone is encountered, the needle is withdrawn into the subcutaneous tissues and redirected superiorly. The contents of the syringe is then gently injected. There should be little resistance to injection. If resistance is encountered, the needle is probably in a ligament or tendon and should be advanced or withdrawn slightly until the injection can proceed without significant resistance. The needle is then removed, and a sterile pressure dressing and ice pack are applied to the injection site.

COMPLICATIONS AND PITFALLS

The major complication of injection is infection, although this should be exceedingly rare if strict aseptic technique is followed. Approximately 25% of patients complain of a transient increase in pain after injection of the medial collateral ligament, and they should be warned of this possibility.

Clinical Pearls

Patients with injury to the medial collateral ligament are best examined with the knee in the slightly flexed position. The clinician may want to examine the nonpainful knee first to reduce the patient's anxiety and to ascertain the findings of a normal examination. The injection technique described is extremely effective in the treatment of pain secondary to medial collateral ligament syndrome. Coexistent bursitis, tendinitis, arthritis, and internal derangement of the knee may contribute to the patient's pain, necessitating additional treatment with more localized injection of local anesthetic and methylprednisolone.

Chapter 86

Jumper's Knee

ICD-9 CODE **726.90**

THE CLINICAL SYNDROME

Jumper's knee is characterized by pain at the inferior or superior pole of the patella. It occurs in up to 20% of jumping athletes at some point in their careers. It may affect one or both knees; males are affected twice as commonly as females when just one knee is involved. Jumper's knee is usually the result of overuse or misuse of the knee joint caused by running, jumping, or overtraining on hard surfaces or direct trauma to the quadriceps or patellar tendon, such as from kicks or head butts during football or kickboxing (Fig. 86-1).

The quadriceps tendon is made up of fibers from the four muscles that constitute the quadriceps muscle: vastus lateralis, vastus intermedius, vastus medialis, and rectus femoris. These muscles are the primary extensors of the lower extremity at the knee. The tendons of these muscles converge and unite to form a single, exceedingly strong tendon (Figs. 86-2). The patella functions as a sesamoid bone within the quadriceps tendon, with fibers of the tendon expanding around the patella and forming the medial and lateral patella retinacula, which strengthen the knee joint. The patellar tendon extends from the patella to the tibial tuberosity. Weak or poor quadriceps and hamstring muscle flexibility; congenital variants in knee anatomy, such as patella alta or baja; and limb length discrepancies have been implicated as risk factors for the development of jumper's knee. Interestingly, it is postulated that the strong eccentric contraction of the quadriceps muscle to strengthen the knee joint during landing is the inciting factor rather than the jump itself.

SIGNS AND SYMPTOMS

Patients with jumper's knee present with pain over the superior or inferior pole (or both) of the sesamoid. Jumper's knee can affect both the medial and lateral sides of both the quadriceps and the patellar tendons. Patients

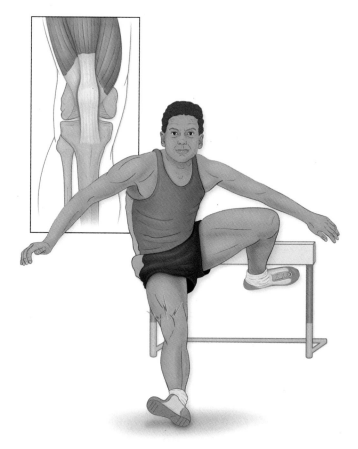

Figure 86–1. Jumper's knee—characterized by pain at the inferior or superior pole of the patella—occurs in up to 20% of jumping athletes at some point in their careers.

note increased pain on walking down slopes or down stairs. Activity using the knee, especially jumping, makes the pain worse, whereas rest and heat provide some relief. The pain is constant and is characterized as aching in nature; it may interfere with sleep. On physical examination, there is tenderness of the quadriceps or patellar tendon (or both), and a joint effusion may be present. Active resisted extension of the knee reproduces the pain. Coexistent suprapatellar and infrapatellar bursitis, tendinitis, arthritis, or internal derangement of the knee

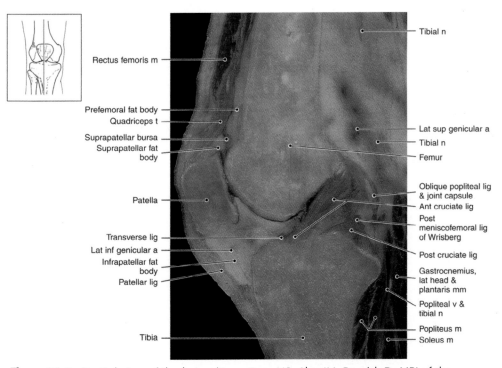

Figure 86-2. Sagittal view of the knee. (From Kang HS, Ahn JM, Resnick D: MRI of the Extremities: An Anatomic Atlas, 2nd ed. Philadelphia, Saunders, 2002, p 341.)

may confuse the clinical picture after trauma to the knee.

TESTING

Plain radiographs are indicated in all patients who present with knee pain. Magnetic resonance imaging of the knee is indicated if jumper's knee is suspected, because it readily demonstrates tendinosis of the quadriceps or patellar tendon (Fig. 86-3). Bone scan may be useful to identify occult stress fractures involving the joint, especially if trauma has occurred. Based on the patient's clinical presentation, additional testing may be indicated, including a complete blood count, erythrocyte sedimentation rate, and antinuclear antibody testing.

DIFFERENTIAL DIAGNOSIS

Jumper's knee is a repetitive stress disorder that causes tendinosis of the quadriceps and patellar tendons and is a distinct clinical entity from tendinitis of those tendons or quadriceps expansion syndrome, which may coexist with jumper's knee and confuse the clinical picture. Quadriceps expansion syndrome has a predilection for the medial side of the superior pole of the patella. The quadriceps tendon is also subject to acute calcific tendinitis, which may coexist with acute strain injuries and the more chronic changes of jumper's knee. Calcific tendinitis of the quadriceps has a characteristic

radiographic appearance of whiskers on the anterosuperior patella. The suprapatellar, infrapatellar, and prepatellar bursae also may become inflamed with dysfunction of the quadriceps tendon.

TREATMENT

Initial treatment of the pain and functional disability associated with jumper's knee includes a combination of nonsteroidal anti-inflammatory drugs or cyclooxygenase-2 inhibitors and physical therapy. A nighttime splint to protect the knee may also help relieve the symptoms. For patients who do not respond to these treatment modalities, injection with local anesthetic and steroid is a reasonable next step.

To perform the injection, the patient is placed in the supine position with a rolled blanket underneath the knee to gently flex the joint. If only the quadriceps tendon is affected, the skin overlying the medial aspect of the knee joint is prepared with antiseptic solution. A sterile syringe containing 2 mL of 0.25% preservative-free bupivacaine and 40 mg methylprednisolone is attached to a 1½-inch, 25-gauge needle using strict aseptic technique. The superior margin of the medial patella is identified (Fig. 86-4). Just above this point, the needle is inserted horizontally to slide just beneath the quadriceps tendon (Fig. 86-5). If the needle strikes the femur, it is withdrawn slightly and redirected with a

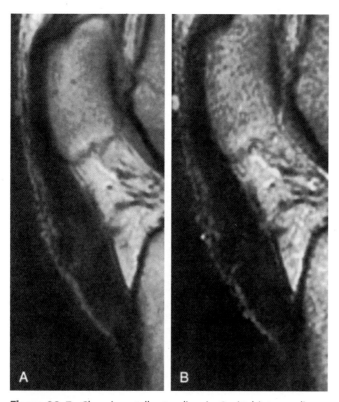

Figure 86–3. Chronic patellar tendinosis. Sagittal intermediate-weighted **(A)** and T2-weighted **(B)** spin echo magnetic resonance images show marked thickening of the entire patellar tendon that is more pronounced in the middle and distal segments. The anterior margin of the tendon is indistinct. There is no increase in signal intensity within the patellar tendon in **B**. (From Resnick D: Diagnosis of Bone and Joint Disorders, 4th ed. Philadelphia, Saunders, 2002, p 3236.)

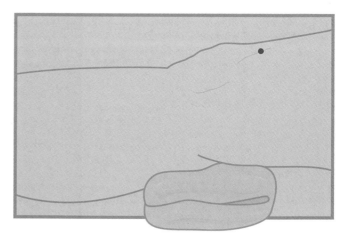

Figure 86–4. Identification of the superior margin of the medial patella. (From Waldman SD: Atlas of Pain Management Injection Techniques. Philadelphia, Saunders, 2000, p 269.)

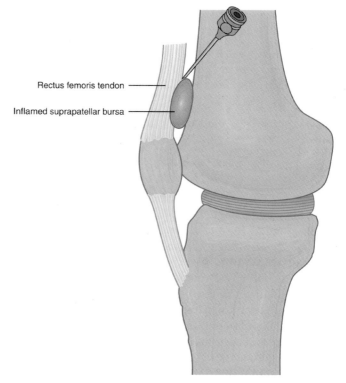

Rectus femoris tendon

Inflamed suprapatellar bursa

Figure 86–5. Correct needle placement for injection of the suprapatellar bursa. (From Waldman SD: Atlas of Pain Management Injection Techniques. Philadelphia, Saunders, 2000, p 269.)

more anterior trajectory. When the needle is in position just below the quadriceps tendon, the contents of the syringe is gently injected. There should be little resistance to injection. If resistance is encountered, the needle is probably in a ligament or tendon and should be advanced or withdrawn slightly until the injection can proceed without significant resistance. The needle is removed, and a sterile pressure dressing and ice pack are applied to the injection site.

If only the patellar tendon is affected, the skin overlying the medial portion of the lower margin of the patella is prepared with antiseptic solution. A sterile syringe containing 2 mL of 0.25% preservative-free bupivacaine and 40 mg methylprednisolone is attached to a 1½-inch, 25-gauge needle using strict aseptic technique. The medial lower margin of the patella is identified (Fig. 86-6). Just below this point, the needle is inserted at a right angle to the patella to slide beneath the patellar ligament into the deep infrapatellar bursa (Fig. 86-7). If the needle strikes the patella, it is withdrawn slightly and redirected with a more inferior trajectory. When the

needle is in position in proximity to the deep infrapatellar bursa, the contents of the syringe are gently injected. There should be little resistance to injection. If resistance is encountered, the needle is probably in a ligament or tendon and should be advanced or withdrawn slightly until the injection can proceed without significant resis-

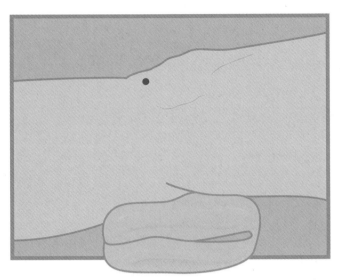

Figure 86–6. Identification of the medial lower margin of the patella. (From Waldman SD: Atlas of Pain Management Injection Techniques. Philadelphia, Saunders, 2000, p 278.)

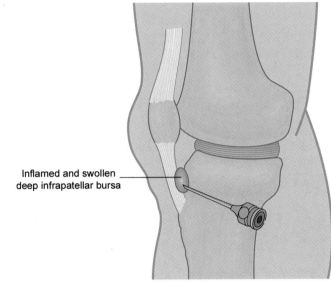

Inflamed and swollen deep infrapatellar bursa

Figure 86–7. Correct needle placement for injection of the deep infrapatellar bursa. (From Waldman SD: Atlas of Pain Management Injection Techniques. Philadelphia, Saunders, 2000, p 278.)

tance. The needle is removed, and a sterile pressure dressing and ice pack are applied to the injection site.

If both the quadriceps and patellar tendons are affected, both injections should be performed.

Physical modalities, including local heat and gentle range-of-motion exercises, should be introduced several days after the patient undergoes injection. Vigorous exercises should be avoided, because they will exacerbate the patient's symptoms. Simple analgesics and non-steroidal anti-inflammatory drugs can be used concurrently with this injection technique.

COMPLICATIONS AND PITFALLS

Failure to identify primary or metastatic tumor of the distal femur or knee joint that is causing the patient's pain can have disastrous results. The injection technique is safe if careful attention is paid to the clinically relevant anatomy. The major complication of injection is infec-

tion, although it should be exceedingly rare if strict aseptic technique is followed. Approximately 25% of patients complain of a transient increase in pain after injection, and they should be warned of this possibility.

Clinical Pearls

Coexistent bursitis, tendinitis, arthritis, and internal derangement of the knee may contribute to the patient's pain, necessitating additional treatment with more localized injection of local anesthetic and methylprednisolone. The injection technique described is extremely effective in treating the pain of jumper's knee.

Chapter 87

Runner's Knee

ICD-9 CODE 726.90

THE CLINICAL SYNDROME

Runner's knee, also known as iliotibial band friction syndrome, is a common cause of lateral knee pain. The iliotibial band is an extension of the fascia lata, which inserts at the lateral condyle of the tibia. The iliotibial band bursa lies between the iliotibial band and the lateral condyle of the femur. Runner's knee is an overuse syndrome caused by friction injury to the iliotibial band as it rubs back and forth across the lateral epicondyle of the femur during running (Figs. 87-1 and 87-2); this rubbing can also irritate the iliotibial bursa beneath it. If inflammation of the iliotibial band becomes chronic, calcification may occur.

Runner's knee is a distinct clinical entity from iliotibial bursitis, although these two painful conditions frequently coexist. Runner's knee occurs more commonly in patients with genu varum and planus feet, although worn-out jogging shoes have also been implicated in the development of this syndrome.

SIGNS AND SYMPTOMS

Patients with runner's knee present with pain over the lateral side of the distal femur just over the lateral femoral epicondyle. Compared with iliotibial bursitis, the pain tends to be a little less localized, and there is rarely an effusion. The onset of runner's knee frequently occurs after long-distance biking or jogging with worn-out shoes that lack proper cushioning (Fig. 87-3). Activity, especially that involving resisted abduction and passive adduction of the lower extremity, makes the pain worse, whereas rest and heat provide some relief. Flexion of the affected knee reproduces the pain in many patients with runner's knee. Often, patients are unable to kneel or walk down stairs. The pain is constant and is characterized as aching in nature; it may interfere with sleep. Coexistent bursitis, tendinitis, arthritis, or internal derangement of the knee may confuse the clinical picture after trauma to the knee.

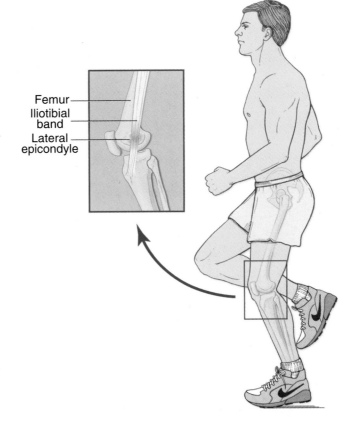

Femur
Iliotibial band
Lateral epicondyle

Figure 87–1. Runner's knee is an overuse syndrome caused by friction injury to the iliotibial band as it rubs back and forth across the lateral epicondyle of the femur. (From Waldman SD: Atlas of Pain Management Injection Techniques, 2nd ed. Philadelphia, Saunders, 2000, p 476.)

Physical examination may reveal point tenderness over the lateral epicondyle of the femur just above the tendinous insertion of the iliotibial band (see Fig. 87-1). If iliotibial bursitis is also present, there may be swelling and fluid accumulation around the bursa. Palpation of this area while the patient flexes and extends the knee may result in a creaking or "catching" sensation. Active resisted abduction of the lower extremity reproduces the pain, as does passive adduction. Sudden release of resistance during this maneuver causes a marked increase

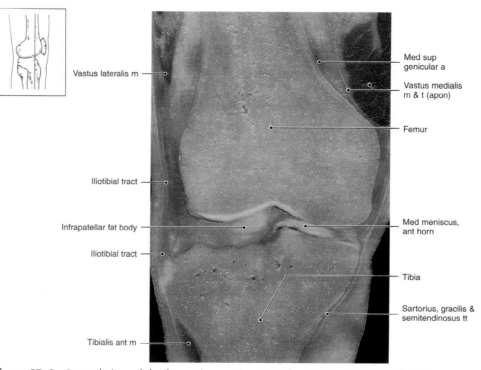

Figure 87–2. Coronal view of the knee. (From Kang HS, Ahn JM, Resnick D: MRI of the Extremities: An Anatomic Atlas, 2nd ed. Philadelphia, Saunders, 2002, p 307.)

in pain. Pain is exacerbated when the patient stands with all his or her weight on the affected extremity and then flexes the affected knee 30 to 40 degrees.

TESTING

Plain radiographs of the knee may reveal calcification of the bursa and associated structures, including the iliotibial band tendon, consistent with chronic inflammation. Magnetic resonance imaging is indicated if runner's knee, iliotibial band bursitis, internal derangement, occult mass, or tumor of the knee is suspected (Fig. 87-4). Electromyography can distinguish iliotibial band bursitis from neuropathy, lumbar radiculopathy, and plexopathy. Bone scan may be useful to identify occult stress fractures involving the joint, especially if trauma has occurred.

DIFFERENTIAL DIAGNOSIS

The iliotibial, suprapatellar, infrapatellar, and prepatellar bursae may become inflamed with dysfunction of the iliotibial band. The patellar tendon, which extends from the patella to the tibial tuberosity, is also subject to tendinitis, which may confuse the clinical picture. Internal derangement of the knee joint may coexist with iliotibial band bursitis.

TREATMENT

Initial treatment of the pain and functional disability associated with runner's knee includes a combination of nonsteroidal anti-inflammatory drugs or cyclooxygenase-2 inhibitors and physical therapy. A nighttime splint to protect the knee may also relieve the symptoms. For patients who fail to respond to these treatment modalities, injection with local anesthetic and steroid is a reasonable next step.

To perform the injection, the patient is placed in the supine position with a rolled blanket underneath the knee to gently flex the joint. The skin over the lateral epicondyle of the femur is prepared with antiseptic solution. A sterile syringe containing 2 mL of 0.25% preservative-free bupivacaine and 40 mg methylprednisolone is attached to a 1½-inch, 25-gauge needle using strict aseptic technique. The iliotibial band bursa is identified by locating the point of maximal tenderness over the lateral condyle of the femur. At this point, the needle is inserted at a 45-degree angle to the femoral condyle, passing through the skin, subcutaneous tissues, and iliotibial band into the iliotibial band bursa. If the needle strikes the femur, it is withdrawn slightly into the substance of the bursa. When the needle is positioned in proximity to the iliotibial band bursa, the contents of the syringe are gently injected. There should be little resistance to pain can have disastrous results. The injection technique is safe if careful attention is paid to the clinically relevant anatomy. The major complication of injection is infection, although this should be exceedingly rare if strict aseptic technique is followed. Approximately 25% of patients complain of a transient increase in pain after injection, and they should be warned of this possibility.

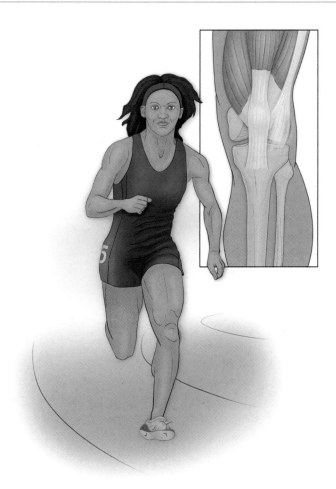

Figure 87–3. Patients with runner's knee present with pain over the lateral side of the distal femur, just over the lateral femoral epicondyle. It is often associated with running or jogging using worn-out shoes.

injection. If resistance is encountered, the needle is probably in a ligament or tendon and should be advanced or withdrawn slightly until the injection can proceed without significant resistance. The needle is removed, and a sterile pressure dressing and ice pack are applied to the injection site.

Physical modalities, including local heat and gentle range-of-motion exercises, should be introduced several days after the patient undergoes injection. Vigorous exercises should be avoided, because they will exacerbate the patient's symptoms. Simple analgesics and nonsteroidal anti-inflammatory drugs can be used concurrently with this injection technique.

COMPLICATIONS AND PITFALLS

Failure to identify primary or metastatic tumor of the distal femur or knee joint that is causing the patient's

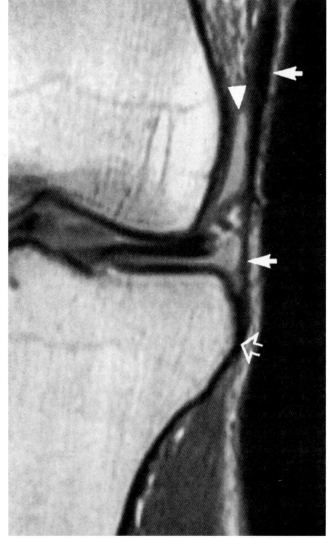

Figure 87–4. Normal iliotibial tract. Coronal, intermediate-weighted, spin echo magnetic resonance image shows the iliotibial tract *(solid arrows)* attaching to Gerdy's tubercle *(open arrow)* in the tibia. A small joint effusion is evident just medial to the iliotibial tract *(arrowhead).* (From Resnick D: Diagnosis of Bone and Joint Disorders, 4th ed. Philadelphia, Saunders, 2002, p 3231.)

Clinical Pearls

Coexistent bursitis, tendinitis, arthritis, and internal derangement of the knee may contribute to the patient's pain, necessitating additional treatment with more localized injection of local anesthetic and methylprednisolone. The injection technique described is extremely effective in treating the pain of runner's knee.

Suprapatellar Bursitis

THE CLINICAL SYNDROME

The suprapatellar bursa extends superiorly from beneath the patella under the quadriceps femoris muscle and its tendon. The bursa is held in place by a small portion of the vastus intermedius muscle called the articularis genus muscle. The suprapatellar bursa may exist as a single bursal sac or, in some patients, as a multisegmented series of loculated sacs. The suprapatellar bursa is vulnerable to injury from both acute trauma and repeated microtrauma. Acute injuries may be caused by direct trauma to the bursa during falls onto the knee or patellar fractures. Overuse injuries may result from running on soft or uneven surfaces or from jobs that require crawling on the knees, such as carpet laying. If inflammation of the suprapatellar bursa becomes chronic, calcification may occur.

SIGNS AND SYMPTOMS

Patient suffering from suprapatellar bursitis complain of pain in the anterior knee above the patella that may radiate superiorly into the distal anterior thigh. Often, patients are unable to kneel or walk down stairs (Fig. 88-1). Patients may also complain of a sharp "catching" sensation with range of motion of the knee, especially on first arising. Suprapatellar bursitis often coexists with arthritis and tendinitis of the knee, confusing the clinical picture.

Physical examination may reveal point tenderness in the anterior knee just above the patella. Passive flexion and active resisted extension of the knee reproduce the pain. Sudden release of resistance during this maneuver causes a marked increase in pain. There may be swelling in the suprapatellar region, with a boggy feeling to palpation. Occasionally, the suprapatellar bursa becomes infected, causing systemic symptoms such as fever and malaise, as well as local symptoms such as rubor, color, and dolor.

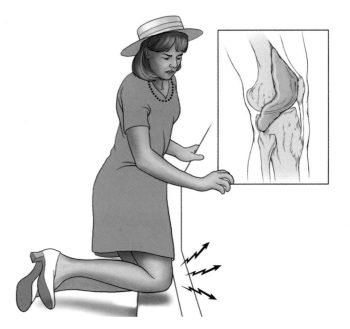

Figure 88–1. Suprapatellar bursitis is usually the result of direct trauma from either acute injury or repeated microtrauma, such as prolonged kneeling.

TESTING

Plain radiographs and magnetic resonance imaging (MRI) of the knee may reveal calcification of the bursa and associated structures, including the quadriceps tendon, consistent with chronic inflammation (Fig. 88-2). MRI is indicated if internal derangement, occult mass, or tumor of the knee is suspected. Electromyography can distinguish suprapatellar bursitis from femoral neuropathy, lumbar radiculopathy, and plexopathy. The injection technique described later serves as both a diagnostic and a therapeutic maneuver. A complete blood count, automated chemistry profile including uric acid level, erythrocyte sedimentation rate, and antinuclear antibody testing are indicated if collagen vascular disease is suspected. If infection is a possibility, aspiration, Gram stain, and culture of bursal fluid should be performed on an emergency basis.

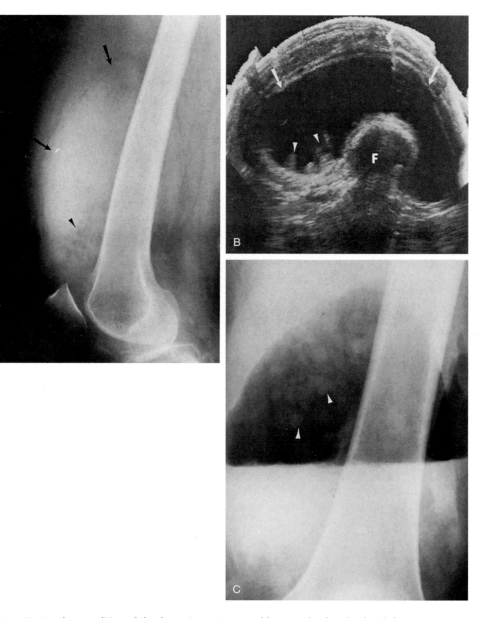

Figure 88–2. Abnormalities of the knee in a 54-year-old man who has had ankylosing spondylitis for approximately 25 years. Multiple episodes of painless swelling of the suprapatellar region were followed by spontaneous resolution. At the time of these imaging studies, aspiration of fluid in the distended suprapatellar pouch produced 3000 cells/mm³ and no growth of organisms. Over a period of several weeks, the swelling resolved. **A,** Lateral radiograph demonstrates massive distention of the suprapatellar pouch *(arrows)* and multiple nodular radiolucent shadows *(arrowhead)*. **B,** On a transverse sonogram, note the distended bursa *(arrows)* containing nodular synovial excrescences *(arrowheads)*. F, femur. **C,** Upright frontal image during double contrast arthrography documents nodular synovial hyperplasia *(arrowheads)* in the distended suprapatellar pouch. (From Resnick D: Diagnosis of Bone and Joint Disorders, 4th ed. Philadelphia, Saunders, 2002, p 1058.)

DIFFERENTIAL DIAGNOSIS

Owing to the anatomy of the region, the associated tendons and other bursae of the knee can become inflamed along with the suprapatellar bursa, confusing the diagnosis. Both the quadriceps tendon and the supra-

patellar bursa are subject to inflammation from overuse, misuse, or direct trauma. The tendon fibers, called expansions, are vulnerable to strain, and the tendon proper is subject to the development of tendinitis. The suprapatellar, infrapatellar, and prepatellar bursae may also become inflamed with dysfunction of the quadriceps tendon. It should be remembered that anything that alters the normal biomechanics of th e knee can result in inflammation of the suprapatellar bursa.

TREATMENT

A short course of conservative therapy consisting of simple analgesics, nonsteroidal anti-inflammatory drugs, or cyclooxygenase-2 inhibitors and a knee brace to prevent further trauma is the first step in the treatment of suprapatellar bursitis. If patients do not experience rapid improvement, injection is a reasonable next step.

To perform the injection, the patient is placed in the supine position with a rolled blanket underneath the knee to gently flex the joint. The skin overlying the medial aspect of the knee joint is prepared with antiseptic solution. A sterile syringe containing 2 mL of 0.25% preservative-free bupivacaine and 40 mg methylprednisolone is attached to a 1½-inch, 25-gauge needle using strict aseptic technique. The superior margin of the medial patella is identified. Just above this point, the needle is inserted horizontally to slide beneath the quadriceps tendon. If the needle strikes the femur, it is withdrawn slightly and redirected with a more anterior trajectory. When the needle is in position just below the quadriceps tendon, the contents of the syringe is gently injected. There should be little resistance to injection. If resistance is encountered, the needle is probably in a ligament or tendon and should be advanced or withdrawn slightly until the injection can proceed without significant resistance. The needle is removed, and a sterile pressure dressing and ice pack are applied to the injection site.

Physical modalities, including local heat and gentle range-of-motion exercises, should be introduced several days after the patient undergoes injection. Vigorous exercises should be avoided, because they will exacerbate the patient's symptoms. Simple analgesics and nonsteroidal anti-inflammatory drugs can be used concurrently with this injection technique.

COMPLICATIONS AND PITFALLS

Failure to identify primary or metastatic tumor of the distal femur or knee joint that is causing the patient's pain can have disastrous results. The injection technique is safe if careful attention is paid to the clinically relevant anatomy. The major complication of injection is infection, although this should be exceedingly rare if strict aseptic technique is followed. Approximately 25% of patients complain of a transient increase in pain after injection, and they should be warned of this possibility.

Clinical Pearls

Coexistent bursitis, tendinitis, arthritis, and internal derangement of the knee may contribute to the patient's pain, necessitating additional treatment with more localized injection of local anesthetic and methylprednisolone. The injection technique described is extremely effective in treating the pain of suprapatellar bursitis.

Chapter 89

Prepatellar Bursitis

ICD-9 CODE 726.65

THE CLINICAL SYNDROME

The prepatellar bursa lies between the subcutaneous tissues and the patella. It is held in place by the patellar ligament. The prepatellar bursa may exist as a single bursal sac or, in some patients, as a multisegmented series of loculated sacs. The prepatellar bursa is vulnerable to injury from both acute trauma and repeated microtrauma. Acute injuries are caused by direct trauma to the bursa during falls onto the knee or patellar fracture. Overuse injuries may be caused by running on soft or uneven surfaces or jobs that require crawling or kneeling, such as carpet laying or scrubbing floors—hence the other name for prepatellar bursitis: housemaid's knee (Fig. 89-1). If inflammation of the prepatellar bursa becomes chronic, calcification may occur.

SIGNS AND SYMPTOMS

Patients suffering from prepatellar bursitis complain of pain and swelling in the anterior knee over the patella that can radiate superiorly and inferiorly into the surrounding area. Often, patients are unable to kneel or walk down stairs. Patients may also complain of a sharp "catching" sensation with range of motion of the knee, especially on first arising. Prepatellar bursitis often coexists with arthritis and tendinitis of the knee, confusing the clinical picture.

TESTING

Plain radiographs and magnetic resonance imaging (MRI) of the knee may reveal calcification of the bursa and associated structures, including the quadriceps tendon, consistent with chronic inflammation (Fig. 89-2). MRI is indicated if internal derangement, occult mass, or tumor of the knee is suspected. Electromyography can distinguish prepatellar bursitis from femoral neuropathy, lumbar radiculopathy, and plexopathy. The injection

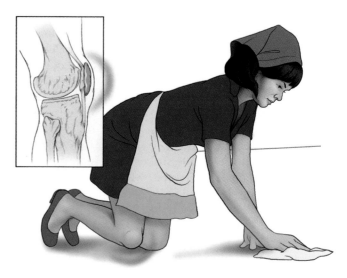

Figure 89-1. Prepatellar bursitis is also known as housemaid's knee because of its prevalence among people whose work requires prolonged crawling or kneeling.

technique described serves as both a diagnostic and a therapeutic maneuver. Antinuclear antibody testing is indicated if collagen vascular disease is suspected. If infection is a possibility, aspiration, Gram stain, and culture of bursal fluid should be performed on an emergency basis.

DIFFERENTIAL DIAGNOSIS

Owing to the anatomy of the region, the associated tendons and other bursae of the knee can become inflamed along with the prepatellar bursa, confusing the diagnosis. Both the quadriceps tendon and the prepatellar bursa are subject to inflammation from overuse, misuse, or direct trauma. The tendon fibers, called expansions, are vulnerable to strain, and the tendon proper is subject to the development of tendinitis. The suprapatellar, infrapatellar, and prepatellar bursae may also become inflamed with dysfunction of the quadriceps tendon. It should be remembered that anything that alters the normal biomechanics of the knee can result in inflammation of the prepatellar bursa.

TREATMENT

A short course of conservative therapy consisting of simple analgesics, nonsteroidal anti-inflammatory drugs, or cyclooxygenase-2 inhibitors and a knee brace to prevent further trauma is the first step in the treatment of prepatellar bursitis. If patients do not experience rapid improvement, injection is a reasonable next step.

To perform the injection, the patient is placed in the supine position with a rolled blanket underneath the knee to gently flex the joint. The skin overlying the patella is prepared with antiseptic solution. A sterile syringe containing 2 mL of 0.25% preservative-free bupivacaine and 40 mg methylprednisolone is attached to a 1½-inch, 25-gauge needle using strict aseptic technique. The center of the medial patella is identified. Just above this point, the needle is inserted horizontally to slide subcutaneously into the prepatellar bursa (Fig. 89-3). If the needle strikes the patella, it is withdrawn slightly and redirected with a more anterior trajectory. When the needle is positioned in proximity to the prepatellar bursa, the contents of the syringe is gently injected. There should be little resistance to injection. If resistance is encountered, the needle is probably in a ligament or tendon and should be advanced or withdrawn slightly until the injection can proceed without significant resistance. The needle is removed, and a sterile pressure dressing and ice pack are applied to the injection site.

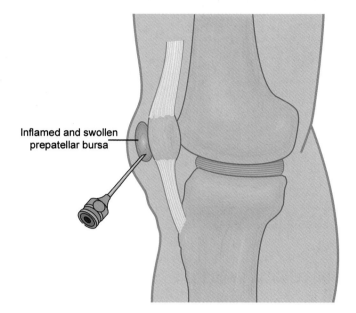

Figure 89–3. Correct needle placement for injection of the prepatellar bursa. (From Waldman SD: Atlas of Pain Management Injection Techniques. Philadelphia, Saunders, 2000.)

Physical modalities, including local heat and gentle range-of-motion exercises, should be introduced several days after the patient undergoes injection. Vigorous exercises should be avoided, because they will exacerbate the patient's symptoms. Simple analgesics and nonsteroidal anti-inflammatory drugs can be used concurrently with this injection technique.

COMPLICATIONS AND PITFALLS

Failure to identify primary or metastatic tumor of the distal femur or knee joint that is causing the patient's pain can have disastrous results. The injection technique is safe if careful attention is paid to the clinically relevant anatomy. The major complication of injection is infection, although this should be exceedingly rare if strict aseptic technique is followed. Approximately 25% of patients complain of a transient increase in pain after injection, and they should be warned of this possibility.

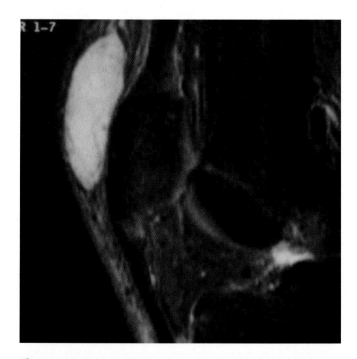

Figure 89–2. Prepatellar bursitis. Sagittal, short tau inversion recovery, magnetic resonance image shows fluid and synovial tissue in the prepatellar bursa. (From Resnick D: Diagnosis of Bone and Joint Disorders, 4th ed. Philadelphia, Saunders, 2002, p 4257.)

Clinical Pearls

Coexistent bursitis, tendinitis, arthritis, and internal derangement of the knee may contribute to the patient's pain, necessitating additional treatment with more localized injection of local anesthetic and methylprednisolone. The injection technique described is extremely effective in treating the pain of prepatellar bursitis.

Chapter 90

Superficial Infrapatellar Bursitis

ICD-9 CODE 726.69

THE CLINICAL SYNDROME

The superficial infrapatellar bursa lies between the subcutaneous tissues and the upper part of the patellar ligament. This bursa may exist as a single bursal sac or, in some patients, as a multisegmented series of loculated sacs. The superficial infrapatellar bursa is vulnerable to injury from both acute trauma and repeated microtrauma. Acute injuries are caused by direct trauma to the bursa during falls onto the knee or patellar fracture. Overuse injuries are caused by running on soft or uneven surfaces or doing jobs that require crawling or kneeling, such as carpet laying or scrubbing floors (Fig. 90-1). If inflammation of the superficial infrapatellar bursa becomes chronic, calcification may occur.

SIGNS AND SYMPTOMS

Patients with superficial infrapatellar bursitis complain of pain and swelling in the anterior knee over the patella that can radiate superiorly and inferiorly into the surrounding area. Often, patients are unable to kneel or walk down stairs. Patients may also complain of a sharp "catching" sensation with range of motion of the knee, especially on first arising. Superficial infrapatellar bursitis often coexists with arthritis and tendinitis of the knee, confusing the clinical picture.

TESTING

Plain radiographs and magnetic resonance imaging (MRI) of the knee may reveal calcification of the bursa and associated structures, including the quadriceps and patellar tendons, consistent with chronic inflammation (Fig. 90-2). MRI is indicated if internal derangement, occult mass, or tumor of the knee is suspected. Electromyography can distinguish superficial infrapatellar bursitis from femoral neuropathy, lumbar radiculopathy, and plexopathy. The injection technique described later serves as both a diagnostic and a therapeutic maneuver. Antinu-

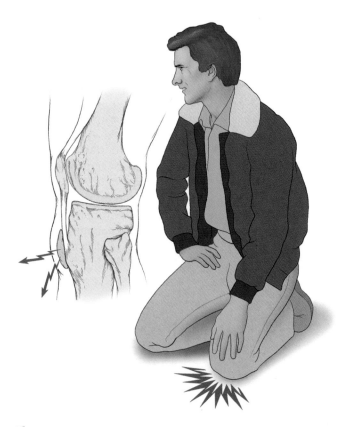

Figure 90–1. Infrapatellar bursitis is a common cause of inferior knee pain.

clear antibody testing is indicated if collagen vascular disease is suspected. If infection is a possibility, aspiration, Gram stain, and culture of bursal fluid should be performed on an emergency basis.

DIFFERENTIAL DIAGNOSIS

Owing to the anatomy of the region, the associated tendons and other bursae of the knee can become inflamed along with the superficial infrapatellar bursa, confusing the diagnosis. Both the quadriceps tendon and the superficial infrapatellar bursa are subject to inflammation from overuse, misuse, or direct trauma. The tendon fibers, called expansions, are vulnerable to strain,

314

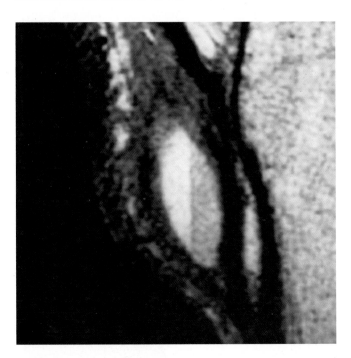

Figure 90–2. Superficial infrapatellar bursitis. A fluid level within the bursa is evident on this sagittal fast spin echo image. (From Resnick D: Diagnosis of Bone and Joint Disorders, 4th ed. Philadelphia, Saunders, 2002, p 4257.)

and the tendon proper is subject to the development of tendinitis. The suprapatellar, infrapatellar, and prepatellar bursae may also become inflamed with dysfunction of the quadriceps tendon. It should be remembered that anything that alters the normal biomechanics of the knee can result in inflammation of the superficial infrapatellar bursa.

TREATMENT

A short course of conservative therapy consisting of simple analgesics, nonsteroidal anti-inflammatory drugs, or cyclooxygenase-2 inhibitors, and a knee brace to prevent further trauma is the first step in the treatment of superficial infrapatellar bursitis. If patients do not experience rapid improvement, injection is a reasonable next step.

To inject the superficial infrapatellar bursa, the patient is placed in the supine position with a rolled blanket underneath the knee to gently flex the joint. The skin overlying the patella is prepared with antiseptic solution. A sterile syringe containing 2 mL of 0.25% preservative-free bupivacaine and 40 mg methylprednisolone is attached to a 1½-inch, 25-gauge needle using strict aseptic technique. The center of the lower pole of the patella is identified. Just below this point, the needle is inserted at a 45-degree angle to slide subcutaneously into the superficial infrapatellar bursa. If the needle strikes the patella, it is withdrawn slightly and redirected with a more inferior trajectory. When the needle is positioned in proximity to the superficial infrapatellar bursa, the contents of the syringe is gently injected. There should be little resistance to injection. If resistance is encountered, the needle is probably in a ligament or tendon and should be advanced or withdrawn slightly until the injection can proceed without significant resistance. The needle is removed, and a sterile pressure dressing and ice pack are applied to the injection site.

Physical modalities, including local heat and gentle range-of-motion exercises, should be introduced several days after the patient undergoes injection. Vigorous exercises should be avoided, because they will exacerbate the patient's symptoms. Simple analgesics and nonsteroidal anti-inflammatory drugs can be used concurrently with this injection technique.

COMPLICATIONS AND PITFALLS

Failure to identify primary or metastatic tumor of the distal femur or knee joint that is causing the patient's pain can have disastrous results. The injection technique is safe if careful attention is paid to the clinically relevant anatomy. The major complication of injection is infection, although this should be exceedingly rare if strict aseptic technique is followed. Approximately 25% of patients complain of a transient increase in pain after injection, and they should be warned of this possibility.

Clinical Pearls

Coexistent bursitis, tendinitis, arthritis, and internal derangement of the knee may contribute to the patient's pain, necessitating additional treatment with more localized injection of local anesthetic and methylprednisolone. The injection technique described is extremely effective in treating the pain of superficial infrapatellar bursitis.

Chapter 91

Deep Infrapatellar Bursitis

ICD-9 CODE 726.69

THE CLINICAL SYNDROME

The deep infrapatellar bursa lies between the patellar ligament and the tibia. This bursa may exist as a single bursal sac or, in some patients, as a multisegmented series of loculated sacs. The deep infrapatellar bursa is vulnerable to injury from both acute trauma and repeated microtrauma. Acute injuries are caused by direct trauma to the bursa during falls onto the knee (Fig. 91-1) or patellar fracture. Overuse injuries are caused by running on soft or uneven surfaces or jobs that require crawling and kneeling, such as carpet laying or scrubbing floors. If inflammation of the deep infrapatellar bursa becomes chronic, calcification may occur.

SIGNS AND SYMPTOMS

Patients with deep infrapatellar bursitis complain of pain and swelling in the anterior knee below the patella that can radiate inferiorly into the surrounding area. Often, patients are unable to kneel or walk down stairs. They may also complain of a sharp "catching" sensation with range of motion of the knee, especially on first arising. Infrapatellar bursitis often coexists with arthritis and tendinitis of the knee, confusing the clinical picture.

Physical examination may reveal point tenderness in the anterior knee just below the patella. Swelling and fluid accumulation surrounding the lower patella are often present. Passive flexion and active resisted extension of the knee reproduce the pain. Sudden release of resistance during this maneuver causes a marked increase in pain. The deep infrapatellar bursa is not as susceptible to infection as the superficial infrapatellar bursa is.

TESTING

Plain radiographs and magnetic resonance imaging (MRI) of the knee may reveal calcification of the bursa and associated structures, including the quadriceps tendon, consistent with chronic inflammation (Fig. 91-2). MRI is

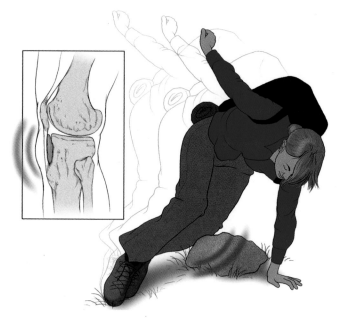

Figure 91–1. Deep infrapatellar bursitis may result from direct trauma, such as falling on the knee.

indicated if internal derangement, occult mass, or tumor of the knee is suspected. Electromyography can distinguish deep infrapatellar bursitis from femoral neuropathy, lumbar radiculopathy, and plexopathy. The injection technique described later serves as both a diagnostic and a therapeutic maneuver. Antinuclear antibody testing is indicated if collagen vascular disease is suspected. If infection is a possibility, aspiration, Gram stain, and culture of bursal fluid should be performed on an emergency basis.

DIFFERENTIAL DIAGNOSIS

Owing to the anatomy of the region, the associated tendons and other bursae of the knee can become inflamed along with the deep infrapatellar bursa, confusing the diagnosis. Both the quadriceps tendon and the deep infrapatellar bursa are subject to inflammation from overuse, misuse, or direct trauma. The tendon fibers,

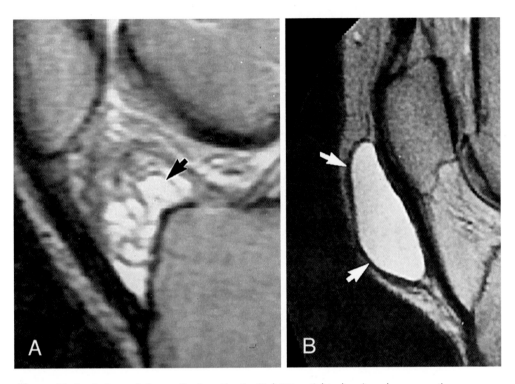

Figure 91–2. A, Deep infrapatellar bursitis. Sagittal, T2-weighted, spin echo magnetic resonance image shows fluid of high signal intensity *(arrow)* in the deep infrapatellar bursa. **B,** Prepatellar bursitis. Sagittal, T2-weighted, spin echo magnetic resonance image shows fluid of high signal intensity *(arrows)* in the prepatellar bursa. (From Resnick D: Diagnosis of Bone and Joint Disorders, 4th ed. Philadelphia, Saunders, 2002, p 3285.)

called expansions, are vulnerable to strain, and the tendon proper is subject to the development of tendinitis. The suprapatellar, infrapatellar, and prepatellar bursae may also become inflamed with dysfunction of the quadriceps tendon. It should be remembered that anything that alters the normal biomechanics of the knee can result in inflammation of the deep infrapatellar bursa.

TREATMENT

A short course of conservative therapy consisting of simple analgesics, nonsteroidal anti-inflammatory drugs, or cyclooxygenase-2 inhibitors, and a knee brace to prevent further trauma is the first step in the treatment of deep infrapatellar bursitis. If patients do not experience rapid improvement, injection is a reasonable next step.

To inject the deep infrapatellar bursa, the patient is placed in the supine position with a rolled blanket underneath the knee to gently flex the joint. The skin overlying the medial portion of the lower margin of the patella is prepared with antiseptic solution. A sterile syringe containing 2 mL of 0.25% preservative-free bupivacaine and 40 mg methylprednisolone is attached to a 1½-inch, 25-gauge needle using strict aseptic technique. The medial lower margin of the patella is identified. Just below this point, the needle is inserted at a right angle to the patella to slide beneath the patellar ligament into the deep infrapatellar bursa. If the needle strikes the patella, it is withdrawn slightly and redirected with a more inferior trajectory. When the needle is positioned in proximity to the deep infrapatellar bursa, the contents of the syringe is gently injected. There should be little resistance to injection. If resistance is encountered, the needle is probably in a ligament or tendon and should be advanced or withdrawn slightly until the injection can proceed without significant resistance. The needle is removed, and a sterile pressure dressing and ice pack are applied to the injection site.

Physical modalities, including local heat and gentle range-of-motion exercises, should be introduced several days after the patient undergoes injection. Vigorous exercises should be avoided, because they will exacerbate the patient's symptoms. Simple analgesics and nonsteroidal anti-inflammatory drugs can be used concurrently with this injection technique.

COMPLICATIONS AND PITFALLS

Failure to identify primary or metastatic tumor of the distal femur or knee joint that is causing the patient's pain can have disastrous results. The injection technique is safe if careful attention is paid to the clinically relevant anatomy. The major complication of injection is infection, although this should be exceedingly rare if strict aseptic technique is followed. Approximately 25% of patients complain of a transient increase in pain after injection, and they should be warned of this possibility.

Clinical Pearls

Coexistent bursitis, tendinitis, arthritis, and internal derangement of the knee may contribute to the patient's pain, necessitating additional treatment with more localized injection of local anesthetic and methylprednisolone. The injection technique described is extremely effective in treating the pain of deep infrapatellar bursitis.

Chapter 92

Baker's Cyst

ICD-9 CODE 727.51

THE CLINICAL SYNDROME

When bursae become inflamed, they may overproduce synovial fluid, which can become trapped in a saclike cyst. Because of a one-way valve effect, this cyst gradually expands. Baker's cyst is the result of an abnormal accumulation of synovial fluid in the medial aspect of the popliteal fossa. Often, a tear of the medial meniscus or tendinitis of the medial hamstring is responsible for the development of a Baker's cyst. Patients suffering from rheumatoid arthritis are especially susceptible to the development of Baker's cysts.

SIGNS AND SYMPTOMS

Patients with Baker's cysts complain of a feeling of fullness behind the knee. They may notice a lump behind the knee that becomes more apparent when they flex the knee. The cyst may continue to enlarge and dissect inferiorly into the calf (Fig. 92-1). Patients suffering from rheumatoid arthritis are prone to this phenomenon, and the pain associated with dissection into the calf may be confused with thrombophlebitis, leading to inappropriate treatment with anticoagulants. Occasionally, a Baker's cyst spontaneously ruptures, usually after frequent squatting. In this case, there may be rubor and color in the calf, again mimicking thrombophlebitis; however, Homan's sign is negative, and no cords are palpable.

On physical examination, patients with Baker's cysts have a cystic swelling in the medial aspect of the popliteal fossa that may be quite large. Activity that includes squatting or walking makes the pain worse, whereas rest and heat provide some relief. The pain is constant and is characterized as aching in nature; it may interfere with sleep.

TESTING

Plain radiographs and magnetic resonance imaging (MRI) of the knee are indicated for all patients who present

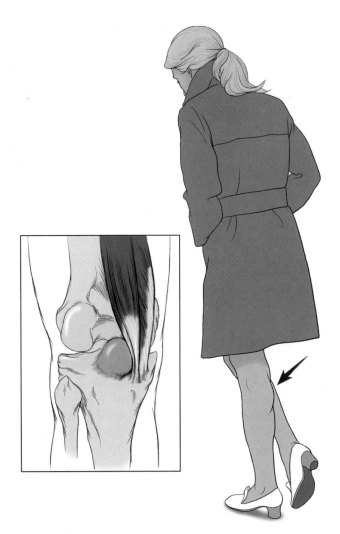

Figure 92–1. Patients with Baker's cyst often complain of a sensation of fullness or a lump behind the knee.

with Baker's cyst (Fig. 92-2). MRI can also detect internal derangement or occult mass or tumor. Based on the patient's clinical presentation, additional testing may be warranted, including a complete blood count, erythrocyte sedimentation rate, and antinuclear antibody testing.

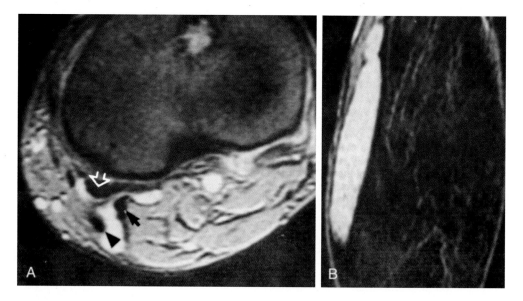

Figure 92–2. Synovial cyst of the knee. **A,** Transaxial, MPGR magnetic resonance image shows the site of origin of the synovial cyst. Note fluid of high signal intensity passing posterior to the semimembranosus tendon *(open arrow),* medial to the tendon of the medial head of the gastrocnemius muscle *(closed arrow),* and lateral to the semitendinosus tendon *(arrowhead).* **B,** Coronal, T2-weighted, spin echo magnetic resonance image in the same patient shows the more distal extent of the synovial cyst, which is superficial to the medial head of the gastrocnemius muscle. (From Resnick D: Diagnosis of Bone and Joint Disorders, 4th ed. Philadelphia, Saunders, 2002, p 4256.)

DIFFERENTIAL DIAGNOSIS

As mentioned, Baker's cysts may rupture spontaneously, leading to a misdiagnosis of thrombophlebitis. Occasionally, tendinitis of the medial hamstring or injury to the medial meniscus is confused with Baker's cyst. Primary or metastatic tumors in the region, though rare, must also be considered in the differential diagnosis.

TREATMENT

Although surgery is often required to treat Baker's cyst, a short trial of conservative therapy consisting of an elastic bandage and nonsteroidal anti-inflammatory drugs or cyclooxygenase-2 inhibitors is warranted. If these conservative measures fail, injection is a reasonable next step.

To inject a Baker's cyst, the patient is placed in the prone position with the anterior ankle resting on a folded towel to slightly flex the knee. The middle of the popliteal fossa is identified, and at a point two finger breadths medial and two finger breadths below the popliteal crease, the skin is prepared with antiseptic solution. A syringe containing 2 mL of 0.25% preservative-free bupivacaine and 40 mg methylprednisolone is attached to a 2-inch, 22-gauge needle. The needle is carefully advanced through the previously identified point at a 45-degree angle from the medial border of the popliteal fossa directly toward the Baker's cyst. While continuously aspirating, the clinician advances the needle very slowly to avoid trauma to the tibial nerve or popliteal artery or vein. When the cyst is entered, synovial fluid suddenly appears in the syringe. At this point, if there is no paresthesia in the distribution of the common peroneal or tibial nerve, the contents of the syringe is gently injected. There should be minimal resistance to injection. A pressure dressing is placed over the cyst to prevent fluid reaccumulation.

COMPLICATIONS AND PITFALLS

Failure to diagnose primary knee pathology, such as tears of the medial meniscus, may lead to further pain and disability. Because of the proximity to the common peroneal and tibial nerves, as well as the popliteal artery and vein, it is imperative that injection of Baker's cysts be performed only by those familiar with the regional anatomy and experienced in the technique. Many patients complain of a transient increase in pain after injection, and infection, though rare, may occur.

Clinical Pearls

The injection technique described is extremely effective in treating the pain and swelling of Baker's cysts. Coexistent semimembranosus bursitis, medial hamstring tendinitis, and internal derangement of the knee may contribute to the patient's pain, necessitating additional treatment with more localized injection of local anesthetic and methylprednisolone.

Chapter 93

Pes Anserine Bursitis

ICD-9 CODE 726.61

THE CLINICAL SYNDROME

The pes anserine bursa lies beneath the pes anserine tendon, which is the insertional tendon of the sartorius, gracilis, and semitendinous muscles on the medial side of the tibia. This bursa may exist as a single bursal sac or, in some patients, as a multisegmented series of loculated sacs. The pes anserine bursa is prone to the development of inflammation from overuse, misuse, or direct trauma. If inflammation of the pes anserine bursa becomes chronic, calcification may occur. Rarely, the pes anserine bursa becomes infected.

With trauma to the medial knee, the medial collateral ligament is often involved, along with the pes anserine bursa. This broad, flat, bandlike ligament runs from the medial condyle of the femur to the medial aspect of the shaft of the tibia, where it attaches just above the groove of the semimembranosus muscle; it also attaches to the edge of the medial semilunar cartilage. The medial collateral ligament is crossed at its lower part by the tendons of the sartorius, gracilis, and semitendinosus muscles.

SIGNS AND SYMPTOMS

Patients with pes anserine bursitis present with pain over the medial knee joint and increased pain on passive valgus and external rotation of the knee. Activity, especially that involving flexion and external rotation of the knee, makes the pain worse, whereas rest and heat provide some relief. Often, patients are unable to kneel or walk down stairs (Fig. 93-1). The pain of pes anserine bursitis is constant and is characterized as aching in nature; it may interfere with sleep. Coexistent bursitis, tendinitis, arthritis, or internal derangement of the knee may confuse the clinical picture after trauma to the knee.

Physical examination may reveal point tenderness in the anterior knee just below the medial knee joint at the

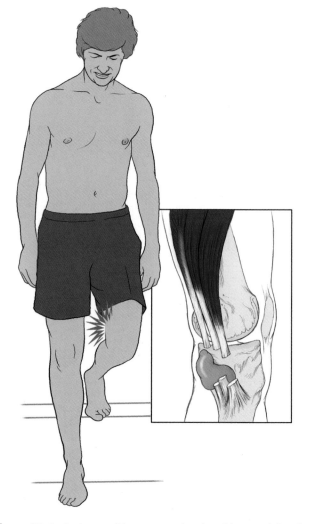

Figure 93–1. Patients with pes anserine bursitis complain of medial knee pain that is made worse with kneeling or walking down stairs.

tendinous insertion of the pes anserine. Swelling and fluid accumulation surrounding the bursa are often present. Active resisted flexion of the knee reproduces the pain. Sudden release of resistance during this maneuver causes a marked increase in pain.

TESTING

Plain radiographs of the knee may reveal calcification of the bursa and associated structures, including the pes anserine tendon, consistent with chronic inflammation. Magnetic resonance imaging (MRI) is indicated if internal derangement, occult mass, or tumor of the knee is suspected. Electromyography can distinguish pes anserine bursitis from neuropathy, lumbar radiculopathy, and plexopathy. The injection technique described later serves as both a diagnostic and a therapeutic maneuver.

DIFFERENTIAL DIAGNOSIS

Pes anserine spurs may coexist with pes anserine bursitis, confusing the clinical picture (Fig. 93-2). Because of the unique anatomic relationships present in the medial knee, it is often difficult to make an accurate clinical diagnosis with regard to which structure is responsible for the patient's pain. MRI can rule out lesions that may require surgical intervention, such as tears of the medial meniscus. It should be remembered that anything that alters the normal biomechanics of the knee can result in inflammation of the pes anserine bursa.

TREATMENT

A short course of conservative therapy consisting of simple analgesics, nonsteroidal anti-inflammatory drugs or cyclooxygenase-2 inhibitors, and a knee brace to prevent further trauma is the first step in the treatment of pes anserine bursitis. If patients do not experience rapid improvement, injection is a reasonable next step.

To inject the pes anserine bursa, the patient is placed in the supine position with a rolled blanket underneath the knee to gently flex the joint. The skin just below the medial knee joint is prepared with antiseptic solution. A sterile syringe containing 2 mL of 0.25% preservative-free bupivacaine and 40 mg methylprednisolone is attached to a 1½-inch, 25-gauge needle using strict aseptic technique. The pes anserine tendon is identified by having the patient strongly flex his or her leg against resistance. The pes anserine bursa is located at a point distal to the medial joint space where the pes anserine tendon attaches to the tibia. The bursa can usually be identified by point tenderness. At that point, the needle is inserted at a 45-degree angle to the tibia, passing through the skin and subcutaneous tissues into the pes anserine bursa. If the needle strikes the tibia, it is

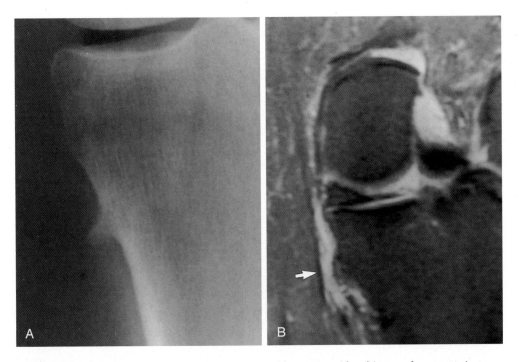

Figure 93–2. Pes anserine spurs. In this 65-year-old woman with a history of pes anserine bursitis, a conventional radiograph **(A)** reveals a small excrescence in the medial portion of the tibia. On a coronal, fat-suppressed, fast spin echo magnetic resonance image **(B),** fluid of high signal intensity *(arrow)* is seen about the bone outgrowth. (From Resnick D: Diagnosis of Bone and Joint Disorders, 4th ed. Philadelphia, Saunders, 2002, p 3898.)

withdrawn slightly into the substance of the bursa. When the needle is positioned in proximity to the pes anserine bursa, the contents of the syringe are gently injected. There should be little resistance to injection. If resistance is encountered, the needle is probably in a ligament or tendon and should be advanced or withdrawn slightly until the injection can proceed without significant resistance. The needle is removed, and a sterile pressure dressing and ice pack are applied to the injection site.

Physical modalities, including local heat and gentle range-of-motion exercises, should be introduced several days after the patient undergoes injection. Vigorous exercises should be avoided, because they will exacerbate the patient's symptoms. Simple analgesics and nonsteroidal anti-inflammatory drugs can be used concurrently with this injection technique.

COMPLICATIONS AND PITFALLS

Failure to identify primary or metastatic tumor of the distal femur or knee joint that is causing the patient's pain can have disastrous results. The injection technique is safe if careful attention is paid to the clinically relevant anatomy. The major complication of injection is infection, although this should be exceedingly rare if strict aseptic technique is followed. Approximately 25% of patients complain of a transient increase in pain after injection, and they should be warned of this possibility.

Clinical Pearls

Coexistent bursitis, tendinitis, arthritis, and internal derangement of the knee may contribute to the patient's pain, necessitating additional treatment with more localized injection of local anesthetic and methylprednisolone. The injection technique described is extremely effective in treating the pain of pes anserine bursitis.

Section 15

Pain Syndromes of the Ankle

Chapter 94

Arthritis Pain of the Ankle

ICD-9 CODE 715.97

THE CLINICAL SYNDROME

Arthritis of the ankle is a common condition. The ankle joint is susceptible to the development of arthritis from a variety of conditions that have the ability to damage the joint cartilage. Osteoarthritis is the most common form of arthritis that results in ankle pain; rheumatoid arthritis and post-traumatic arthritis are also common causes of ankle pain. Less common causes include the collagen vascular diseases, infection, villonodular synovitis, and Lyme disease. Acute infectious arthritis is usually accompanied by significant systemic symptoms, including fever and malaise, and should be easily recognized; it is treated with culture and antibiotics rather than injection therapy. Collagen vascular disease generally presents as a polyarthropathy rather than a monoarthropathy limited to the ankle joint, although ankle pain secondary to collagen vascular disease responds exceedingly well to the treatment modalities described here.

SIGNS AND SYMPTOMS

The majority of patients complain of pain localized around the ankle and distal lower extremity. Activity makes the pain worse, whereas rest and heat provide some relief. The pain is constant and is characterized as aching in nature; it may interfere with sleep. Some patients complain of a grating or popping sensation with use of the joint, and crepitus may be present on physical examination.

In addition to pain, patients with arthritis of the ankle often experience a gradual decrease in functional ability because of reduced ankle range of motion, making simple everyday tasks such as walking and climbing stairs and ladders quite difficult (Fig. 94-1). With continued disuse, muscle wasting may occur, and a frozen ankle due to adhesive capsulitis may develop.

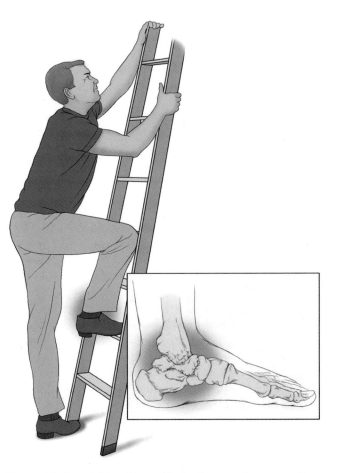

Figure 94–1. Arthritis of the ankle is often made worse with activity.

TESTING

Plain radiographs are indicated in all patients who present with ankle pain. Magnetic resonance imaging of the ankle is indicated in the case of trauma, if the diagnosis is in question, or if an occult mass or tumor is suspected. Based on the patient's clinical presentation, additional testing may be warranted, including a complete blood count, erythrocyte sedimentation rate, and antinuclear antibody testing.

DIFFERENTIAL DIAGNOSIS

Lumbar radiculopathy may mimic the pain and disability of arthritis of the ankle; however, the ankle examination is negative. Bursitis of the ankle and entrapment neuropathies such as tarsal tunnel syndrome may also confuse the diagnosis; both these conditions may coexist with arthritis of the ankle. Primary and metastatic tumors of the distal tibia and fibula and spine, as well as occult fractures, may also present in a manner similar to arthritis of the ankle.

TREATMENT

Initial treatment of the pain and functional disability associated with arthritis of the ankle includes a combination of nonsteroidal anti-inflammatory drugs or cyclooxygenase-2 inhibitors and physical therapy. The local application of heat and cold may also be beneficial. Avoidance of repetitive activities that aggravate the patient's symptoms, as well as short-term immobilization of the ankle joint, may provide relief. For patients who do not respond to these treatment modalities, intra-articular injection of local anesthetic and steroid is a reasonable next step.

To perform intra-articular injection of the ankle, the patient is placed in the supine position, and the skin overlying the ankle joint is prepared with antiseptic solution. A sterile syringe containing 2 mL of 0.25% preservative-free bupivacaine and 40 mg methylprednisolone is attached to a 1½-inch, 25-gauge needle using strict aseptic technique. With the foot in the neutral position, the junction of the tibia and fibula just above the talus is identified. At this point, a triangular indentation indicating the joint space is easily palpable (Fig. 94-2). The needle is carefully advanced through the skin, subcutaneous tissues, and joint capsule and into the joint. If bone is encountered, the needle is withdrawn into the subcutaneous tissues and redirected superiorly and slightly more medially. After the joint space is entered, the contents of the syringe is gently injected. There should be little resistance to injection. If resistance is encountered, the needle is probably in a ligament or tendon and should be advanced slightly into the joint space until the injection can proceed without significant resistance. The needle is removed, and a sterile pressure dressing and ice pack are applied to the injection site.

Physical modalities, including local heat and gentle range-of-motion exercises, should be introduced several days after the patient undergoes injection. Vigorous exercises should be avoided, because they will exacerbate the patient's symptoms.

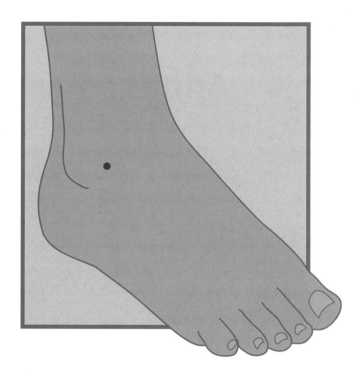

Figure 94–2. With the foot in the neutral position, the junction of the tibia and fibula just above the talus can be identified. At this point, a triangular indentation indicating the joint space is easily palpable. (From Waldman SD: Atlas of Pain Management Injection Techniques. Philadelphia, Saunders, 2000, p 301.)

COMPLICATIONS AND PITFALLS

Failure to identify primary or metastatic tumor of the ankle that is causing the patient's pain can have disastrous results. The injection technique is safe if careful attention is paid to the clinically relevant anatomy. The major complication of intra-articular injection of the ankle is infection, although this should be exceedingly rare if strict aseptic technique is followed. Approximately 25% of patients complain of a transient increase in pain after injection, and they should be warned of this possibility.

Clinical Pearls

Coexistent bursitis and tendinitis may contribute to the patient's ankle pain, necessitating additional treatment with more localized injection of local anesthetic and methylprednisolone. The injection technique described is extremely effective in treating the pain of arthritis of the ankle joint.

Chapter 95

Arthritis Pain of the Midtarsal Joint

ICD-9 CODE 715.97

THE CLINICAL SYNDROME

Arthritis of the midtarsal joints is a common condition. The midtarsal joints are susceptible to the development of arthritis from a variety of conditions that have the ability to damage the joint cartilage. Osteoarthritis is the most common form of arthritis that results in midtarsal joint pain; rheumatoid arthritis and post-traumatic arthritis are also common causes of midtarsal pain. Less common causes include the collagen vascular diseases, infection, and Lyme disease. Acute infectious arthritis is usually accompanied by significant systemic symptoms, including fever and malaise, and should be easily recognized; it is treated with culture and antibiotics rather than injection therapy. Collagen vascular disease generally presents as a polyarthropathy rather than a monoarthropathy limited to the midtarsal joint, although midtarsal pain secondary to collagen vascular disease responds exceedingly well to the treatment modalities described here.

SIGNS AND SYMPTOMS

The majority of patients present with pain localized to the dorsum of the foot. Activity, especially that involving inversion and adduction of the midtarsal joint, makes the pain worse (Fig. 95-1), whereas rest and heat provide some relief. The pain is constant and is characterized as aching in nature; it may interfere with sleep. Some patients complain of a grating or popping sensation with use of the joints, and crepitus may be present on physical examination. In addition to pain, patients with arthritis of the midtarsal joint often experience a gradual decrease in functional ability because of reduced midtarsal range of motion, making simple everyday tasks such as walking and climbing stairs quite difficult.

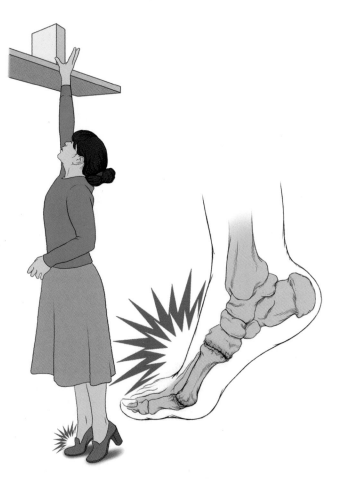

Figure 95–1. Arthritis of the midtarsal joint presents as pain in the dorsum of the foot that is made worse with inversion and adduction of the affected joint.

TESTING

Plain radiographs are indicated for all patients who present with midtarsal pain (Fig. 95-2). Magnetic resonance imaging of the midtarsal joint is indicated if aseptic necrosis, occult mass, or tumor is suspected. Based on the patient's clinical presentation, additional testing may be warranted, including a complete blood count,

329

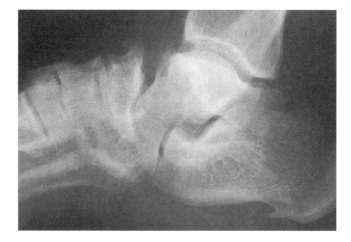

Figure 95–2. Lateral view of the tarsal bones shows osteoarthritis secondary to a vertical talus. (From Brower AC, Flemming DJ: Arthritis in Black and White, 2nd ed. Philadelphia, Saunders, 1997.)

erythrocyte sedimentation rate, and antinuclear antibody testing.

DIFFERENTIAL DIAGNOSIS

Primary pathology of the foot, including gout and occult fractures, may mimic the pain and disability of arthritis of the midtarsal joint. Bursitis and plantar fasciitis of the foot, as well as entrapment neuropathies such as tarsal tunnel syndrome, may also confuse the diagnosis; these conditions may coexist with arthritis of the midtarsal joint. Primary and metastatic tumors of the foot may also present in a manner similar to arthritis of the midtarsal joint.

TREATMENT

Initial treatment of the pain and functional disability associated with arthritis of the midtarsal joint includes a combination of nonsteroidal anti-inflammatory drugs or cyclooxygenase-2 inhibitors and physical therapy. The local application of heat and cold may also be beneficial. Avoidance of repetitive activities that aggravate the patient's symptoms, as well as short-term immobilization of the midtarsal joint, may provide relief. For patients who do not respond to these treatment modalities, intra-articular injection of local anesthetic and steroid is a reasonable next step.

To perform midtarsal injection, the patient is placed in the supine position, and the skin overlying the most tender midtarsal joint is prepared with antiseptic solution. A sterile syringe containing 2 mL of 0.25% preservative-free bupivacaine and 40 mg methylprednisolone is attached to a ⅝-inch, 25-gauge needle using strict aseptic technique. The affected joint space is identified. At this point, the needle is carefully advanced at a right angle to the dorsal aspect of the ankle through the skin, subcutaneous tissues, and joint capsule and into the joint. If bone is encountered, the needle is withdrawn into the subcutaneous tissues and redirected superiorly. After the joint space is entered, the contents of the syringe is gently injected. There should be little resistance to injection. If resistance is encountered, the needle is probably in a ligament or tendon and should be advanced slightly into the joint space until the injection can proceed without significant resistance. The needle is removed, and a sterile pressure dressing and ice pack are applied to the injection site.

Physical modalities, including local heat and gentle range-of-motion exercises, should be introduced several days after the patient undergoes injection. Vigorous exercises should be avoided, because they will exacerbate the patient's symptoms.

COMPLICATIONS AND PITFALLS

Failure to identify primary or metastatic tumor of the midtarsal joint that is causing the patient's pain can have disastrous results. The injection technique is safe if careful attention is paid to the clinically relevant anatomy. The major complication of intra-articular injection of the midtarsal joint is infection, although this should be exceedingly rare if strict aseptic technique is followed. Approximately 25% of patients complain of a transient increase in pain after injection, and they should be warned of this possibility.

Clinical Pearls

Coexistent bursitis and tendinitis may contribute to the patient's pain, necessitating additional treatment with more localized injection of local anesthetic and methlyprednisolone. The injection technique described is extremely effective in treating the pain of arthritis of the midtarsal joint.

Chapter 96

Deltoid Ligament Strain

ICD-9 CODE 845.01

THE CLINICAL SYNDROME

The deltoid ligament is exceptionally strong and is not as easily strained as the anterior talofibular ligament is. However, the deltoid ligament is susceptible to strain from acute injury due to sudden overpronation of the ankle or to repetitive microtrauma to the ligament from overuse or misuse, such as long-distance running on soft or uneven surfaces. The deltoid ligament has two layers, both of which attach to the medial malleolus above (Fig. 96-1). The deep layer attaches below to the medial body of the talus, and the superficial fibers attach to the medial talus, the sustentaculum tali of the calcaneus, and the navicular tuberosity.

SIGNS AND SYMPTOMS

Patients with deltoid ligament strain complain of pain just below the medial malleolus. Plantar flexion and eversion of the ankle joint exacerbate the pain. Often, patients with injury to the deltoid ligament note a "pop," followed by significant swelling and the inability to walk (Fig. 96-2).

On physical examination, there is point tenderness over the medial malleolus. With acute trauma, ecchymosis over the ligament may be noted. Patients with deltoid ligament strain have a positive eversion test, which is performed by passively everting and plantar-flexing the affected ankle joint (Fig. 96-3). Coexistent bursitis and arthritis of the ankle and subtalar joint may also be present, confusing the clinical picture.

TESTING

Plain radiographs are indicated for all patients who present with ankle pain. Magnetic resonance imaging (MRI) of the ankle is indicated if disruption of the deltoid ligament, joint instability, occult mass, or tumor is suspected. Radionuclide bone scanning should be performed if occult fracture is suspected. Based on the patient's clinical presentation, additional testing may be warranted, including a complete blood count, erythrocyte sedimentation rate, and antinuclear antibody testing.

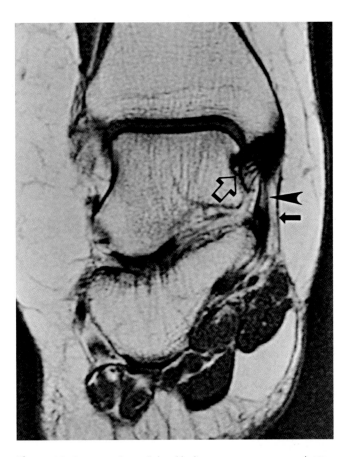

Figure 96–1. Normal medial ankle ligaments on a coronal, T1-weighted magnetic resonance image. The two layers of the deltoid (medial) ligament are seen. The deep tibiotalar ligament is striated *(open arrow)*. The more superficial tibiocalcaneal ligament *(arrowhead)* may have vertical striations as well. The thin, vertical, low-signal structure superficial to the tibiocalcaneal ligament is the flexor retinaculum *(solid arrow)*. (From Kaplan PA, Helms CA, Dussault R, et al: Musculoskeletal MRI. Philadelphia, Saunders, 2001, p 835.)

DIFFERENTIAL DIAGNOSIS

Avulsion fracture of the calcaneus, talus, medial malleolus, or base of the fifth metatarsal can mimic deltoid

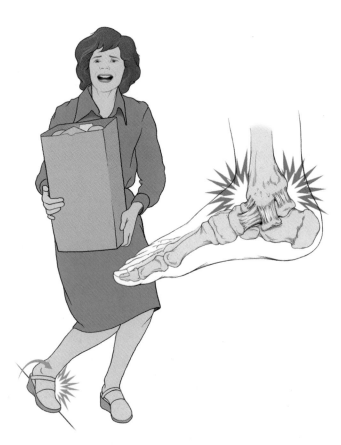

Figure 96–2. With deltoid ligament strain, patients may notice a "pop," followed by significant swelling.

ligament pain. Bursitis, tendinitis, and gout of the midtarsal joints may coexist with deltoid ligament strain, confusing the diagnosis. Tarsal tunnel syndrome may occur after ankle trauma, further complicating the clinical picture.

TREATMENT

Initial treatment of the pain and functional disability associated with deltoid ligament strain includes a combination of nonsteroidal anti-inflammatory drugs or cyclooxygenase-2 inhibitors and physical therapy. The local application of heat and cold may also be beneficial. Avoidance of repetitive activities that aggravate the patient's symptoms, as well as short-term immobilization of the ankle joint, may provide relief. For patients who do not respond to these treatment modalities, injection is a reasonable next step.

To perform deltoid ligament injection, the patient is placed in the supine position, and the skin overlying the area of the medial malleolus is prepared with antiseptic solution. A sterile syringe containing 2 mL of 0.25% preservative-free bupivacaine and 40 mg methylprednisolone is attached to a 1½-inch, 25-gauge needle using strict

aseptic technique. With the lower extremity slightly abducted, the lower margin of the medial malleolus is identified. At this point, the needle is carefully advanced at a 30-degree angle to the ankle through the skin and subcutaneous tissues to impinge on the lower margin of the medial malleolus. The needle is then withdrawn slightly, and the contents of the syringe are gently injected. There should be slight resistance to injection. If significant resistance is encountered, the needle is probably in the ligament and should be withdrawn slightly until the injection can proceed without significant resistance. The needle is removed, and a sterile pressure dressing and ice pack are applied to the injection site.

Physical modalities, including local heat and gentle range-of-motion exercises, should be introduced several days after the patient undergoes injection. Vigorous exercises should be avoided, because they will exacerbate the patient's symptoms. Simple analgesics and nonsteroidal anti-inflammatory drugs can be used concurrently with this injection technique.

COMPLICATIONS AND PITFALLS

Failure to identify occult fractures of the ankle and foot may result in significant morbidity; therefore,

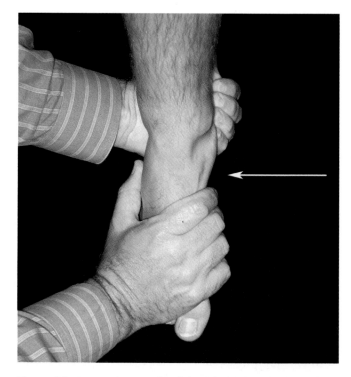

Figure 96–3. Eversion test for deltoid ligament insufficiency. (From Waldman SD: Physical Diagnosis of Pain: An Atlas of Signs and Symptoms. Philadelphia, Saunders, 2006, p 369.)

radionuclide bone scanning and MRI should be performed in all patients with unexplained ankle and foot pain, especially if trauma is present. The major complication of injection is infection, although this should be exceedingly rare if strict aseptic technique is followed. Approximately 25% of patients complain of a transient increase in pain after injection, and they should be warned of this possibility. A gentle technique should always be used when injecting around strained ligaments to avoid further damage to the already compromised ligament.

Clinical Pearls

It is estimated that approximately 25,000 people sprain an ankle every day. Although the public generally views this as a minor injury, ankle sprains can result in significant permanent pain and disability. The injection technique described is extremely effective in treating the pain of deltoid ligament strain. Coexistent arthritis, bursitis, and tendinitis may contribute to medial ankle pain, necessitating additional treatment with more localized injection of local anesthetic and methylprednisolone.

Chapter 97

Anterior Tarsal Tunnel Syndrome

ICD-9 CODE 355.5

THE CLINICAL SYNDROME

Anterior tarsal tunnel syndrome is caused by compression of the deep peroneal nerve as it passes beneath the superficial fascia of the ankle. The most common cause of this compression is trauma to the dorsum of the foot. Severe, acute plantar flexion of the foot has been implicated in anterior tarsal tunnel syndrome, as has the wearing of tight shoes or squatting and bending forward, such as when planting flowers (Fig. 97-1). Anterior tarsal

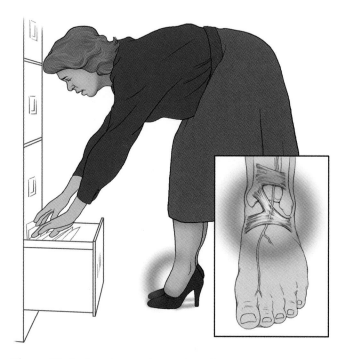

Figure 97–1. Anterior tarsal tunnel syndrome presents as deep, aching pain in the dorsum of the foot, weakness of the extensor digitorum brevis, and numbness in the distribution of the deep peroneal nerve.

tunnel syndrome is much less common than posterior tarsal tunnel syndrome.

SIGNS AND SYMPTOMS

This entrapment neuropathy presents primarily as pain, numbness, and paresthesias in the dorsum of the foot that radiate into the first dorsal web space; these symptoms may also radiate proximal to the entrapment, into the anterior ankle. There is no motor involvement unless the distal lateral division of the deep peroneal nerve is involved. Nighttime foot pain analogous to that of carpal tunnel syndrome is often present. Patients may report that holding the foot in the everted position decreases the pain and paresthesias.

Physical findings include tenderness over the deep peroneal nerve at the dorsum of the foot. A positive Tinel's sign just medial to the dorsalis pedis pulse over the deep peroneal nerve as it passes beneath the fascia is usually present (Fig. 97-2). Active plantar flexion often reproduces the symptoms of anterior tarsal tunnel syndrome. Weakness of the extensor digitorum brevis may be present if the lateral branch of the deep peroneal nerve is affected.

TESTING

Electromyography can distinguish lumbar radiculopathy and diabetic polyneuropathy from anterior tarsal tunnel syndrome. Plain radiographs are indicated in all patients who present with foot or ankle pain to rule out occult bony pathology. Magnetic resonance imaging of the ankle and foot is indicated if joint instability or a space-occupying lesion is suspected. Based on the patient's clinical presentation, additional testing may be warranted, including a complete blood count, uric acid level, erythrocyte sedimentation rate, and antinuclear antibody testing. The injection technique described later serves as both a diagnostic and a therapeutic maneuver.

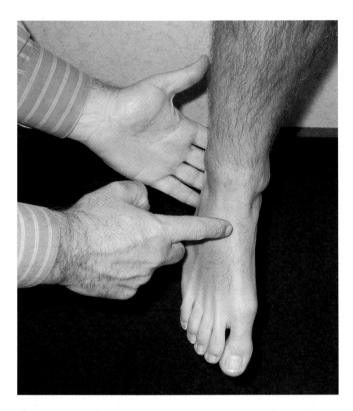

Figure 97–2. Eliciting Tinel's sign for anterior tarsal tunnel synrome. (From Waldman SD: Physical Diagnosis of Pain: An Atlas of Signs and Symptoms. Philadelphia, Saunders, 2006, p 373.)

DIFFERENTIAL DIAGNOSIS

Anterior tarsal tunnel syndrome is often misdiagnosed as arthritis of the ankle joint, lumbar radiculopathy, or diabetic polyneuropathy. Patients with arthritis of the ankle, however, have radiographic evidence of arthritis. Most patients suffering from lumbar radiculopathy have reflex, motor, and sensory changes associated with back pain, whereas patients with anterior tarsal tunnel syndrome have no reflex changes or motor deficits, and sensory changes are limited to the distribution of the distal deep peroneal nerve. It should be remembered, however, that lumbar radiculopathy and deep peroneal nerve entrapment may coexist as the "double crush" syndrome. Diabetic polyneuropathy generally presents as a symmetrical sensory deficit involving the entire foot rather than being limited to the distribution of the deep peroneal nerve. When anterior tarsal tunnel syndrome occurs in diabetic patients, diabetic polyneuropathy is usually present as well.

TREATMENT

Mild cases of tarsal tunnel syndrome usually respond to conservative therapy; surgery should be reserved for severe cases. Initial treatment of tarsal tunnel syndrome consists of simple analgesics, nonsteroidal anti-inflammatory drugs, or cyclooxygenase-2 inhibitors and splinting of the ankle. At a minimum, the splint should be worn at night, but 24 hours a day is ideal. Avoidance of repetitive activities that may be responsible for the development of tarsal tunnel syndrome, such as prolonged squatting or wearing shoes that are too tight, can also ameliorate the symptoms. If patients fail to respond to these conservative measures, injection of the tarsal tunnel with local anesthetic and steroid is a reasonable next step.

Tarsal tunnel injection is performed by placing the patient in the supine position with the leg extended. The extensor hallucis longus tendon is identified by having the patient extend his or her big toe against resistance. A point just medial to the tendon at the skin crease of the ankle is identified and prepared with antiseptic solution. A 1½-inch, 25-gauge needle is advanced through this point very slowly toward the tibia until a paresthesia is elicited in the web space between the first and second toes, usually at a needle depth of ¼ to ½ inch. The patient should be warned to expect this paresthesia and instructed to say "There!" as soon as it is felt. If no paresthesia is elicited, the needle is withdrawn and redirected slightly more posteriorly until a paresthesia is induced. The needle is then withdrawn 1 mm, and the patient is observed to ensure that he or she is not experiencing any persistent paresthesia. After careful aspiration, a total of 6 mL of 1% preservative-free lidocaine and 40 mg methylprednisolone is slowly injected. Care must be taken not to advance the needle into the substance of the nerve and inadvertently inject the solution intraneurally. After injection, pressure is applied to the injection site to decrease the incidence of ecchymosis and hematoma formation.

COMPLICATIONS AND PITFALLS

Failure to adequately treat tarsal tunnel syndrome can result in permanent pain, numbness, and functional disability; these problems can be exacerbated if coexistent reflex sympathetic dystrophy is not treated aggressively with sympathetic neural blockade. The main complications of deep peroneal nerve block are ecchymosis and hematoma, which can be avoided by applying pressure to the injection site. Because a paresthesia is elicited with this technique, needle-induced trauma to the common peroneal nerve is a possibility. By advancing the needle slowly and then withdrawing it slightly away from the nerve, needle-induced trauma can be avoided.

Clinical Pearls

It should be remembered that the most common cause of pain radiating into the lower extremity is herniated lumbar disk or nerve impingement secondary to degenerative arthritis of the spine, not disorders involving the common or deep peroneal nerve. Lesions above the origin of the common peroneal nerve, such as lesions of the sciatic nerve, or lesions at the point where the common peroneal nerve winds around the head of the fibula, may be confused with deep peroneal nerve entrapment. Electromyography and magnetic resonance imaging of the lumbar spine, combined with the clinical history and physical examination, can determine the cause of distal lower extremity and foot pain. Diabetics and others with vulnerable nerve syndrome may be more susceptible to the development of anterior tarsal tunnel syndrome.

The injection technique described is useful in the treatment of anterior tarsal tunnel syndrome. Careful preinjection neurologic assessment is important to identify preexisting neurologic deficits that might later be attributed to the deep peroneal nerve block. These assessments are especially important in patients who have sustained trauma to the ankle or foot and in those suffering from diabetic neuropathy in whom deep peroneal nerve block is being used for acute pain control.

Chapter 98

Posterior Tarsal Tunnel Syndrome

ICD-9 CODE 355.5

THE CLINICAL SYNDROME

Posterior tarsal tunnel syndrome is caused by compression of the posterior tibial nerve as it passes through the posterior tarsal tunnel. The posterior tarsal tunnel is made up of the flexor retinaculum, the bones of the ankle, and the lacunate ligament. In addition to the posterior tibial nerve, the tunnel contains the posterior tibial artery and a number of flexor tendons that are subject to tenosynovitis. The most common cause of compression of the posterior tibial nerve at this location is trauma to the ankle, including fracture, dislocation, and crush injury. Thrombophlebitis involving the posterior tibial artery has also been implicated in the development of posterior tarsal tunnel syndrome. Patients with rheumatoid arthritis have a higher incidence of posterior tarsal tunnel syndrome than does the general population. Posterior tarsal tunnel syndrome is much more common than anterior tarsal tunnel syndrome.

SIGNS AND SYMPTOMS

Posterior tarsal tunnel syndrome presents in a manner analogous to carpal tunnel syndrome. Patients complain of pain, numbness, and paresthesias in the sole of the foot; these symptoms may also radiate proximal to the entrapment, into the medial ankle (Fig. 98-1). Patients may note weakness of the toe flexors and instability of the foot due to weakness of the lumbrical muscles. Nighttime foot pain analogous to that of carpal tunnel syndrome is often present.

Physical findings include tenderness over the posterior tibial nerve at the medial malleolus. A positive Tinel's sign just below and behind the medial malleolus over the posterior tibial nerve is usually present. Active inversion of the ankle often reproduces the symptoms of posterior tarsal tunnel syndromes. Medial and lateral plantar divi-

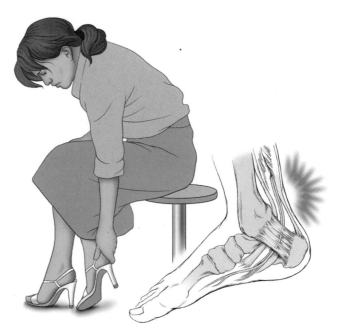

Figure 98–1. Posterior tarsal tunnel syndrome is characterized by pain, numbness, and paresthesias of the sole of the foot.

sions of the posterior tibial nerve provide motor innervation to the intrinsic muscles of the foot; thus, weakness of the flexor digitorum brevis and the lumbrical muscles may be present if these branches of the nerve are affected.

TESTING

Electromyography can distinguish lumbar radiculopathy and diabetic polyneuropathy from posterior tarsal tunnel syndrome. Plain radiographs and magnetic resonance imaging (MRI) are indicated for all patients who present with posterior tarsal tunnel syndrome to rule out occult bony pathology (Fig. 98-2). MRI of the ankle and foot is also indicated if joint instability or a space-occupying lesion is suspected. Based on the patient's clinical

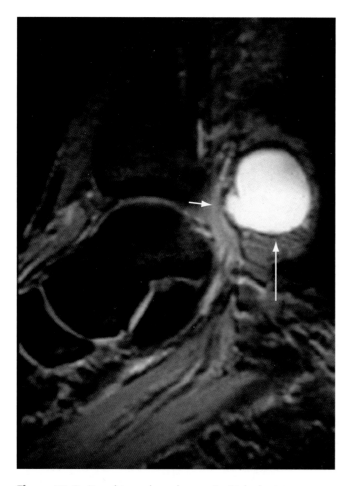

Figure 98-2. Tarsal tunnel syndrome. Sagittal, short tau inversion recovery magnetic resonance image shows a ganglion cyst *(arrow)* compressing the neurovascular bundle in the tarsal tunnel *(arrowhead)*. (From Edelman RR, Hessellink JR, Zlatkin MB, Crues JV: Clinical Magnetic Resonance Imaging, 3rd ed. Philadelphia, Saunders, 2006, p 3454.)

presentation, additional testing may be warranted, including a complete blood count, uric acid level, erythrocyte sedimentation rate, and antinuclear antibody testing. The injection technique described later serves as both a diagnostic and a therapeutic maneuver.

DIFFERENTIAL DIAGNOSIS

Posterior tarsal tunnel syndrome is often misdiagnosed as arthritis of the ankle joint, lumbar radiculopathy, or diabetic polyneuropathy. Patients with arthritis of the ankle, however, have radiographic evidence of arthritis. Most patients suffering from lumbar radiculopathy have reflex, motor, and sensory changes associated with back pain, whereas those with posterior tarsal tunnel syndrome have no reflex changes, and motor and sensory

changes are limited to the distribution of distal posterior tibial nerve. It should be remembered, however, that lumbar radiculopathy and posterior tibial nerve entrapment may coexist as the "double crush" syndrome. Diabetic polyneuropathy generally presents as a symmetrical sensory deficit involving the entire foot rather than being limited to the distribution of the posterior tibial nerve. When posterior tarsal tunnel syndrome occurs in diabetic patients, diabetic polyneuropathy is usually present as well.

TREATMENT

Mild cases of tarsal tunnel syndrome usually respond to conservative therapy; surgery should be reserved for severe cases. Initial treatment of tarsal tunnel syndrome consists of simple analgesics, nonsteroidal anti-inflammatory drugs, or cyclooxygenase-2 inhibitors and splinting of the ankle. At a minimum, the splint should be worn at night, but 24 hours a day is ideal. Avoidance of repetitive activities that may be responsible for the development of tarsal tunnel syndrome can also ameliorate the symptoms. If patients fail to respond to these conservative measures, injection of the tarsal tunnel with local anesthetic and steroid is a reasonable next step.

Posterior tarsal tunnel injection is performed with the patient in the lateral position and the affected leg in the dependent position and slightly flexed. The posterior tibial artery is palpated, and the area between the medial malleolus and the Achilles tendon is identified and prepared with antiseptic solution. A 1½-inch, 25-gauge needle is inserted at this level and directed anteriorly toward the pulsation of the posterior tibial artery. If the arterial pulsation cannot be identified, the needle is directed toward the posterior superior border of the medial malleolus. The needle is advanced slowly toward the tibial nerve, which lies in the posterior groove of the medial malleolus, until a paresthesia is elicited in the distribution of the tibial nerve, usually after the needle is advanced ½ to ¾ inch. The patient should be warned to expect this paresthesia and instructed to say "There!" as soon as it is felt. If no paresthesia is elicited, the needle is withdrawn and redirected slightly more cephalad until a paresthesia is induced. The needle is then withdrawn 1 mm, and the patient is observed to ensure that he or she is not experiencing any persistent paresthesia. After careful aspiration, a total of 6 mL of 1% preservative-free lidocaine and 40 mg methylprednisolone is slowly injected. Care must be taken not to advance the needle into the substance of the nerve and inadvertently inject the solution intraneurally. After injection, pressure is applied to the injection site to decrease the incidence of ecchymosis and hematoma formation.

COMPLICATIONS AND PITFALLS

Failure to adequately treat tarsal tunnel syndrome can result in permanent pain, numbness, and functional disability; these problems can be exacerbated if coexistent reflex sympathetic dystrophy is not treated aggressively with sympathetic neural blockade. The main complications of injection are ecchymosis and hematoma, which can be avoided by applying pressure to the injection site. Because a paresthesia is elicited, needle-induced trauma to the nerve is a possibility. By advancing the needle slowly and then withdrawing it slightly away from the nerve, needle-induced trauma can be avoided.

Clinical Pearls

It should be remembered that the most common cause of pain radiating into the lower extremity is herniated lumbar disk or nerve impingement secondary to degenerative arthritis of the spine, not disorders involving the tibial, common, or deep peroneal nerve. Lesions above the origin of the tibial or common peroneal nerve may be confused with posterior tarsal tunnel syndrome. Electromyography and MRI of the lumbar spine, combined with the clinical history and physical examination, can determine the cause of distal lower extremity and foot pain.

Chapter 99

Achilles Tendinitis

ICD-9 CODE 727.00

THE CLINICAL SYNDROME

Achilles tendinitis has become more common as jogging has increased in popularity. The Achilles tendon is susceptible to the development of tendinitis both at its insertion on the calcaneus and at its narrowest part—a point approximately 5 cm above its insertion. The Achilles tendon is subjected to repetitive motion that may result in microtrauma, which heals poorly owing to the tendon's avascular nature. Running is often the inciting factor in acute Achilles tendinitis, which frequently coexists with bursitis, causing additional pain and functional disability. Calcium deposition around the tendon may occur if inflammation persists, making subsequent treatment more difficult. Continued trauma to the inflamed tendon may ultimately result in tendon rupture.

SIGNS AND SYMPTOMS

The onset of Achilles tendinitis is usually acute, occurring after overuse or misuse of the ankle joint. Inciting activities include running with sudden stops and starts, such as when playing tennis. Improper stretching of the gastrocnemius and Achilles tendon before exercise has also been implicated in Achilles tendinitis as well as acute tendon rupture. The pain of Achilles tendinitis is constant and severe and is localized in the posterior ankle (Fig. 99-1). Significant sleep disturbance is often reported. Patients may attempt to splint the inflamed Achilles tendon by adopting a flatfooted gait to avoid plantar-flexing the tendon. Pain is induced with resisted plantar flexion of the foot, and a creaking or grating sensation may be palpated when passively plantar-flexing the foot (Fig. 99-2). A chronically inflamed Achilles tendon may suddenly rupture with stress or during injection into the tendon itself.

TESTING

Plain radiographs and magnetic resonance imaging (MRI) are indicated in all patients who present with posterior

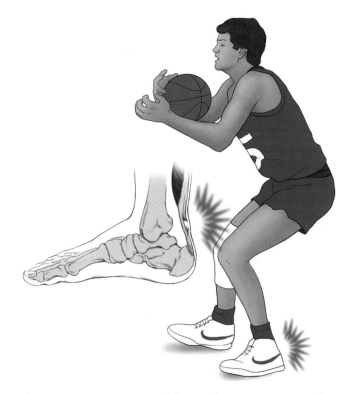

Figure 99–1. The pain of Achilles tendinitis is constant and severe and is localized to the posterior ankle.

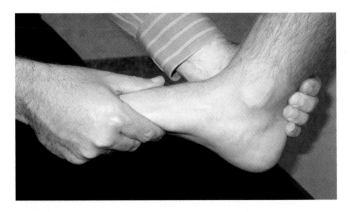

Figure 99–2. Eliciting the creak sign for Achilles tendinitis. (From Waldman SD: Physical Diagnosis of Pain: An Atlas of Signs and Symptoms. Philadelphia, Saunders, 2006, p 377.)

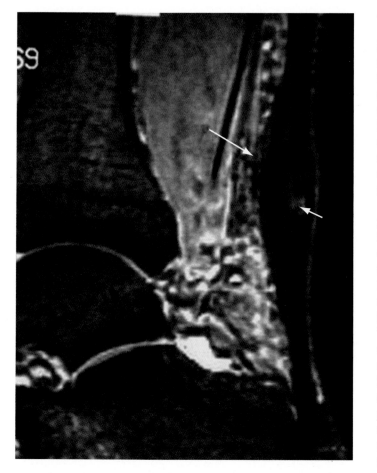

Figure 99–3. Chronic Achilles tendinosis. Sagittal, short tau inversion recovery magnetic resonance image shows fusiform thickening of the Achilles tendon *(long arrow),* with a focal area of increased signal intensity *(short arrow).* Note the diffuse peritendinitis of Kager's fat triangle. (From Edelman RR, Hessellink JR, Zlatkin MB, Crues JV: Clinical Magnetic Resonance Imaging, 3rd ed. Philadelphia, Saunders, 2006, p 3451.)

ankle pain (Fig. 99-3). MRI of the ankle is also indicated if joint instability is suspected. Radionuclide bone scanning is useful to identify stress fractures not seen on plain radiographs. Based on the patient's clinical presentation, additional testing may be warranted, including a complete blood count, erythrocyte sedimentation rate, and antinuclear antibody testing. The injection technique described later serves as both a diagnostic and a therapeutic maneuver.

DIFFERENTIAL DIAGNOSIS

Achilles tendinitis is usually easily identified on clinical grounds. However, if the bursa located between the Achilles tendon and the base of the tibia and the upper posterior calcaneus is inflamed, coexistent bursitis may confuse the diagnosis. Stress fractures of the ankle may also mimic Achilles tendinitis.

TREATMENT

Initial treatment of the pain and functional disability associated with Achilles tendinitis includes a combination of nonsteroidal anti-inflammatory drugs or cyclooxygenase-2 inhibitors and physical therapy. The local application of heat and cold may also be beneficial. Repetitive activities thought to be responsible for the development of tendinitis, such as jogging, should be avoided. For patients who do not respond to these treatment modalities, injection with local anesthetic and steroid is a reasonable next step.

Injection for Achilles tendinitis is carried out by placing the patient in the prone position with the affected foot hanging off the end of the table. The foot is gently dorsiflexed to facilitate identification of the margin of the tendon, because injection directly into the tendon should be avoided. The tender point at the tendinous insertion or at its narrowest part approximately 5 cm above the insertion is identified and marked with a sterile marker. The skin overlying this point is prepared with antiseptic solution. A sterile syringe containing 2 mL of 0.25% preservative-free bupivacaine and 40 mg methylprednisolone is attached to a 1½-inch, 25-gauge needle using strict aseptic technique. The previously marked point is palpated, and the needle is carefully advanced at this point along the tendon and through the skin and subcutaneous tissues, taking care not to enter the substance of the tendon. The contents of the syringe is gently injected while slowly withdrawing the needle. There should be minimal resistance to injection. If there is significant resistance, the needle tip is probably in the substance of the Achilles tendon and should be withdrawn slightly until the injection can proceed without significant resistance. The needle is removed, and a sterile pressure dressing and ice pack are applied to the injection site.

Physical modalities, including local heat and gentle range-of-motion exercises, should be introduced several days after the patient undergoes injection. Vigorous exercises should be avoided, because they will exacerbate the patient's symptoms. Simple analgesics and nonsteroidal anti-inflammatory drugs can be used concurrently with this injection technique.

COMPLICATIONS AND PITFALLS

Trauma to the Achilles tendon from the injection itself is an ever-present possibility. Tendons that are highly inflamed or previously damaged are subject to rupture if they are injected directly. This complication can be avoided if the clinician uses gentle technique and stops injecting immediately if significant resistance is encountered. Approximately 25% of patients complain of a transient increase in pain after injection, and they should be warned of this possibility.

Clinical Pearls

Although the Achilles tendon is the thickest and strongest tendon in the body, it is susceptible to inflammation or even rupture. It begins at the midcalf and continues downward, narrowing as it goes, to attach to the posterior calcaneus; it becomes narrowest approximately 5 cm above its calcaneal insertion. At these two points, tendinitis is most likely to develop. The injection technique described is extremely effective in treating Achilles tendinitis. Coexistent bursitis and arthritis may contribute to the patient's symptoms, necessitating additional treatment with more localized injection of local anesthetic and methylprednisolone.

Section 16

Pain Syndromes of the Foot

Chapter 100

Arthritis Pain of the Toes

ICD-9 CODE **715.97**

THE CLINICAL SYNDROME

The toe joint is susceptible to the development of arthritis from a variety of conditions that have the ability to damage the joint cartilage. Osteoarthritis is the most common form of arthritis that results in toe joint pain; rheumatoid arthritis and post-traumatic arthritis are also common causes of toe pain. Less common causes include the collagen vascular diseases, infection, and Lyme disease. Acute infectious arthritis is usually accompanied by significant systemic symptoms, including fever and malaise, and should be easily recognized; it is treated with culture and antibiotics rather than injection therapy. Collagen vascular disease generally presents as a polyarthropathy rather than a monoarthropathy limited to the toe joint, although toe pain secondary to collagen vascular disease responds exceedingly well to the intra-articular injection technique described here.

SIGNS AND SYMPTOMS

The majority of patients present with pain localized to the affected joint of the foot, most commonly the great toe. Activity, especially flexion of the toe joints, makes the pain worse (Fig. 100-1), whereas rest and heat provide some relief. The pain is constant and is characterized as aching in nature; it may interfere with sleep. Some patients complain of a grating or popping sensation with use of the joint, and crepitus may be present on physical examination. In addition to pain, patients often experience a gradual decrease in functional ability because of reduced toe range of motion, making simple everyday tasks such as walking, standing on tiptoes, and climbing stairs quite difficult.

TESTING

Plain radiographs are indicated in all patients who present with toe joint pain. Magnetic resonance imaging of the

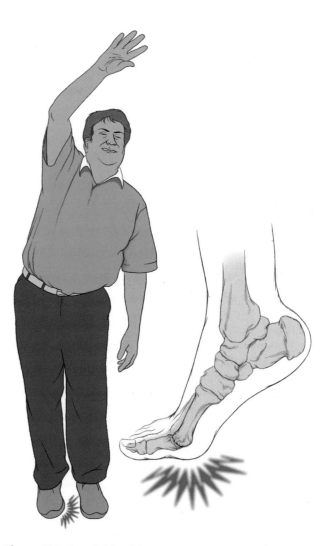

Figure 100–1. Arthritis of the toe presents as pain that is made worse with weight-bearing activity.

toe is indicated if joint instability, occult mass, or tumor is suspected. Based on the patient's clinical presentation, additional testing may be warranted, including a complete blood count, erythrocyte sedimentation rate, and antinuclear antibody testing.

DIFFERENTIAL DIAGNOSIS

Bursitis and tendinitis of the foot, as well as entrapment neuropathies such as tarsal tunnel syndrome, may confuse the diagnosis; these conditions may coexist with arthritis of the toes. Primary and metastatic tumors of the foot, occult fractures of the tarsals and metatarsals, and fractures of the sesamoid bones of the foot may present in a manner similar to arthritis of the toes.

TREATMENT

Initial treatment of the pain and functional disability associated with arthritis of the toes includes a combination of nonsteroidal anti-inflammatory drugs or cyclooxygenase-2 inhibitors and physical therapy. The local application of heat and cold may also be beneficial. Avoidance of repetitive activities that aggravate the patient's symptoms, as well as short-term immobilization of the toe joints, may provide relief. For patients who do not respond to these treatment modalities, intra-articular injection with local anesthetic and steroid is a reasonable next step.

To perform intra-articular injection of the toes, the patient is placed in the supine position, and the skin overlying the affected toe joint is prepared with antiseptic solution. A sterile syringe containing 1.5 mL of 0.25% preservative-free bupivacaine and 40 mg methylprednisolone is attached to a ⅝-inch, 25-gauge needle using strict aseptic technique. The affected toe is distracted to open the joint space, which is identified. At this point, the needle is carefully advanced perpendicular to the joint space next to the extensor tendons through the skin, subcutaneous tissues, and joint capsule and into the joint. If bone is encountered, the needle is withdrawn into the subcutaneous tissues and redirected superiorly. Once the needle is in the joint space, the contents of the syringe is gently injected. There should be little resistance to injection. If resistance is encountered, the needle is probably in a ligament or tendon and should be advanced slightly into the joint space until the injection can proceed without significant resistance. The needle is removed, and a sterile pressure dressing and ice pack are applied to the injection site.

Physical modalities, including local heat and gentle range-of-motion exercises, should be introduced several days after the patient undergoes injection. Vigorous exercises should be avoided, because they will exacerbate the patient's symptoms.

COMPLICATIONS AND PITFALLS

Failure to identify primary or metastatic tumor of the foot that is causing the patient's pain can have disastrous results. The injection technique is safe if careful attention is paid to the clinically relevant anatomy. The major complication of injection is infection, although this should be exceedingly rare if strict aseptic technique is followed. Approximately 25% of patients complain of a transient increase in pain after injection, and they should be warned of this possibility.

Clinical Pearls

Coexistent bursitis and tendinitis may contribute to the patient's pain, necessitating additional treatment with more localized injection of local anesthetic and methylprednisolone. The injection technique described is extremely effective in treating the pain of arthritis of the toe joints.

Chapter 101

Bunion Pain

ICD-9 CODE 727.1

THE CLINICAL SYNDROME

Bunion is one of the most common causes of foot pain. The term *bunion* refers to soft tissue swelling over the first metatarsophalangeal joint associated with abnormal angulation of the joint that results in a prominent first metatarsal head and overlapping of the first and second toes, called the hallux valgus deformity. The first metatarsophalangeal joint may ultimately subluxate, causing the overlapping of the first and second toes to worsen. An inflamed adventitious bursa may accompany bunion formation. The most common cause of bunions is the wearing of narrow-toed shoes, and high heels may exacerbate the problem (Fig. 101-1); thus, bunions are more common in females.

SIGNS AND SYMPTOMS

The majority of patients present with pain localized to the affected first metatarsophalangeal joint and complain of being unable to get shoes to fit. Walking makes the pain worse, whereas rest and heat provide some relief. The pain is constant and is characterized as aching in nature; it may interfere with sleep. Some patients complain of a grating or popping sensation with use of the joint, and crepitus may be present on physical examination. In addition to pain, patients with bunions develop the characteristic hallux valgus deformity, with a prominent first metatarsal head, improper angulation of the joint, and overlapping first and second toes.

TESTING

Plain radiographs are indicated in all patients who present with bunion pain (Fig. 101-2). Magnetic resonance imaging of the toe is indicated if joint instability, occult mass, or tumor is suspected. Based on the patient's clinical presentation, additional testing may be warranted, including a complete blood count, erythrocyte sedimentation rate, and antinuclear antibody testing.

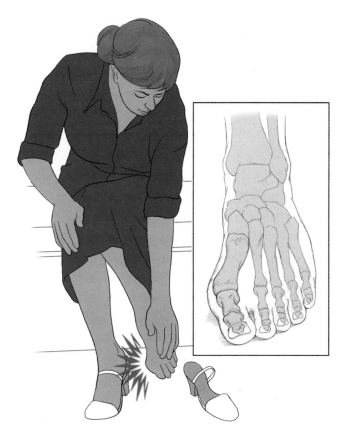

Figure 101–1. Narrow-toed shoes are implicated in the development of bunions.

DIFFERENTIAL DIAGNOSIS

The diagnosis of bunion is usually obvious on clinical grounds alone. Bursitis and tendinitis of the foot and ankle often coexist with bunion pain. In addition, stress fractures of the metatarsals, phalanges, or sesamoid bones may confuse the diagnosis and require specific treatment.

TREATMENT

Initial treatment of the pain and functional disability associated with bunion includes a combination of nonsteroidal anti-inflammatory drugs or cyclooxygenase-2

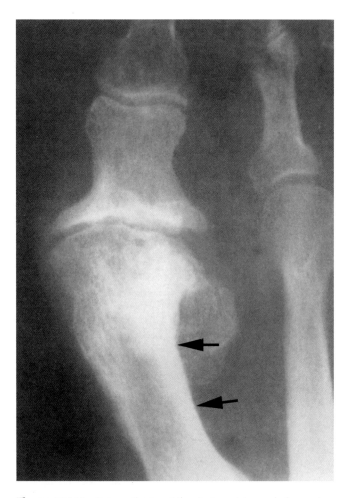

Figure 101-2. Osteoarthritis of the first metatarsophalangeal joint in a patient with hallux valgus deformity. The sesamoids are lateral to the metatarsal head. There is narrowing of the joint space, with subchondral bone and osteophyte formation. Marked thickening of the lateral cortex of the metatarsal shaft *(arrows)* is evident. (From Brower AC, Flemming DJ: Arthritis in Black and White, 2nd ed. Philadelphia, Saunders, 1997.)

inhibitors and physical therapy. The local application of heat and cold may also be beneficial. Avoidance of repetitive activities that aggravate the patient's symptoms, avoidance of narrow-toed or high-heeled shoes, and short-term immobilization of the affected toes may also provide relief. For patients who do not respond to these treatment modalities, injection with local anesthetic and steroid is a reasonable next step.

To inject the bunion deformity, the patient is placed in the supine position, and the skin overlying the bunion is prepared with antiseptic solution. A sterile syringe containing 1.5 mL of 0.25% preservative-free bupivacaine and 40 mg methylprednisolone is attached to a ⅝-inch, 25-gauge needle using strict aseptic technique. The bunion is identified, and the needle is carefully advanced against the first metatarsal head. It is then withdrawn slightly out of the periosteum, and the contents of the syringe is gently injected. There should be little resistance to injection. If resistance is encountered, the needle is probably in a ligament or tendon and should be advanced or withdrawn slightly until the injection can proceed without significant resistance. The needle is removed, and a sterile pressure dressing and ice pack are applied to the injection site.

Physical modalities, including local heat and gentle range-of-motion exercises, should be introduced several days after the patient undergoes injection.

COMPLICATIONS AND PITFALLS

Failure to identify primary or metastatic tumor of the foot that is causing the patient's pain can have disastrous results. The injection technique is safe if careful attention is paid to the clinically relevant anatomy. The major complication of injection is infection, although this should be exceedingly rare if strict aseptic technique is followed. Approximately 25% of patients complain of a transient increase in pain after injection, and they should be warned of this possibility.

Clinical Pearls

Coexistent bursitis and tendinitis may contribute to the patient's foot pain, necessitating additional treatment with more localized injection of local anesthetic and methylprednisolone. The injection technique described is extremely effective in treating bunion pain. Narrow-toed and high-heeled shoes should be avoided, because they will exacerbate the patient's symptoms.

Chapter 102

Morton's Neuroma

ICD-9 CODE 355.6

THE CLINICAL SYNDROME

Morton's neuroma is one of the most common pain syndromes affecting the forefoot. It is characterized by tenderness and burning pain in the plantar surface of the forefoot, with painful paresthesias in the two affected toes. This pain syndrome is thought to be caused by perineural fibrosis of the interdigital nerves. Although the nerves between the third and fourth toes are affected most commonly, the second and third toes and, rarely, the fourth and fifth toes can be affected as well (Fig. 102-1). Patients may feel like they are walking with a stone in the shoe. The pain of Morton's neuroma worsens with prolonged standing or walking for long distances and is exacerbated by poorly fitting or improperly padded shoes. As with bunion and hammer toe deformities, Morton's neuroma is associated with the wearing of tight, narrow-toed shoes.

SIGNS AND SYMPTOMS

On physical examination, pain can be reproduced by performing Mulder's maneuver: firmly squeezing the two metatarsal heads together with one hand while placing firm pressure on the interdigital space with the other (Fig. 102-2). In contrast to metatarsalgia, in which the tender area is over the metatarsal heads, with Morton's neuroma, the tender area is localized to only the plantar surface of the affected interspace, with paresthesias radiating into the two affected toes. Patients with Morton's neuroma often exhibit an antalgic gait in an effort to reduce weight bearing during walking.

TESTING

Plain radiographs and magnetic resonance imaging (MRI) are indicated in all patients who present with Morton's neuroma to rule out fractures and to identify sesamoid bones that may have become inflamed (Fig. 102-3). MRI of the metatarsal bones is also indicated if joint instability, occult mass, or tumor is suspected. Radionuclide

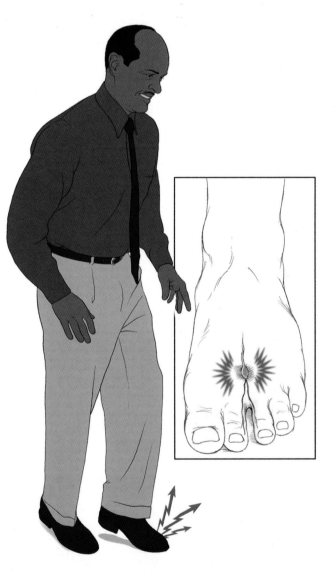

Figure 102–1. The pain of Morton's neuroma is made worse with prolonged standing or walking.

bone scanning may be useful to identify stress fractures of the metatarsal or sesamoid bones that may be missed on plain radiographs. Based on the patient's clinical presentation, additional testing may be warranted, including a complete blood count, erythrocyte sedimentation rate, and antinuclear antibody testing.

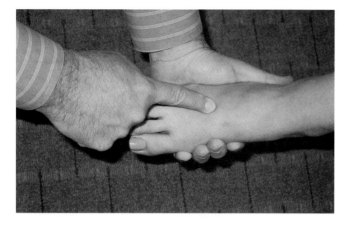

Figure 102–2. Eliciting Mulder's sign for Morton's neuroma. (From Waldman SD: Physical Diagnosis of Pain: An Atlas of Signs and Symptoms. Philadelphia, Saunders, 2006, p 381.)

DIFFERENTIAL DIAGNOSIS

Fractures of the sesamoid bones of the foot are often confused with Morton's neuroma; although the pain of sesamoid fracture is localized to the plantar surface of the foot, it is less neuritic in character than that of Morton's neuroma. Tendinitis, bursitis, and stress fractures of the foot can also mimic the pain of Morton's neuroma.

TREATMENT

Initial treatment of the pain and functional disability associated with Morton's neuroma includes a combination of nonsteroidal anti-inflammatory drugs or cyclooxygenase-2 inhibitors and physical therapy. The local application of heat and cold may also be beneficial. Avoidance of repetitive activities that aggravate the patient's symptoms, avoidance of narrow-toed or high-heeled shoes, and short-term immobilization of the

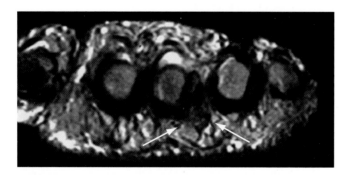

Figure 102–3. Morton's neuroma. Coronal (short axis) T2-weighted image through the forefoot demonstrates a hypointense lesion located between the third and fourth metatarsal heads *(arrows)*. (From Edelman RR, Hessellink JR, Zlatkin MB, Crues JV: Clinical Magnetic Resonance Imaging, 3rd ed. Philadelphia, Saunders, 2006, p 4355.)

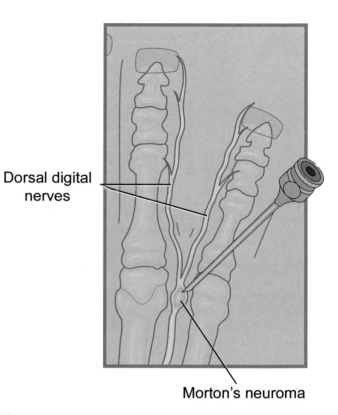

Dorsal digital nerves

Morton's neuroma

Figure 102–4. Proper needle placement for injection of Morton's neuroma. (From Waldman SD: Atlas of Pain Management Injection Techniques. Philadelphia, Saunders, 2000.)

affected foot may also provide relief. For patients who do not respond to these treatment modalities, injection with local anesthetic and steroid is a reasonable next step.

To inject Morton's neuroma, the patient is placed in the supine position with a pillow under the knee to slightly flex the leg. A total of 3 mL non-epinephrine-containing local anesthetic and 40 mg methylprednisolone is drawn up in a 12-mL sterile syringe. The affected interdigital space is identified, the dorsal surface of the foot at this point is marked with a sterile marker, and the skin is prepared with antiseptic solution. At a point proximal to the metatarsal head, a 1½-inch, 25-gauge needle is inserted between the two metatarsal bones in the area to be blocked (Fig. 102-4). While the clinician is slowly injecting, the needle is advanced from the dorsal surface of the foot toward the palmar surface. Because the plantar digital nerve is situated on the dorsal side of the flexor retinaculum, the needle must be advanced almost to the palmar surface of the foot. The needle is removed, and pressure is applied to the injection site to avoid hematoma formation.

Physical modalities, including local heat and gentle range-of-motion exercises, should be introduced several days after the patient undergoes injection.

COMPLICATIONS AND PITFALLS

Failure to identify primary or metastatic tumor of the foot that is causing the patient's pain can have disastrous results. The major complication of injection is infection, although this should be exceedingly rare if strict aseptic technique is followed. Because of the confined space of the soft tissues surrounding the metatarsals and digits, mechanical compression of the blood supply after injection is a possibility. To prevent vascular insufficiency and gangrene from occurring, the clinician must avoid rapidly injecting a large volume of solution into these confined spaces; epinephrine-containing solutions should not be used, for the same reasons. Approximately 25% of patients complain of a transient increase in pain after injection, and they should be warned of this possibility.

Clinical Pearls

Coexistent bursitis and tendinitis may contribute to the patient's foot pain, necessitating additional treatment with more localized injection of local anesthetic and methylprednisolone. The injection technique described is extremely effective in treating the pain of Morton's neuroma; however, patients often require shoe orthoses and shoes with a wider toe box to take pressure off the affected interdigital nerves.

Chapter 103

Plantar Fasciitis

ICD-9 CODE 728.71

THE CLINICAL SYNDROME

Plantar fasciitis is characterized by pain and tenderness over the plantar surface of the calcaneus. It is twice as common in women as in men. Plantar fasciitis is thought to be caused by inflammation of the plantar fascia, which can occur alone or as part of a systemic inflammatory condition such as rheumatoid arthritis, Reiter's syndrome, or gout. Obesity seems to predispose patients to the development of plantar fasciitis, as does going barefoot or wearing house slippers for prolonged periods (Fig. 103-1). High-impact aerobic exercise has also been implicated as a causative factor.

SIGNS AND SYMPTOMS

The pain of plantar fasciitis is most severe when first walking after a period of non–weight bearing and is made worse by prolonged standing or walking. On physical examination, patients exhibit a positive calcaneal jump sign, which consists of point tenderness over the plantar medial calcaneal tuberosity (Fig. 103-2). Patients may also have tenderness along the plantar fascia as it moves anteriorly. Pain is increased by dorsiflexing the toes, which pulls the plantar fascia taut, and then palpating along the fascia from the heel to the forefoot.

TESTING

Plain radiographs and magnetic resonance imaging are indicated in all patients who present with pain thought to be caused by plantar fasciitis to rule out occult bony pathology and tumor (Figs. 103-3 and 103-4). Although characteristic radiographic changes are lacking in plantar fasciitis, radionuclide bone scanning may show increased uptake where the plantar fascia attaches to the medial calcaneal tuberosity; it can also rule out stress fractures not visible on plain radiographs. Based on the patient's clinical presentation, additional testing may be

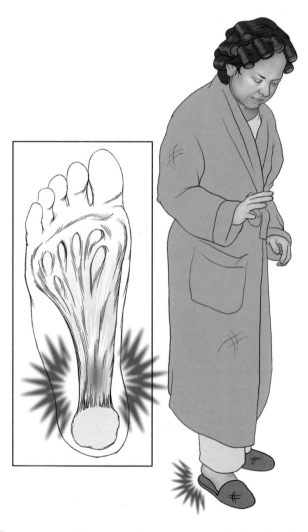

Figure 103–1. The pain of plantar fasciitis is localized to the hindfoot and can cause significant functional disability.

warranted, including a complete blood count, prostate-specific antigen level, erythrocyte sedimentation rate, and antinuclear antibody testing. The injection technique described later serves as both a diagnostic and a therapeutic maneuver.

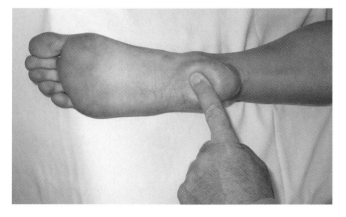

Figure 103-2. Eliciting the calcaneal jump sign for plantar fasciitis. (From Waldman SD: Physical Diagnosis of Pain: An Atlas of Signs and Symptoms. Philadelphia, Saunders, 2006, p 379.)

DIFFERENTIAL DIAGNOSIS

The pain of plantar fasciitis may be confused with that of Morton's neuroma or sesamoiditis; however, the characteristic pain on dorsiflexion of the toes associated with plantar fasciitis should help distinguish these conditions. Stress fractures of the metatarsal or sesamoid bones, bursitis, and tendinitis may also confuse the clinical picture.

TREATMENT

Initial treatment of the pain and functional disability associated with plantar fasciitis includes a combination

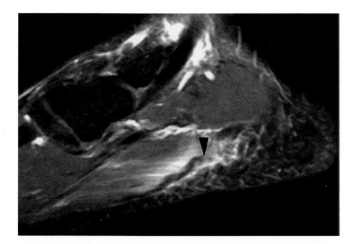

Figure 103-3. Rupture of the central cord of the plantar fascia. Sagittal, short tau inversion recovery image demonstrates discontinuity of the plantar fascia, with extensive edema of the flexor digitorum brevis muscle *(arrowhead)*. (From Edelman RR, Hessellink JR, Zlatkin MB, Crues JV: Clinical Magnetic Resonance Imaging, 3rd ed. Philadelphia, Saunders, 2006, p 3456.)

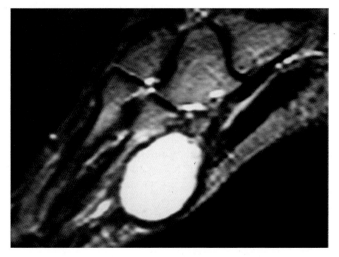

Figure 103-4. Synovial sarcoma. Sagittal, T2-weighted image demonstrates a large soft tissue mass in the plantar aspect of the foot. The mass is homogeneous and exhibits a thick capsule, simulating a fluid collection. (From Edelman RR, Hessellink JR, Zlatkin MB, Crues JV: Clinical Magnetic Resonance Imaging, 3rd ed. Philadelphia, Saunders, 2006, p 3456.)

of nonsteroidal anti-inflammatory drugs or cyclooxygenase-2 inhibitors and physical therapy. The local application of heat and cold may also be beneficial. Avoidance of repetitive activities that aggravate the patient's symptoms, avoidance of walking barefoot or with shoes that do not provide good support, and short-term immobilization of the affected foot may provide relief. For patients who do not respond to these treatment modalities, injection with local anesthetic and steroid is a reasonable next step.

To perform an injection for plantar fasciitis, the patient is placed in the supine position. The medial aspect of the heel is identified by palpation, and the skin overlying this point is prepared with antiseptic solution. A syringe containing 2 mL of 0.25% preservative-free bupivacaine and 40 mg methylprednisolone is attached to a 1½-inch, 25-gauge needle. The needle is slowly advanced through the previously identified point at a right angle to the skin, directly toward the center of the medial aspect of the calcaneus, until the needle impinges on bone. The needle is then withdrawn slightly out of the periosteum, and the contents of the syringe are gently injected as the needle is slowly withdrawn. There should be slight resistance to injection, given the closed nature of the heel.

Physical modalities, including local heat and gentle stretching exercises, should be introduced several days after the patient undergoes injection. Vigorous exercises should be avoided, because they will exacerbate the patient's symptoms. Heel pads or molded orthotic devices may also be of value. Simple analgesics, nonsteroidal anti-inflammatory drugs, and antimyotonic agents such as tizanidine can be used concurrently with this injection technique.

COMPLICATIONS AND PITFALLS

Most complications of injection are related to needle-induced trauma at the injection site and in the underlying tissues. Many patients complain of a transient increase in pain after injection, which can be minimized by injecting gently and slowly. Infection, though rare, may occur if sterile technique is not followed.

Clinical Pearls

The injection technique described is extremely effective in treating the pain of plantar fasciitis. It is a safe procedure if careful attention is paid to the clinically relevant anatomy, sterile technique is used to avoid infection, and universal precautions are implemented to minimize any risk to the operator.

Chapter 104

Calcaneal Spur Syndrome

ICD-9 CODE 726.73

THE CLINICAL SYNDROME

Calcaneal spurs are a common cause of heel pain. They can occur anywhere along the calcaneal tuberosity but are most frequent at the insertion of the plantar fascia (Fig. 104-1). Calcaneal spurs are usually asymptomatic, but when they are painful it is generally the result of inflammation of the insertional fibers of the plantar fascia at the medial tuberosity; symptomatic calcaneal spurs are often found in association with plantar fasciitis. Like plantar fasciitis, calcaneal spurs can occur alone or may be part of a systemic inflammatory condition such as rheumatoid arthritis, Reiter's syndrome, or gout. In some patients, the cause seems to be entirely mechanical, and such patients often exhibit an abnormal gait with excessive heel strike. High-impact aerobic exercise has also been implicated in the development of calcaneal spur syndrome (Fig. 104-2).

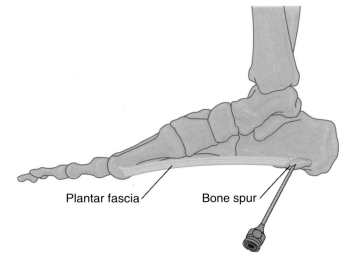

Figure 104–1. Calcaneal spurs commonly form at the insertion of the plantar fascia on the medial calcaneal tuberosity. (From Waldman SD: Atlas of Pain Management Injection Techniques, 2nd ed. Philadelphia, Saunders, 2007, p 554.)

Plantar fascia · Bone spur

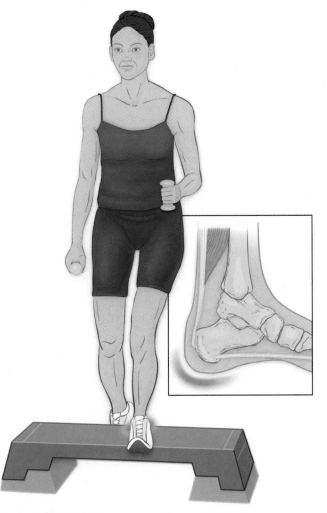

Figure 104–2. High-impact aerobic exercise has been implicated in the development of calcaneal spurs.

SIGNS AND SYMPTOMS

The pain of calcaneal spurs is most severe when first walking after a period of non–weight bearing and is made worse by prolonged standing or walking. On physical examination, patients exhibit point tenderness over the plantar medial calcaneal tuberosity; there may also be tenderness along the plantar fascia as it moves anteriorly. The pain of calcaneal spurs is increased by weight bearing and relieved by padding of the affected heel.

TESTING

Plain radiographs are indicated in all patients who present with pain thought to be caused by calcaneal spurs to rule out occult bony pathology and tumor. Characteristic radiographic changes are lacking, but radionuclide bone scanning may show increased uptake at the point of attachment of the plantar fascia to the medial calcaneal tuberosity. Magnetic resonance imaging (MRI) of the foot is indicated if calcaneal spurs, occult mass, or tumor is suspected (Fig. 104-3). MRI and radionuclide bone scanning may also be useful to rule out stress fractures not visible on plain radiographs (Fig. 104-4). Based on

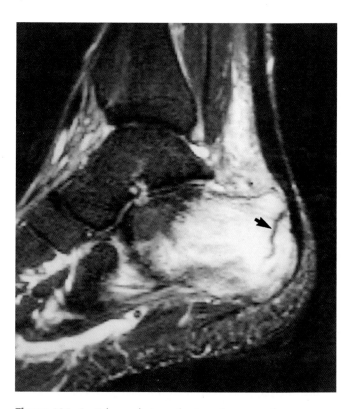

Figure 104–4. Calcaneal stress fracture. In a marathon runner, a sagittal, short tau inversion recovery magnetic resonance image shows a fatigue fracture *(arrow)* of the calcaneus, with extensive marrow edema and slight thickening of the Achilles tendon. Abnormal high signal intensity anterior to this tendon indicates peritendinitis. (From Resnick D: Diagnosis of Bone and Joint Disorders, 4th ed. Philadelphia, Saunders, 2002, p 2661.)

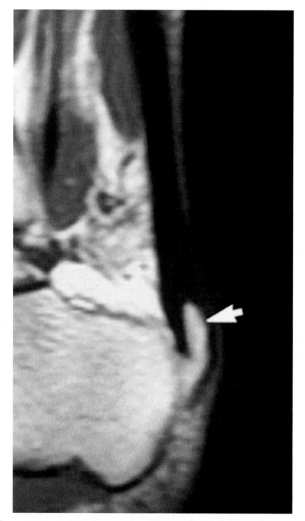

Figure 104–3. Sagittal, T1-weighted, spin echo magnetic resonance image shows a large marrow-containing calcaneal enthesophyte arising at the insertion of the Achilles tendon *(arrow)*. (From Resnick D: Diagnosis of Bone and Joint Disorders, 4th ed. Philadelphia, Saunders, 2002, p 555.)

the patient's clinical presentation, additional testing may be warranted, including a complete blood count, prostate-specific antigen level, erythrocyte sedimentation rate, and antinuclear antibody testing. The injection technique described later serves as both a diagnostic and a therapeutic maneuver.

DIFFERENTIAL DIAGNOSIS

The pain of calcaneal spurs is often confused with that of plantar fasciitis; however, the characteristic pain on dorsiflexion of the toes associated with plantar fasciitis should distinguish these conditions. Stress fractures of the calcaneus, bursitis, and tendinitis can also confuse the clinical picture.

TREATMENT

Initial treatment of the pain and functional disability associated with calcaneal spur syndrome includes a combination of nonsteroidal anti-inflammatory drugs or cyclooxygenase-2 inhibitors and physical therapy. The local application of heat and cold may also be beneficial. Avoidance of repetitive activities that aggravate the patient's symptoms, combined with short-term immobilization of the affected heel, may provide relief. For patients who do not respond to these treatment modalities, injection with local anesthetic and steroid is a reasonable next step.

To inject the calcaneal spur, the patient is placed in the supine position. The painful area of the heel overlying the calcaneal spur is identified by palpation, and the skin overlying this point is prepared with antiseptic solution. A syringe containing 2 mL of 0.25% preservative-free bupivacaine and 40 mg methylprednisolone is attached to a 1½-inch, 25-gauge needle. The needle is slowly advanced through the previously identified point at a right angle to the skin, directly toward the center of the painful area (Fig. 104-5), until it impinges on bone. The needle is then withdrawn slightly out of the periosteum, and the contents of the syringe are gently injected as the needle is slowly withdrawn. There should be slight resistance to injection, given the closed nature of the heel.

Physical modalities, including local heat and gentle range-of-motion exercises, should be introduced several days after the patient undergoes injection.

COMPLICATIONS AND PITFALLS

Failure to identify primary or metastatic tumor of the foot that is causing the patient's pain can have disastrous results. The major complication of injection is infection, although this should be exceedingly rare if strict aseptic technique is followed. Approximately 25% of patients complain of a transient increase in pain after injection, and they should be warned of this possibility.

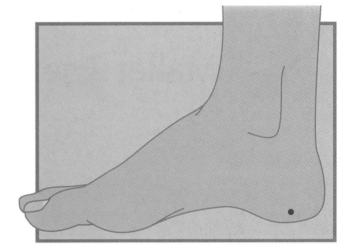

Figure 104–5. The pain of calcaneal spurs can be relieved by injecting the painful area of the heel overlying the spur. (From Waldman SD: Atlas of Pain Management Injection Techniques, 2nd ed. Philadelphia, Saunders, 2007, p 555.)

Clinical Pearls

Coexistent bursitis, plantar fasciitis, and tendinitis may contribute to the patient's foot pain, necessitating additional treatment with more localized injection of local anesthetic and methylprednisolone. The injection technique described is extremely effective in treating the pain of calcaneal spur syndrome, and it is safe if careful attention is paid to the clinically relevant anatomy.

Chapter 105

Mallet Toe

ICD-9 CODE 735.4

THE CLINICAL SYNDROME

Mallet toe is a painful flexion deformity of the distal interphalangeal joint (Fig. 105-1). The second toe is affected most commonly. Mallet toe is usually the result of a jamming injury to the toe, although, like bunion and hammer toe, the wearing of tight, narrow-toed shoes has also been implicated (Fig. 105-2); also like bunion, mallet toe occurs more commonly in females than in males. An inflamed adventitious bursa may accompany mallet toe, contributing to the patient's pain. A callus or ulcer overlying the tip of the affected toe may be present as well. High-heeled shoes may exacerbate the problem.

SIGNS AND SYMPTOMS

The majority of patients complain of pain localized to the distal interphalangeal joint and an inability to get

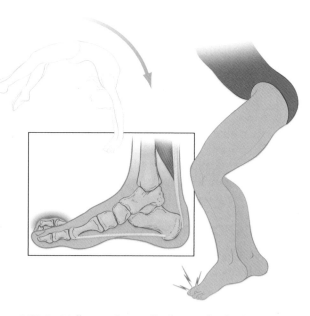

Figure 105–2. Mallet toe is usually the result of a jamming injury to the second toe. It is often seen in gymnasts, although the wearing of tight, narrow-toed shoes has also been implicated in its development.

shoes to fit. Walking makes the pain worse, whereas rest and heat provide some relief. The pain is constant and is characterized as aching in nature. Some patients complain of a grating or popping sensation with use of the joint, and crepitus may be present on physical examination. In addition to pain, patients with mallet toe develop a characteristic flexion deformity of the distal interphalangeal joint. Unlike with bunion, alignment of the toes is relatively normal.

TESTING

Plain radiographs are indicated in all patients who present with mallet toe. Magnetic resonance imaging of the toe is indicated if joint instability, occult mass, or tumor is suspected. Based on the patient's clinical presentation, additional testing may be warranted, including a

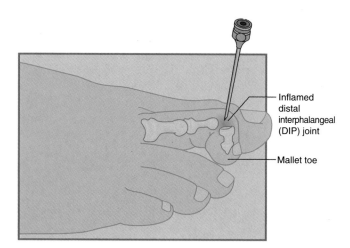

Inflamed distal interphalangeal (DIP) joint

Mallet toe

Figure 105–1. Mallet toe is a painful flexion deformity of the distal interphalangeal joint. (From Waldman SD: Atlas of Pain Management Injection Techniques. Philadelphia, Saunders, 2000, p 357.)

complete blood count, erythrocyte sedimentation rate, and antinuclear antibody testing.

DIFFERENTIAL DIAGNOSIS

The diagnosis of mallet toe is usually obvious on clinical grounds alone. Bursitis and tendinitis of the foot and ankle frequently coexist with mallet toe. In addition, stress fractures of the metatarsals, phalanges, or sesamoid bones may confuse the clinical diagnosis and require specific treatment.

TREATMENT

Initial treatment of the pain and functional disability associated with mallet toe includes a combination of nonsteroidal anti-inflammatory drugs or cyclooxygenase-2 inhibitors and physical therapy. The local application of heat and cold may also be beneficial. Avoidance of repetitive activities that aggravate the patient's symptoms, avoidance of narrow-toed or high-heeled shoes, and short-term immobilization of the affected toes may provide relief. For patients who do not respond to these treatment modalities, injection with local anesthetic and steroid is a reasonable next step.

To inject mallet toe, the patient is placed in the supine position, and the skin overlying the affected toe is prepared with antiseptic solution. A sterile syringe containing 1.5 mL of 0.25% preservative-free bupivacaine and 40 mg methylprednisolone is attached to a $^5/_8$-inch, 25-gauge needle using strict aseptic technique. The mallet toe is identified, and the needle is carefully advanced against the affected distal phalanges (see Fig. 105-1). The needle is then withdrawn slightly out of the periosteum, and the contents of the syringe is gently injected. There should be little resistance to injection. If resistance is encountered, the needle is probably in a ligament or tendon and should be advanced or withdrawn slightly until the injection can proceed without significant resistance. The needle is removed, and a sterile pressure dressing and ice pack are applied to the injection site.

COMPLICATIONS AND PITFALLS

Failure to identify primary or metastatic tumor of the foot that is causing the patient's pain can have disastrous results. The major complication of injection is infection, although this should be exceedingly rare if strict aseptic technique is followed. Approximately 25% of patients complain of a transient increase in pain after injection, and they should be warned of this possibility.

Physical modalities, including local heat and gentle range-of-motion exercises, should be introduced several days after the patient undergoes injection.

Clinical Pearls

Coexistent bursitis and tendinitis may contribute to the patient's foot pain, necessitating additional treatment with more localized injection of local anesthetic and methylprednisolone. The injection technique described is extremely effective in treating the pain of mallet toe, and it is safe if careful attention is paid to the clinically relevant anatomy. Narrow-toed and high-heeled shoes should be avoided, because they will exacerbate the patient's symptoms.

Chapter 106

Hammer Toe

ICD-9 CODE 735.3

THE CLINICAL SYNDROME

Hammer toe is a painful flexion deformity of the proximal interphalangeal joint in which the middle and distal phalanges are flexed down onto the proximal phalange (Fig. 106-1). The second toe is affected most often, and the condition is usually bilateral. Like hallux valgus deformity, hammer toe is usually the result of wearing shoes that are too tight in the toe box, although trauma has also been implicated (Fig. 106-2). As with bunion, hammer toe deformity occurs more commonly in females than in males. An inflamed adventitious bursa may accompany hammer toe, contributing to the patient's pain. A callus overlying the plantar surface of these bony prominences is usually present as well. High-heeled shoes may exacerbate the problem.

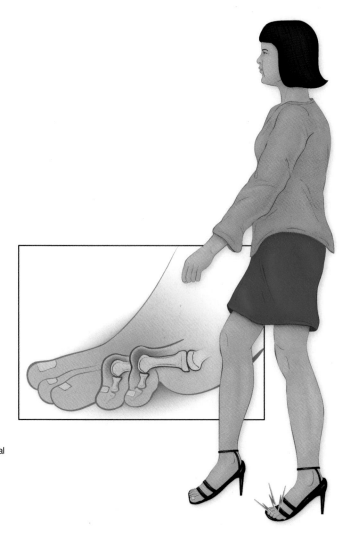

Figure 106–2. Hammer toe deformity is usually the result of wearing shoes that are too tight in the toe box, although trauma has also been implicated.

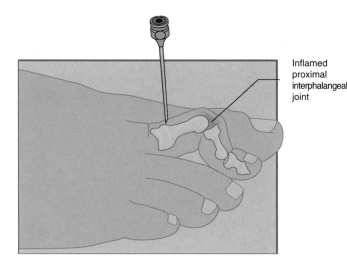

Inflamed proximal interphalangeal joint

Figure 106–1. Hammer toe is a painful flexion deformity of the proximal interphalangeal joint in which the middle and distal phalanges are flexed down onto the proximal phalanx. (From Waldman SD: Atlas of Pain Management Injection Techniques. Philadelphia, Saunders, 2000, p 359.)

SIGNS AND SYMPTOMS

The majority of patients complain of pain localized to the proximal interphalangeal joint and an inability to get shoes to fit. Walking makes the pain worse, whereas rest and heat provide some relief. The pain is constant and is characterized as aching in nature; it may interfere with sleep. Some patients complain of a grating or popping sensation with use of the joint, and crepitus may be present on physical examination. In addition to pain, patients with hammer toe develop a characteristic flexion deformity of the proximal interphalangeal joint.

TESTING

Plain radiographs are indicated in all patients who present with hammer toe. Magnetic resonance imaging of the toe is indicated if joint instability, occult mass, or tumor is suspected. Based on the patient's clinical presentation, additional testing may be warranted, including a complete blood count, erythrocyte sedimentation rate, and antinuclear antibody testing.

DIFFERENTIAL DIAGNOSIS

The diagnosis of hammer toe is usually obvious on clinical grounds alone. Bursitis and tendinitis of the foot and ankle frequently coexist with hammer toe. In addition, stress fractures of the metatarsals, phalanges, or sesamoid bones may confuse the clinical diagnosis and require specific treatment.

TREATMENT

Initial treatment of the pain and functional disability associated with hammer toe includes a combination of nonsteroidal anti-inflammatory drugs or cyclooxygenase-2 inhibitors and physical therapy. The local application of heat and cold may also be beneficial. Avoidance of repetitive activities that aggravate the patient's symptoms, avoidance of narrow-toed or high-heeled shoes, and short-term immobilization of the affected toes may provide relief. For patients who do not respond to these treatment modalities, injection with local anesthetic and steroid is a reasonable next step.

To inject hammer toe, the patient is placed in the supine position, and the skin overlying the affected toe is prepared with antiseptic solution. A sterile syringe containing 1.5 mL of 0.25% preservative-free bupivacaine and 40 mg methylprednisolone is attached to a $^5/_8$-inch, 25-gauge needle using strict aseptic technique. The hammer toe is identified, and the needle is carefully advanced against the second metatarsal head (see Fig. 106-1). The needle is then withdrawn slightly out of the periosteum, and the contents of the syringe is gently injected. There should be little resistance to injection. If resistance is encountered, the needle is probably in a ligament or tendon and should be advanced or withdrawn slightly until the injection can proceed without significant resistance. The needle is removed, and a sterile pressure dressing and ice pack are applied to the injection site.

Physical modalities, including local heat and gentle range-of-motion exercises, should be introduced several days after the patient undergoes injection.

COMPLICATIONS AND PITFALLS

Failure to identify primary or metastatic tumor of the foot that is causing the patient's pain can have disastrous results. The major complication of injection is infection, although this should be exceedingly rare if strict aseptic technique is followed. Approximately 25% of patients complain of a transient increase in pain after injection, and they should be warned of this possibility.

Clinical Pearls

Coexistent bursitis and tendinitis may contribute to the patient's foot pain, necessitating additional treatment with more localized injection of local anesthetic and methylprednisolone. The injection technique described is extremely effective in treating the pain of hammer toe, and it is safe if careful attention is paid to the clinically relevant anatomy. Narrow-toed and high-heeled shoes should be avoided, because they will exacerbate the patient's symptoms.

Index